A Short Tex

PSYCHI

A Short Textbook of
PSYCHIATRY

Seventh Edition

Niraj Ahuja MBBS MD MRCPsych
Consultant Psychiatrist
Newcastle Upon Tyne, UK
Formerly
Associate Professor (Psychiatry)
GB Pant Hospital and
Associated Maulana Azad Medical College (MAMC) and
Lok Nayak Hospital, New Delhi, India
Formerly also at
Department of Psychiatry
Jawaharlal Institute of Postgraduate Medical Education and Research (JIPMER), Pondicherry
Lady Hardinge Medical College (LHMC) and Smt. SK Hospital, New Delhi
All India Institute of Medical Sciences (AIIMS), New Delhi, India

Contributing Editor
Savita Ahuja MBBS DGO DFSRH DRCOG

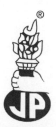

JAYPEE BROTHERS MEDICAL PUBLISHERS (P) LTD

New Delhi • St Louis (USA) • Panama City (Panama) • London (UK) • Ahmedabad • Bengaluru
Chennai • Hyderabad • Kochi • Kolkata • Lucknow • Mumbai • Nagpur

Published by
Jitendar P Vij
Jaypee Brothers Medical Publishers (P) Ltd

Corporate Office
4838/24 Ansari Road, Daryaganj, New Delhi - 110002, India,
Phone: +91-11-43574357, Fax: +91-11-43574314

Registered Office
B-3 EMCA House, 23/23B Ansari Road, Daryaganj, New Delhi - 110 002, India
Phones: +91-11-23272143, +91-11-23272703, +91-11-23282021
+91-11-23245672, Rel: +91-11-32558559, Fax: +91-11-23276490, +91-11-23245683
e-mail: jaypee@jaypeebrothers.com, Website: www.jaypeebrothers.com

Offices in India
- **Ahmedabad,** Phone: Rel: +91-79-32988717, e-mail: ahmedabad@jaypeebrothers.com
- **Bengaluru,** Phone: Rel: +91-80-32714073, e-mail: bangalore@jaypeebrothers.com
- **Chennai,** Phone: Rel: +91-44-32972089, e-mail: chennai@jaypeebrothers.com
- **Hyderabad,** Phone: Rel:+91-40-32940929, e-mail: hyderabad@jaypeebrothers.com
- **Kochi,** Phone: +91-484-2395740, e-mail: kochi@jaypeebrothers.com
- **Kolkata,** Phone: +91-33-22276415, e-mail: kolkata@jaypeebrothers.com
- **Lucknow,** Phone: +91-522-3040554, e-mail: lucknow@jaypeebrothers.com
- **Mumbai,** Phone: Rel: +91-22-32926896, e-mail: mumbai@jaypeebrothers.com
- **Nagpur,** Phone: Rel: +91-712-3245220, e-mail: nagpur@jaypeebrothers.com

Overseas Offices
- **North America Office, USA,** Ph: 001-636-6279734, e-mail: jaypee@jaypeebrothers.com,
  anjulav@jaypeebrothers.com
- **Central America Office, Panama City, Panama,** Ph: 001-507-317-0160, e-mail: cservice@jphmedical.com,
  Website: www.jphmedical.com
- **Europe Office, UK,** Ph: +44 (0) 2031708910, e-mail: info@jpmedpub.com

A Short Textbook of Psychiatry

© 2011, Niraj Ahuja

This book has been published in good faith that the material provided by author is original. Every effort is made to ensure accuracy of material, but the publisher, printer and author will not be held responsible for any inadvortent orror (s). In case of any dispute, all legal matters are to be settled under Delhi jurisdiction only.

First Edition: 1990
Second Edition: 1992
Third Edition: 1995
Fourth Edition: 1999
Fifth Edition: 2002
Sixth Edition: 2006
Reprint: 2009
Seventh Edition: 2011

ISBN: 978-93-80704-66-1

Typeset at JPBMP typesetting unit
Printed at Rajkamal Electric Press, Plot No. 2, Phase-IV, Kundli, Haryana.

For
Manisha
and
Neha

Preface to the Seventh Edition

It is rather humbling to consider that it has been two decades that the *Short Textbook of Psychiatry* has enjoyed a wide distribution among the undergraduate medical students, interns, junior residents, postgraduate psychiatry students, nursing students, psychology and psychiatric social work students, occupational therapy and physiotherapy students, general medical practitioners, other physicians and health professionals in India and some other countries. I am really indebted to the many astute readers who have provided a very constructive and useful feedback, along with encouraging comments regarding the existing format and the contents of the book.

The seventh edition of the *Short Textbook of Psychiatry* has been once again extensively revised and updated. Significant changes have been made in almost all the chapters, especially in chapters on diagnosis and classification, psychoactive substance use disorders, psychopharmacology, schizophrenia, mood disorders and other biological methods of treatment. Coloured-shaded boxes have been added at various places in the text to highlight the important points in tables and figures. The chapter on psychiatric history and examination contains a summary of laboratory tests in psychiatry, in additions to other significant changes. The appendices have been revised and contain a glossary of common psychiatric terms.

The *Short Textbook of Psychiatry* sincerely hopes to retain its original aim of providing a brief yet comprehensive account of the psychiatric disorders and their allied aspects in a 'user-friendly' and 'easy-to-follow' manner.

I am grateful to Shri Jitendar P Vij, Chairman and Managing Director, Jaypee Brothers Medical Publishers (P) Ltd for his exquisite control over the production and distribution of the *Short Textbook of Psychiatry* over the last 20 years.

I hope you enjoy reading the book and I warmly welcome critical comments and constructive suggestions. Please send your comments by email to STBPsy@gmail.com.

July 2010   Niraj Ahuja

Preface to the First Edition

Psychiatry, as a branch of Medicine, has been cold-shouldered by physicians for a long time. There are various reasons for such an attitude. But, the most important exposition is an unfamiliarity with the psychiatric disorders and their treatment. This is easy to understand in the light of the fact that an easily comprehensible, non-intimidating and concise text on psychiatry was not earlier available.

Recently too, the various postgraduate entrance examinations have laid an increasing emphasis on psychiatry and its related branches. Keeping this in mind, the *Medical Examination Review—Psychiatry* (Multiple Choice Questions with Explanatory Answers) was written, the new edition of which appears this year. Its tremendous success during the last four years and encouraging suggestions from the readers have been a source of stimulation for drafting this text.

The *Short Textbook of Psychiatry* aims to provide a brief yet comprehensive account of psychiatric disorders and their allied aspects. While striving to make the book simple and easy-to-follow, an attempt has been made to keep the book aligned to the most recent developments in classification, terminology and treatment methods.

The *Short Textbook of Psychiatry* is addressed to medical students, interested physicians and other health professionals. A postgraduate student in psychiatry will find the text elementary and basic, although a first year postgraduate will find it useful for a broad introduction to the subject.

I will like to put on record my deep appreciation for Shri Jitendar P Vij, Managing Director; Mr. Pawaninder Vij, Production Manager and their efficient staff at the Jaypee Brothers Medical Publishers (P) Ltd, New Delhi for bringing out this volume in a short time.

I welcome critical comments and constructive suggestions from the readers.

January 1990   Niraj Ahuja

Contents

Chapter 1

Diagnosis and Classification in Psychiatry

Classification is a process by which phenomena are organized into categories so as to bring together those phenomena that most resemble each other and to separate those that differ. Any classification of psychiatric disorders, like that of medical illnesses, should ideally be based on aetiology. For a large majority of psychiatric disorders, no distinct aetiology is known at present, although there are many attractive probabilities for several of them. Therefore, one of the most rational ways to classify psychiatric disorders at present is probably syndromal. A syndrome is defined as a group of symptoms and signs that often occur together, and delineate a recognisable clinical condition.

The syndromal approach of classifying psychiatric disorders, on the basis of their clinical signs and symptoms, is very similar to the historical approach of classification of medical illnesses, when aetiology of a majority of medical illnesses was still obscure.

There are three major purposes of classification of psychiatric disorders:
1. To enable communication regarding the diagnosis of disorders,
2. To facilitate comprehension of the underlying causes of these disorders, and
3. To aid prediction of the prognosis of psychiatric disorders.

This syndromal approach of classification, in the absence of clearly known aetiologies, fulfils these purposes reasonably well.

Before proceeding to look at current classifications of psychiatric disorders, it is important to define what is meant by the term, psychiatric disorder.

DEFINITION OF A PSYCHIATRIC DISORDER

The simplest way to conceptualize a psychiatric disorder is a disturbance of Cognition (i.e. Thought), Conation (i.e. Action), or Affect (i.e. Feeling), or any disequilibrium between the three domains. However, this simple definition is not very useful in routine clinical practice.

Another way to define a psychiatric disorder or mental disorder is as a clinically significant psychological or behavioural syndrome that causes significant (subjective) distress, (objective) disability, or loss of freedom; and which is not merely a socially deviant behaviour or an expected response to a stressful life event (e.g. loss of a loved one). Conflicts between the society and the individual are not considered psychiatric disorders. A psychiatric disorder should be a manifestation of behavioural, psychological, and/or biological dysfunction in that person (Definition modified after DSM-IV-TR, APA).

Although slightly lengthy, this definition defines a psychiatric disorder more accurately.

NORMAL MENTAL HEALTH

According to the World Health Organization (WHO), Health is a state of complete physical, mental and social well-being, and not merely absence of disease or infirmity.

Normal mental health, much like normal health, is a rather difficult concept to define. There are several models available for understanding what may constitute 'normality' (see Table 1.1).

Although, normality is not an easy concept to define, some of the following traits are more commonly found in 'normal' individuals.

1. Reality orientation.
2. Self-awareness and self-knowledge.
3. Self-esteem and self-acceptance.
4. Ability to exercise voluntary control over their behaviour.
5. Ability to form affectionate relationships.
6. Pursuance of productive and goal-directive activities.

CLASSIFICATION IN PSYCHIATRY

Like any growing branch of Medicine, Psychiatry has seen rapid changes in classification to keep up with a conglomeration of growing research data dealing with epidemiology, symptomatology, prognostic factors, treatment methods and new theories for the causation of psychiatric disorders.

Although first attempts to classify psychiatric disorders can be traced back to Ayurveda, Plato (4th century BC) and Asclepiades (1st century BC), classification in Psychiatry has certainly evolved ever since.

At present, there are two major classifications in Psychiatry, namely ICD-10 (1992) and DSM-IV-TR (2000).

ICD-10 (International Classification of Diseases, 10th Revision, 1992) is World Health Organisation's classification for all diseases and related health problems (and not only psychiatric disorders).

Chapter 'F' classifies psychiatric disorders as Mental and Behavioural Disorders (MBDs) and codes them on an alphanumeric system from F00 to F99. ICD-10 is now available in several versions, the most important of which are listed in Table 1.2. There are several versions of ICD-10; some are listed in Table 1.3.

DSM-IV-TR (Diagnostic and Statistical Manual of Mental Disorders, IV Edition, Text Revision, 2000) is the American Psychiatric Association (APA)'s

Table 1.1: Some Models of Normality in Mental Health

1. *Medical Model (Normality as Health)*: Normal mental health is conceptualized as the absence of any psychiatric disorder ('disease') or psychopathology.
2. *Statistical Model (Normality as an Average)*: Statistically normal mental health falls within two standard deviations (SDs) of the normal distribution curve for the population.
3. *Utopian Model (Normality as Utopia)*: In this model, the focus in defining normality is on 'optimal functioning'.
4. *Subjective Model*: According to this model, normality is viewed as an absence of distress, disability, or any help-seeking behaviour resulting thereof. This definition is similar in many ways to the medical model.
5. *Social Model*: A normal person, according to this definition, is expected to behave in a socially 'acceptable' behaviour.
6. *Process Model (Normality as a Process)*: This model views normality as a dynamic and changing process, rather than as a static concept. This model can be combined with any other model mentioned here.
7. *Continuum Model (Normality as a Continuum)*: Normality and mental disorder are considered by this model as falling at the two ends of a continuum, rather than being disparate entities. According to this model, it is the severity (scores above the 'cut-off') that determines whether a particular person's experience constitutes a symptom of a disorder or falls on the healthy side of the continuum.

classification of mental disorders. DSM-IV-TR is a text revision of the DSM-IV which was originally published in 1994.

The next editions of ICD (ICD-11) and DSM (DSM-V) are likely to be available in the years 2012-14.

For the purpose of this book, it is intended to follow the ICD-10 classification. ICD-10 is easy to follow, has been tested extensively all over the world (51 countries; 195 clinical centres), and has been found to be generally applicable across the globe. At some places in the book, DSM-IV-TR diagnostic criteria are also discussed, wherever appropriate.

Table 1.2: Mental and Behavioural Disorders in ICD-10

1. *F00-F09 Organic, Including Symptomatic, Mental Disorders*, such as delirium, dementia, organic amnestic syndrome, and other organic mental disorders.
2. *F10-F19 Mental and Behavioural Disorders due to Psychoactive Substance Use*, such as acute intoxication, harmful use, dependence syndrome, withdrawal state, amnestic syndrome, and psychotic disorders due to psychoactive substance use.
3. *F20-F29 Schizophrenia, Schizotypal and Delusional Disorders*, such as schizophrenia, schizotypal disorder, persistent delusional disorders, acute and transient psychotic disorders, induced delusional disorder, and schizo-affective disorders.
4. *F31-F39 Mood (Affective) Disorders*, such as manic episode, depressive episode, bipolar affective disorder, recurrent depressive disorder, and persistent mood disorder.
5. *F40-F48 Neurotic, Stress-related and Somatoform Disorders* (There is no category with code number F49), such as anxiety disorders, phobic anxiety disorders, obsessive-compulsive disorder, dissociative (conversion) disorders, somatoform disorders, reaction to stress, and adjustment disorders, and other neurotic disorders.
6. *F50-F59 Behavioural Syndromes Associated with Physiological Disturbances and Physical Factors*, such as eating disorders, non-organic sleep disorders, sexual dysfunctions (not caused by organic disorder or disease), mental and behavioural disorders associated with puerperium, and abuse of non-dependence-producing substances.
7. *F60-F69 Disorders of Adult Personality and Behaviour*, such as specific personality disorders, enduring personality changes, habit and impulse disorders, gender-identity disorders, disorders of sexual preference, and psychological and behavioural disorders associated with sexual development and orientation.
8. *F70-F79 Mental Retardation*, including mild, moderate, severe, and profound mental retardation.
9. *F80-F89 Disorders of Psychological Development*, such as specific developmental disorders of speech and language, specific developmental disorders of scholastic skills, specific developmental disorders of motor function, mixed specific developmental disorders, and pervasive developmental disorders.
10. *F90-F98 Behavioural and Emotional Disorders with Onset Usually Occurring in Childhood and Adolescence*, such as hyperkinetic disorders, conduct disorders, mixed disorders of conduct and emotions, tic disorders, and other disorders.
11. *F99 Unspecified Mental Disorder*

Table 1.3: Some Versions of ICD-10

A. Clinical Descriptions and Diagnostic Guidelines (CDDG)
B. Diagnostic Criteria for Research (DCR)
C. Multi-axial Classification Version
D. Primary Care Version

Earlier classifications in psychiatry were based on hierarchies of diagnoses with presence of a diagnosis higher in the hierarchy usually ruling out a diagnosis lower in the hierarchy. This was felt to be in keeping with the teaching of Medicine at large at the time, where there was emphasis on making a single diagnosis of one disease rather than explaining different symptoms by different disease entities.

The presence of a diagnostic hierarchy implied that the conditions higher up in the hierarchy needed to be considered first, before making a diagnosis of those lower down in the hierarchy. For example, it was felt that a current diagnosis of organic mental disorder such as delirium would exclude a diagnosis of anxiety disorder in presence of agitation; and alcohol and drug induced disorders would take precedence over a diagnosis of primary mood disorder.

The current classifications however encourage recording of multiple diagnoses in a given patient (as co-morbidity) regardless of any hierarchy. Although a diagnostic hierarchy makes much clinical sense, consideration and recording of co-morbidity can be helpful in identifying more of patient's needs; for example, a diagnosis of co-morbid anxiety disorder in a patient with bipolar disorder helps identify and treat the anxiety component adequately.

MULTI-AXIAL CLASSIFICATION

The process of making a correct diagnosis is a very useful clinical exercise as evidence-based management can be dependent on making a correct diagnosis. However, sometimes making a clinical diagnosis can lead to labelling of patient and can be stigmatizing. This can also degrade the patient to "just another case" and does not direct attention to the whole individual.

In the last few decades, there has been an upsurge of interest in multi-axial systems for achieving a more comprehensive description of an individual's clinical problems and needs. The pattern adopted by DSM-IV-TR is a very good example of this attempt.

Table 1.4: The Five Axes of DSM-IV-TR

AXIS I:	Clinical Psychiatric Diagnosis
AXIS II:	Personality Disorders and Mental Retardation
AXIS III:	General Medical Conditions
AXIS IV:	Psychosocial and Environmental Problems
AXIS V:	Global Assessment of Functioning: Current and in past one year (Rated on a scale)

In this system, an individual patient is diagnosed on five separate axes, ensuring a more through evaluation of needs (see Table 1.4).

This method helps in making a more holistic, biopsychosocial assessment of an individual patient. Recently, ICD-10 has also brought out its own multi-axial classification version (see Table 1.3).

Chapter 2

Psychiatric History and Examination

Familiarity with the technique of psychiatric assessment is important not only for a psychiatrist but also for a medical practitioner or any mental health professional, since more than one-third of medical patients can present with psychiatric symptoms.

INTERVIEW TECHNIQUE

In no other branch of Medicine is the history taking interview as important as in Psychiatry. All physicians need to communicate with their patients and a skilful interview can clearly help in obtaining better information, making a more accurate diagnosis, establishing a better rapport with patients, and working towards better adherence with management plan.

A psychiatric interview is usually different from the routine medical interview in several ways (Table 2.1). A few important points regarding the interview technique are mentioned below. These serve as pointers towards a technique which clearly has to be mastered over a period of time with repeated examinations.

A consistent scheme should be used each time for recording the interview, although the interview need not (and should not) follow a fixed and rigid method. The interview technique should have flexibility, varying according to appropriate clinical circumstances.

Whenever possible, the patient should be seen first. When the account of historical information given by the patient and the informant(s) is different, it is useful to record them separately.

Table 2.1: Psychiatric vs Medical Interview

A psychiatric interview can be different from a medical interview in several ways, some of which can include:
1. Presence of disturbances in thinking, behaviour and emotions can interfere with meaningful communication
2. Collateral information from significant others can be really important
3. Important to obtain detailed information of personal history and pre-morbid personality
4. Need for more astute observation of patient's behaviour
5. Difficulty in establishing rapport may be encountered more often
6. Patients may lack insight into their illness and may have poor judgement
7. Usually more important to elicit information regarding stressors and social situation

During the interview session(s), the patient should be put at ease and an empathic relationship should be established.

In psychiatric assessment, history taking interview and mental status examination need not always be conducted separately (though they must be recorded individually). During assessment, the interviewer should observe any abnormalities in verbal and non-verbal communication and make note of them.

It is helpful to record patient's responses verbatim rather than only naming the signs (for example, rather than just writing delusion of persecution, it is better to record in addition: "my neighbour is trying to poison me"). It is best done in the patient's own spoken language, whenever possible.

It is useful to ask open-ended and non-directive questions (for example, "how are you feeling today"?) rather than asking direct, leading questions (for example, "are you feeling sad at present"?).

Arguably the most important interviewing skills are listening, and demonstrating that you are interested in listening and attending to the patient. It is important to remember that listening is an active, and not a passive, process.

Confidentiality must always be observed. However, in cases of suicidal/homicidal risk and child abuse, an exception may have to be made (see Chapter 20 for details). Patients suffering from psychiatric disorders are usually no more violent than the general population. However, it is important to ensure safety if any risks are apparent.

A comprehensive psychiatric interview often requires more than one session. The psychiatric assessment can be discussed under the following headings.

IDENTIFICATION DATA

It is best to start the interview by obtaining some identification data which may include Name (including aliases and pet names), Age, Sex, Marital status, Education, Occupation, Income, Residential and Office Address(es), Religion, and Socioeconomic background, as appropriate according to the setting. It is useful to record the source of referral of the patient. In medicolegal cases, in addition, two identification marks should also be recorded.

INFORMANTS

Since sometimes the history provided by the patient may be incomplete, due to factors such as absent insight or uncooperativeness, it is important to take the history from patient's relatives or friends who act as informants and sources of collateral information. It is important to take the patient's consent before taking this collateral history unless the patient does not have capacity to consent.

The informants' identification data should be recorded along with their relationship to the patient, whether they stay with the patient or not, and the duration of stay together.

Finally, a comment should be made regarding the reliability of the information provided. The reliability of the information provided by the informants should be assessed on the following parameters:
1. Relationship with patient,
2. Intellectual and observational ability,
3. Familiarity with the patient and length of stay with the patient, and
4. Degree of concern regarding the patient.

The source of referral (such as a letter from patient's general practitioner or a letter of referral from the referring physician/surgeon in case of a liaison psychiatry referral) often provides valuable information regarding the patient's condition.

PRESENTING (CHIEF) COMPLAINTS

The presenting complaints and/or reasons for consultation should be recorded. Both the patient's and the informant's version should be recorded, if relevant. If the patient has no complaints (due to absent insight) this fact should also be noted.

It is important to use patient's own words and to note the duration of each presenting complaint. Some of the additional points which should be noted include:
1. Onset of present illness/symptom.
2. Duration of present illness/symptom.
3. Course of symptoms/illness.
4. Predisposing factors.
5. Precipitating factors (include life stressors).
6. Perpetuating and/or relieving factors.

HISTORY OF PRESENT ILLNESS

When the patient was last well or asymptomatic should be clearly noted. This provides useful information about the onset as well as duration of illness. Establishing the time of onset is really important as it provides clarity about the duration of illness and symptoms. The symptoms of the illness, from the earliest time at which a change was noticed (the onset) until the present time, should be narrated chronologically, in a coherent manner.

The presenting (chief) complaints should be expanded. In particular, any disturbances in physiological functions such as sleep, appetite and sexual functioning should be enquired. One should always enquire about the presence of suicidal ideation, ideas of self-harm and ideas of harm to others (see Chapter 19 for details), with details about any possible intent and/or plans.

It is also essential to consider and record any important negative history (such as history of alcohol/drug use in new onset psychosis).

A life chart (Fig. 2.1) provides a valuable display of the course of illness, episodic sequence, polarity (if any), severity, frequency, relationship to stressors, and response to treatment, if any.

PAST PSYCHIATRIC AND MEDICAL HISTORY

Any history of any past psychiatric illness should be obtained. Any past history of having received any psychotropic medication, alcohol and drug abuse or dependence, and psychiatric hospitalisation should be enquired.

A past history of any serious medical or neurological illness, surgical procedure, accident or hospitalisation should be obtained. The nature of treatment received, and allergies, if any, should be ascertained.

A past history of relevant aetiological causes such as head injury, convulsions, unconsciousness, diabetes

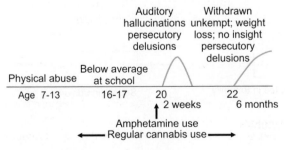

Fig. 2.1: An Example of Life Chart

mellitus, hypertension, coronary artery disease, acute intermittent porphyria, syphilis and HIV positivity (or AIDS) should be explored.

TREATMENT HISTORY

Any treatment received in present and/or previous episode(s) should be asked along with history of treatment adherence, response to treatment received, any adverse effects experienced or any drug allergies which should be prominently noted in medical records.

FAMILY HISTORY

The family history usually includes the 'family of origin' (i.e. the patient's parents, siblings, grandparents, uncles, etc.). The 'family of procreation' (i.e. the patient's spouse, children and grandchildren) is conventionally recorded under the heading of personal history.

Family history is usually recorded under the following headings:

1. *Family structure:* Drawing of a 'family tree' (pedigree chart) can help in recording all the relevant information in very little space which is easily readable. An example of a typical family tree is given in Figure 2.2. It should be noted whether the family is a nuclear, extended nuclear or joint family. Any consanguineous relationships should be noted. The age and cause of death (if any) of family members should be asked.

2. Family history of similar or other psychiatric illnesses, major medical illnesses, alcohol or drug dependence and suicide (and suicidal attempts) should be recorded.

3. *Current social situation:* Home circumstances, per capita income, socioeconomic status, leader of the family (nominal as well as functional) and current attitudes of family members towards the patient's illness should be noted.

The communication patterns in the family, range of affectivity, cultural and religious values, and social support system, should be enquired about, where relevant.

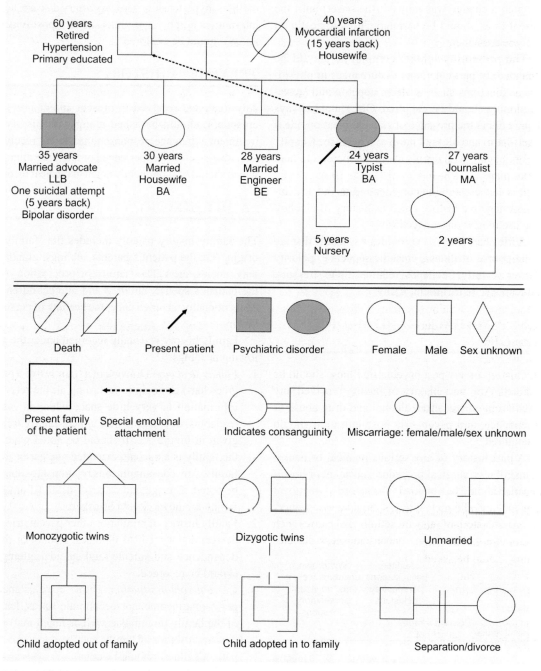

Fig. 2.2: A Typical Family Tree and Common Pedigree Symbols

PERSONAL AND SOCIAL HISTORY

In a younger patient, it is often possible to give more attention to details regarding earlier personal history. In older patients, it is sometimes harder to get a detailed account of the early childhood history. Parents and older siblings, if alive, can often provide much additional information regarding the past personal history. Not all questions need to be asked from all patients and personal history (much like rest of the history taking) should be individualised for each patient.

Personal history can be recorded under the following headings:

Perinatal History

Difficulties in pregnancy (particularly in the first three months of gestation) such as any febrile illness, medications, drugs and/or alcohol use; abdominal trauma, any physical or psychiatric illness should be asked. Other relevant questions may include whether the patient was a wanted or unwanted child, date of birth, whether delivery was normal, any instrumentation needed, where born (hospital or home), any perinatal complications (cyanosis, convulsions, jaundice), APGAR score (if available), birth cry (immediate or delayed), any birth defects, and any prematurity.

Childhood History

Whether the patient was brought up by mother or someone else, breastfeeding, weaning and any history suggestive of maternal deprivation should be asked. The age of passing each important developmental milestone should be noted. The age and ease of toilet training should be asked.

The occurrence of neurotic traits should be noted. These include stuttering, stammering, tics, enuresis, encopresis, night terrors, thumb sucking, nail biting, head banging, body rocking, morbid fears or phobias, somnambulism, temper tantrums, and food fads.

Educational History

The age of beginning and finishing formal education, academic achievements and relationships with peers and teachers, should be asked.

Any school phobia, non-attendance, truancy, any learning difficulties and reasons for termination of studies (if occurs prematurely) should be noted.

Play History

The questions to be asked include, what games were played at what stage, with whom and where. Relationships with peers, particularly the opposite sex, should be recorded. The evaluation of play history is obviously more important in the younger patients.

Puberty

The age at menarche, and reaction to menarche (in females), the age at appearance of secondary sexual characteristics (in both females and males), nocturnal emissions (in males), masturbation and any anxiety related to changes in puberty should be asked.

Menstrual and Obstetric History

The regularity and duration of menses, the length of each cycle, any abnormalities, the last menstrual period, the number of children born, and termination of pregnancy (if any) should be asked for.

Occupational History

The age at starting work; jobs held in chronological order; reasons for changes; job satisfactions; ambitions; relationships with authorities, peers and subordinates; present income; and whether the job is appropriate to the educational and family background, should be asked.

Sexual and Marital History

Sexual information, how acquired and of what kind; masturbation (fantasy and activity); sex play, if any; adolescent sexual activity; premarital and extramarital sexual relationships, if any; sexual practices (normal and abnormal); and any gender identity disorder, are the areas to be enquired about.

The duration of marriage(s) and/or relationship(s); time known the partner before marriage; marriage arranged by parents with or without consent, or by self-choice with or without parental consent; number of marriages, divorces or separations; role in marriage; interpersonal and sexual relations; contraceptive measures used; sexual satisfaction; mode and frequency of sexual intercourse; and psychosexual dysfunction (if any) should be asked.

Conventionally, the details of the 'family of procreation' are recorded here.

Premorbid Personality (PMP)

It is important to elicit details regarding the personality of the individual (*temperament*, if the age is less than 16 years). Instead of using labels such as schizoid or histrionic, it is more useful to describe the personality in some detail.

The following subheadings are often used for the description of premorbid personality.

1. Interpersonal relationship: Interpersonal relationships with family members, friends, and work colleagues; introverted/extroverted; ease of making and maintaining social relationships.
2. Use of leisure time: Hobbies; interests; intellectual activities; critical faculty; energetic/sedentary.
3. Predominant mood: Optimistic/pessimistic; stable/prone to anxiety; cheerful/despondent; reaction to stressful life events.
4. Attitude to self and others: Self-confidence level; self-criticism; self-consciousness; self-centred/thoughtful of others; self-appraisal of abilities, achievements and failures.
5. Attitude to work and responsibility: Decision making; acceptance of responsibility; flexibility; perseverance; foresight.
6. Religious beliefs and moral attitudes: Religious beliefs; tolerance of others' standards and beliefs; conscience; altruism.
7. Fantasy life: Sexual and nonsexual fantasies; daydreaming-frequency and content; recurrent or favourite daydreams; dreams.
8. Habits: Food fads; alcohol; tobacco; drugs; sleep.

One of the most reliable methods of assessment of premorbid personality is interviewing an informant familiar with the patient prior to the onset of illness.

ALCOHOL AND SUBSTANCE HISTORY

Although alcohol and drug history is often elicited as a part of personal history, it is often customary to record it separately. Alcohol and drugs can often contribute to causation of several psychiatric symptoms and are often present co-morbidly alongside many psychiatric diagnoses.

PHYSICAL EXAMINATION

A detailed general physical examination (GPE) and systemic examination is a must in every patient. Physical disease, which is aetiologically important (for causing psychiatric symptomatology), or accidentally co-existent, or secondarily caused by the psychiatric condition or treatment, is often present and can be detected by a good physical examination.

MENTAL STATUS EXAMINATION (MSE)*

Mental status examination is a standardised format in which the clinician records the psychiatric signs and symptoms present at the time of the interview.

MSE should describe all areas of mental functioning (Table 2.2). Some areas, however, may deserve more emphasis according to the clinical impressions that may arise from the history; for example, mood and affect in depression, and cognitive functions in delirium and dementia.

General Appearance and Behaviour

A rich deal of information can be elicited from examination of the general appearance and behaviour. While examining, it is important to remember patient's sociocultural background and personality.

---

*The definitions of some MSE terms are described in Appendix III.

Table 2.2: Mental Status Examination

1. **General Appearance and Behaviour**
   i. General Appearance
   ii. Attitude towards Examiner
   iii. Comprehension
   iv. Gait and Posture
   v. Motor Activity
   vi. Social Manner
   vii. Rapport
2. **Speech**
   i. Rate and Quantity
   ii. Volume and Tone
   iii. Flow and Rhythm
3. **Mood and Affect**
4. **Thought**
   i. Stream and Form
   ii. Content
5. **Perception**
6. **Cognition (Higher Mental Functions)**
   i. Consciousness
   ii. Orientation
   iii. Attention
   iv. Concentration
   v. Memory
   vi. Intelligence
   vii. Abstract thinking
7. **Insight**
8. **Judgement**

Understandably, general appearance and behaviour needs to be given more emphasis in the examination of an uncooperative patient.

General appearance

The important points to be noted are:
Physique and body habitus (build) and physical appearance (approximate height, weight, and appearance),
Looks comfortable/uncomfortable,
Physical health,
Grooming, Hygiene, Self-care,
Dressing (adequate, appropriate, any peculiarities),
Facies (non-verbal expression of mood),
Effeminate/masculine

Attitude towards examiner

Cooperation/guardedness/evasiveness/hostility/combativeness/haughtiness,
Attentiveness,
Appears interested/disinterested/apathetic,
Any ingratiating behaviour,
Perplexity

Comprehension

Intact/impaired (partially/fully)

Gait and posture

Normal or abnormal (way of sitting, standing, walking, lying)

Motor activity

Increased/decreased,
Excitement/stupor,
Abnormal involuntary movements (AIMs) such as tics, tremors, akathisia,
Restlessness/ill at ease,
Catatonic signs (mannerisms, stereotypies, posturing, waxy flexibility, negativism, ambitendency, automatic obedience, stupor, echopraxia, psychological pillow, forced grasping) (see Chapter 5 for details),
Conversion and dissociative signs (pseudoseizures, possession states),
Social withdrawal, Autism,
Compulsive acts, rituals or habits (for example, nail biting),
Reaction time

Social manner and non-verbal behaviour

Increased, decreased, or inappropriate behaviour
Eye contact (gaze aversion, staring vacantly, staring at the examiner, hesitant eye contact, or normal eye contact).

Rapport

Whether a working and empathic relationship can be established with the patient, should be mentioned.

Hallucinatory Behaviour

Smiling or crying without reason, Muttering or talking to self (non-social speech).

Odd gesturing in response to auditory or visual hallucinations.

Speech

Speech can be examined under the following headings:

Rate and quantity of speech

Whether speech is present or absent (mutism),
If present, whether it is spontaneous, whether productivity is increased or decreased,
Rate is rapid or slow (its appropriateness), Pressure of speech or poverty of speech.

Volume and tone of speech

Increased/decreased (its appropriateness),
Low/high/normal pitch

Flow and rhythm of speech

Smooth/hesitant, Blocking (sudden),
Dysprosody, Stuttering/Stammering/Cluttering, Any accent,
Circumstantiality, Tangentiality,
Verbigeration, Stereotypies (verbal),
Flight of ideas, Clang associations.

Mood and Affect

Mood is the pervasive feeling tone which is sustained (lasts for some length of time) and colours the total experience of the person. *Affect*, on the other hand, is the outward objective expression of the immediate, cross-sectional experience of emotion at a given time.

The assessment of *mood* includes testing the quality of mood, which is assessed subjectively ('how do you feel') and objectively (by examination). The other components are stability of mood (over a period of time), reactivity of mood (variation in mood with stimuli), and persistence of mood (length of time the mood lasts).

The *affect* is similarly described under quality of affect, range of affect (of emotional changes displayed over time), depth or intensity of affect (normal, increased or blunted) and appropriateness of affect (in relation to thought and surrounding environment).

Mood is described as general warmth, euphoria, elation, exaltation and/or ecstasy (seen in severe mania) in mania; anxious and restless in anxiety and depression; sad, irritable, angry and/or despaired in depression; and shallow, blunted, indifferent, restricted, inappropriate and/or labile in schizophrenia.

Anhedonia may occur in both schizophrenia and depression.

Thought

Normal thinking is a goal directed flow of ideas, symbols and associations initiated by a problem or a task, characterised by rational connections between successive ideas or thoughts, and leading towards a reality oriented conclusion. Therefore, thought process that is not goal-directed, or not logical, or does not lead to a realistic solution to the problem at hand, is not considered normal.

Traditionally, in the clinical examination, thought is assessed (by the content of speech) under the four headings of stream, form, content and possession of thought. However, since there is widespread disagreement regarding this subdivision, 'thought' is discussed here under the following two headings of 'stream and form', and 'content'.

Stream and form of thought

For obvious reasons, the 'stream of thought' overlaps with examination of 'speech'. Spontaneity, productivity, flight of ideas, prolixity, poverty of content of speech, and thought block should be mentioned here.

The 'continuity' of thought is assessed; Whether the thought processes are relevant to the questions asked; Any loosening of associations, tangentiality, circumstantiality, illogical thinking, perseveration, or verbigeration is noted.

Content of thought

Any preoccupations;
Obsessions (recurrent, irrational, intrusive, ego-dystonic, ego-alien ideas);

Contents of phobias (irrational fears);

Delusions (false, unshakable beliefs) or Over-valued ideas;

Explore for delusions/ideas of persecution, reference, grandeur, love, jealousy (infidelity), guilt, nihilism, poverty, somatic (hypochondriacal) symptoms, hopelessness, helplessness, worthlessness, and suicidal ideation.

Delusions of control, thought insertion, thought withdrawal, and thought broadcasting are Schneiderian first rank symptoms (SFRS). The presence of neologisms should be recorded here.

Perception

Perception is the process of being aware of a sensory experience and being able to recognize it by comparing it with previous experiences.

Perception is assessed under the following headings:

Hallucinations

The presence of hallucinations should be noted. A hallucination is a perception experienced in the absence of an external stimulus. The hallucinations can be in the auditory, visual, olfactory, gustatory or tactile domains.

Auditory hallucinations are commonest types of hallucinations in non-organic psychiatric disorders. It is really important to clarify whether they are elementary (only sounds are heard) or complex (voices heard).

The hallucination is experienced much like a true perception and it seems to come from an external objective space (for example, from outside the ears in the case of an auditory hallucination). If the hallucination does not either appear to be a true perception or comes from a subjective internal space (for example, inside the person's own head in the case of auditory hallucination), then it is called as a *pseudohallucination*.

It should be further enquired what was heard, how many voices were heard, in which part of the day, male or female voices, how interpreted and whether these are second person or third person hallucinations

(i.e. whether the voices were addressing the patient or were discussing him in third person); also enquire about command (imperative) hallucinations (which give commands to the person).

Enquire whether the hallucinations occurred during wakefulness, or were they hypnagogic (occurring while going to sleep) and/or hypnopompic (occurring while getting up from sleep) hallucinations.

Illusions and misinterpretations

Whether visual, auditory, or in other sensory fields; whether occur in clear consciousness or not; whether any steps taken to check the reality of distorted perceptions.

Depersonalisation/derealisation

Depersonalisation and derealisation are abnormalities in the perception of a person's reality and are often described as 'as-if' phenomena.

Somatic passivity phenomenon

Somatic passivity is the presence of strange sensations described by the patient as being imposed on the body by 'some external agency', with the patient being a passive recipient. It is one of the Schneider's first rank symptoms.

Others

Autoscopy, abnormal vestibular sensations, sense of presence should be noted here.

Cognition (Neuropsychiatric) Assessment

Assessment of the cognitive or higher mental functions is an important part of the MSE. A significant disturbance of cognitive functions commonly points to the presence of an organic psychiatric disorder. It is usual to use Folstein's mini mental state examination (MMSE) for a systematic clinical examination of higher mental functions.

Consciousness

The intensity of stimulation needed to arouse the patient should be indicated to demonstrate the level of alertness, for example, by calling patient's name in a normal voice, calling in a loud voice, light touch on the arm, vigorous shaking of the arm, or painful stimulus.

Grade the level of consciousness: conscious/confusion/somnolence/clouding/delirium/stupor/coma. Any disturbance in the level of consciousness should ideally be rated on Glasgow Coma Scale, where a numeric value is given to the best response in each of the three categories (eye opening, verbal, motor).

Orientation

Whether the patient is well oriented to time (test by asking the time, date, day, month, year, season, and the time spent in hospital), place (test by asking the present location, building, city, and country) and person (test by asking his own name, and whether he can identify people around him and their role in that setting). Disorientation in time usually precedes disorientation in place and person.

Attention

Is the attention easily aroused and sustained; Ask the patient to repeat digits forwards and backwards (digit span test; digit forward and backward test), one at a time (for example, patient may be able to repeat 5 digits forward and 3 digits backwards). Start with two digit numbers increasing gradually up to eight digit numbers or till failure occurs on three consecutive occasions.

Concentration

Can the patient concentrate; Is he easily distractible; Ask to subtract serial sevens from hundred (100-7 test), or serial threes from fifty (50-3 test), or to count backwards from 20, or enumerate the names of the months (or days of the week) in the reverse order.

Note down the answers and the time taken to perform the tests.

Memory

a. Immediate Retention and Recall (IR and R)
Use the digit span test to assess the immediate memory; digit forwards and digit backwards subtests

(also used for testing attention; are described under attention).

b. Recent Memory
Ask how did the patient come to the room/hospital; what he ate for dinner the day before or for breakfast the same morning. Give an address to be memorised and ask it to be recalled 15 minutes later or at the end of the interview.

c. Remote Memory
Ask for the date and place of marriage, name and birthdays of children, any other relevant questions from the person's past. Note any amnesia (anterograde/retrograde), or confabulation, if present.

Intelligence

Intelligence is the ability to think logically, act rationally, and deal effectively with environment.

Ask questions about general information, keeping in mind the patient's educational and social background, his experiences and interests, for example, ask about the current and the past prime ministers and presidents of India, the capital of India, and the name of the various states.

Test for reading and writing; Use simple tests of calculation.

Abstract thinking

Abstract thinking is characterised by the ability to:
a. assume a mental set voluntarily,
b. shift voluntarily from one aspect of a situation to another,
c. keep in mind simultaneously the various aspects of a situation,
d. grasp the essentials of a 'whole' (for example, situation or concept), and
e. to break a 'whole' into its parts.

Abstract thinking testing assesses patient's concept formation. The methods used are:
a. Proverb Testing: The meaning of simple proverbs (usually three) should be asked.
b. Similarities (and also the differences) between familiar objects should be asked, such as: table/chair; banana/orange; dog/lion; eye/ear.

The answers may be overly concrete or abstract. The appropriateness of answers is judged. Concretisation of responses or inappropriate answers may occur in schizophrenia.

Insight

Insight is the degree of awareness and understanding that the patient has regarding his illness.

Ask the patient's attitude towards his present state; whether there is an illness or not; if yes, which kind of illness (physical, psychiatric or both); is any treatment needed; is there hope for recovery; what is the cause of illness. Depending on the patient's responses, insight can be graded on a six-point scale (Table 2.3).

Judgement

Judgement is the ability to assess a situation correctly and act appropriately within that situation. Both social and test judgement are assessed.

i. Social judgement is observed during the hospital stay and during the interview session. It includes an evaluation of 'personal judgement'.

ii. Test judgement is assessed by asking the patient what he would do in certain test situations, such as 'a house on fire', or 'a man lying on the road', or 'a sealed, stamped, addressed envelope lying on a street'.

Judgement is rated as Good/Intact/Normal or Poor/Impaired/Abnormal.

INVESTIGATIONS

After a detailed history and examination, investigations (laboratory tests, diagnostic standardised interviews, family interviews, and/or psychological tests) are carried out based on the diagnostic and aetiological possibilities. Some of these investigations are described briefly in Table 2.4.

FORMULATION

After a comprehensive psychiatric assessment, a diagnostic formulation summarises the detailed posi-

Table 2.3: Clinical Rating of Insight

Insight is rated on a 6-point scale from one to six.
1. Complete denial of illness.
2. Slight awareness of being sick and needing help, but denying it at the same time.
3. Awareness of being sick, but it is attributed to external or physical factors.
4. Awareness of being sick, due to something unknown in self.
5. Intellectual Insight: Awareness of being ill and that the symptoms/failures in social adjustment are due to own particular irrational feelings/thoughts; yet does not apply this knowledge to the current/future experiences.
6. True Emotional Insight: It is different from intellectual insight in that the awareness leads to significant basic changes in the future behaviour.

Table 2.4: Some Investigations in Psychiatry

I. Biological Investigations
Medical Screen
Some of the following tests may be useful in screening for the medical disorders causing the psychiatric symptoms. Some examples of indications are stated in front of the tests (these examples are not intended to be comprehensive).
Haemoglobin: Routine screen.
Total and differential leucocyte counts: Routine screen, Treatment with antipsychotics (e.g. clozapine), lithium, carbamazepine.
Mean Corpuscular Volume (MCV): Alcohol dependence (increased).
Urinalysis: Routine screen; Drug screening.
Peripheral smear: Anaemia.
Renal function tests: Treatment with lithium.
Liver function tests: Treatment with carbamazepine, valproate, benzodiazepines. Alcohol dependence.
Serum electrolytes: Dehydration, SIADH, Treatment with carbamazepine, antipsychotics, lithium.
Blood glucose: Routine screen (age > 35 years), treatment with antipsychotics

Contd...

Contd...

Thyroid function tests: Refractory depression, rapid cycling mood disorder. Treatment with lithium, carbamazepine.

Electrocardiogram (ECG): Age > 35 years, Treatment with lithium, antidepressants, ECT, antipsychotics.

HIV testing: Intravenous drug users, suggestive sexual history, AIDS dementia.

VDRL: Suggestive sexual history.

Chest X-ray: Age > 35 years, Treatment with ECT.

Skull X-ray: History of head Injury.

Serum CK: Neuroleptic malignant syndrome (markedly increased levels).

Toxicology Screen

Useful when substance use is suspected; for example, alcohol, cocaine, opiates, cannabis, phencyclidine, benzodiazepines, barbiturates; remember that certain medications can cause false positive results (for example, quetiapine for methadone).

Drug Levels

Drug levels are indicated to test for therapeutic blood levels, for toxic blood levels, and for testing drug compliance. Examples are lithium (0.6-1.0 meq/L), carbamazepine (4-12 mg/ml), valproate (50-100 mg/ml), haloperidol (8-18 ng/ml), tricyclic antidepressants (nortriptyline 50-150 ng/ml; imipramine 200-250 ng/ml), benzodiazepines, barbiturates and clozapine (350-500 μg/L).

Electrophysiological Tests

EEG (Electroencephalogram): Seizures, dementia, pseudoseizures vs. seizures, episodic abnormal behaviour.

BEAM (Brain electrical activity mapping): Provides topographic imaging of EEG data.

Video-Telemetry EEG: Pseudoseizures vs. seizures.

Evoked potentials (e.g. p300): Research tool.

Polysomnography/Sleep studies: Sleep disorders, seizures (occurring in sleep). The various components in sleep studies include EEG, ECG, EOG, EMG, airflow measurement, penile tumescence, oxygen saturation, body temperature, GSR (Galvanic skin response), and body movement.

Holter ECG: Panic disorder.

Brain Imaging Tests (Cranial)

Computed Tomography (CT) Scan: Dementia, delirium, seizures, first episode psychosis.

Magnetic Resonance Imaging (MRI) Scan: Dementia. Higher resolution than CT scan.

Positron Emission Tomography (PET) Scan: Research tool for study of brain function and physiology.

Single Photon Emission Computed Tomography (SPECT) Scan: Research tool.

Magnetic Resonance (MR) Angiography: Research tool

Magnetic Resonance Spectroscopy (MRS): Research tool

Neuroendocrine Tests

Dexamethasone Suppression Test (DST): Research tool in depression (response to antidepressants or ECT). If plasma cortisol is > 5 mg/100 ml following administration of dexamethasone (1 mg, given at 11 PM the night before and plasma cortisol taken at 4 PM and 11 PM the next day), it indicates non-suppression.

TRH Stimulation Test: Lithium-induced hypothyroidism, refractory depression. If the serum TSH is > 35 mIU/ml (following 500 mg of TRH given IV), the test is positive.

Serum Prolactin Levels: Seizures vs. pseudoseizures, galactorrhoea with antipsychotics.

Serum 17-hydroxycorticosteroid: Organic mood (depression) disorder.

Serum Melatonin Levels: Seasonal mood disorders.

Biochemical Tests

5-HIAA: Research tool (depression, suicidal and/or aggressive behaviour).

MHPG: Research tool (depression).

Platelet MAO: Research tool (depression).

Catecholamine levels: Organic anxiety disorder (e.g. pheochromocytoma).

Genetic Tests

Cytogenetic work-up is useful in some cases of mental retardation.

Sexual Disorder Investigations

Papaverine test: Male erectile disorder (intracavernosal injection of papaverine is sometimes used to differentiate organic from non-organic male erectile disorder).

Nocturnal penile tumescence: Male erectile disorder.

Contd...

Contd...

Serum testosterone: Sexual desire disorders, Male erectile disorder.

Penile Doppler: Male erectile disorder.

Miscellaneous Tests

Lactate provocation test: Panic disorders (In about 70% of patients with panic disorders, sodium lactate infusion can provoke a panic attack).

Drug assisted interview (Amytal interview): Useful in catatonia, unexplained mutism, and dissociative stupor. Discussed in Chapter 18.

CSF examination: Meningitis.

II. Psychological Investigations

Objective Tests

These are pen-and-paper objective tests, which are employed to test the various aspects of personality and intelligence in a person.

Objective personality tests: Some examples of objective personality tests are *MMPI (Minnesota multiple personality inventory)* and *16-PF (16 personality factors)*.

Intelligence tests: Some commonly used tests of intelligence are *WAIS (Wechsler adult intelligence scale)*, *Stanford-Binet test* and *Bhatia's battery of intelligence tests*.

Projective Tests

In projective tests, ambiguous stimuli are used which are not clear to the person immediately. Some commonly used projective tests of personality are *Rorschach inkblot test*, *TAT (Thematic apperception test)*, *DAPT (Draw-a-person test)*, and *sentence completion test* (SCT).

Neuropsychological Tests

Some of the commonly used neuropsychological tests are *Wisconsin card sorting test*, *Wechsler memory scale*, *PGI memory scale*, *BG test (Bender Gestalt test)*, *BVRT (Benton visual retention test)*, *Luria-Nabraska neuropsychological test battery*, *Halstead-Reitan neuropsychological test battery*, and *PGI battery of brain dysfunction*.

Rating Scales

Several rating scales are used in psychiatry to quantify the psychopathology observed. Some of the commonly used scales are *BPRS (Brief psychiatric rating scale)*, *SANS (Scale for assessment of negative symptoms)*, *SAPS (Scale for assessment of positive symptoms)*, *HARS (Hamilton's anxiety rating scale)*, *HDRS (Hamilton's depression rating scale)*, and *Y-BOCS (Yale-Brown obsessive-compulsive scale)*.

Diagnostic Standardized Interviews

The use of these instruments makes the diagnostic assessment more standardized. These include *PSE (Present state examination)*, *SCAN (Schedules for clinical assessment in neuropsychiatry)*, *SCID (Structured clinical interview for DSM-IV)*, and *IPDE (International personality disorder examination)*.

tive (and important negative) information regarding the patient under the focus of care, before listing differential diagnosis, prognostic factors, and a management plan.

The diagnostic formulation focuses on aetiological factors based on the biopsychosocial model (Table 2.5; Fig. 2.3). Similarly, it is useful to devise the management plan based on the biopsychosocial model (Table 2.6). It is possible to use specific formulations based on treatment options; for example, a cognitive formulation for CBT and a psychodynamic formulation for psychodynamic psychotherapy.

Thus, psychiatric assessment is an initial step towards diagnosis and management of psychiatric disorders.

Table 2.5: Diagnostic Formulation

	Biological	*Psychological*	*Social*
Predisposing			
Precipitating			
Perpetuating			
Protective			

Table 2.6: Management Plan

	Biological	*Psychological*	*Social*
Short-term			
Medium-term			
Long-term			

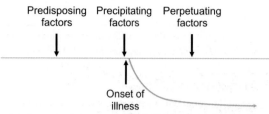

Fig. 2.3: Aetiological Factors Drawn on a Timeline

SPECIAL INTERVIEWS

There are different formats available for detailed evaluation of special populations such as uncooperative patients, hostile and aggressive patients (Chapter 19), suicidal patients (Chapter 19), and children. These formats should be used whenever appropriate.

Chapter 3

Organic (Including Symptomatic) Mental Disorders

It is assumed that all psychological and behavioural processes, whether normal or abnormal, are a result of normal or deranged brain function. A rational corollary would be that all psychiatric disorders are due to abnormal brain functioning and are therefore organic. However, this would be a gross oversimplification.

According to our present knowledge, there are broadly three types of psychiatric disorders:
1. Those due to a known organic cause.
2. Those in whose causation an organic factor has not yet been found or proven.
3. Those primarily due to psychosocial factors.

Only disorders with a known organic cause are called *organic mental disorders*. Thus, organic mental disorders are behavioural or psychological disorders associated with transient or permanent brain dysfunction and include only those mental and behavioural disorders that are due to *demonstrable* cerebral disease or disorder, either *primary* (primary brain pathology) or *secondary* (brain dysfunction due to systemic diseases). The use of term *organic* here does not imply that other psychiatric disorders are 'non-organic' in the sense of having no biological basis. It simply means that the organic mental disorders have a *demonstrable* and *independently diagnosable* cerebral disease or disorder, unlike other psychiatric disorders that do not at present.

Since organic brain illness can mimic any psychiatric disorder, especially in the initial stages, *organic mental disorder should be the first consideration in evaluating a patient with any psychological or behavioural clinical syndrome.* The presence of following features requires a high index of suspicion for an organic mental disorder (or what is loosely called as *organicity*):
1. First episode.
2. Sudden onset.
3. Older age of onset.
4. History of drug and/or alcohol use disorder.
5. Concurrent medical or neurological illness.
6. Neurological symptoms or signs, such as seizures, impairment of consciousness, head injury, sensory or motor disturbance.
7. Presence of confusion, disorientation, memory impairment or soft neurological signs.
8. Prominent visual or other non-auditory (e.g. olfactory, gustatory or tactile) hallucinations.

These disorders can be broadly subcategorised into the following categories:
1. Delirium,
2. Dementia,
3. Organic amnestic syndrome, and
4. Other organic mental disorders.

DELIRIUM

Delirium is the commonest organic mental disorder seen in clinical practice. Five to fifteen percent of all patients in medical and surgical inpatient units are estimated to develop delirium at some time in their lives. This percentage is higher in postoperative patients.

Delirium is the most appropriate substitute for a variety of names used in the past such as acute confusional states, acute brain syndrome, acute organic reaction, toxic psychosis, and metabolic (and other acute) encephalopathies.

Clinical Features

Delirium is characterised by the following features:
1. A relatively acute onset,
2. Clouding of consciousness, characterised by a decreased awareness of surroundings and a decreased ability to respond to environmental stimuli, and
3. Disorientation (most commonly in time, then in place and usually later in person), associated with a decreased attention span and distractibility.

Marked perceptual disturbances such as illusions, misinterpretations, and hallucinations also occur. These are most commonly visual though other perceptual domains can also be involved. There is often a disturbance of sleep-wake cycle; most commonly, insomnia at night with daytime drowsiness. Diurnal variation is marked, usually with worsening of symptoms in the evening and night (called *sun downing*). There is also an impairment of registration and retention of new memories. Psychomotor disturbance, usually in form of agitation and occasionally retardation, is present. Generalised autonomic dysfunction, speech and thought disturbances (such as slurring of speech, incoherence, dysarthria, and fleeting delusions) are often present.

The motor symptoms in delirium can include:
1. Asterixis (flapping tremor),
2. Multifocal myoclonus,
3. *Carphologia* or *floccillation* (picking movements at cover-sheets and clothes),
4. *Occupational delirium* (elaborate pantomimes as if continuing their usual occupation in the hospital bed), and
5. Tone and reflex abnormalities.

Lability of affect is usually present. Motor and verbal perseveration, dysnomia, agraphia and impaired comprehension can also be seen.

Diagnosis

The diagnosis of delirium is frequently missed, as the possibility can be overlooked in medical/surgical settings. It is important to recognize delirium at the earliest possible as delirium often has an underlying aetiology which may be correctable. Any delay in diagnosis, and thus starting treatment, may lead to permanent deficits which can be irreversible.

The diagnosis of delirium is mainly clinical. No ancillary laboratory test is diagnostic, although tests may help in finding the aetiology.

According to ICD-10, for a definite diagnosis of delirium, symptoms (mild or severe) should be present in each one of the five areas described. These include impairment of consciousness and attention (on a continuum from clouding to coma; reduced ability to direct, focus, sustain, and shift attention), global disturbance of cognition, psychomotor disturbances, disturbance of sleep-wake cycle, and emotional disturbances.

The onset is usually rapid, the course diurnally fluctuating, and the total duration of the condition much less than 6 months. The above clinical picture is so characteristic that a fairly confident diagnosis of delirium can be made even if the underlying cause is not clearly established.

A history of underlying physical or brain disease, and/or evidence of cerebral dysfunction (e.g. an abnormal EEG, usually but not always, showing slowing of the background activity) may help in reaching the diagnosis.

Predisposing Factors

Presence of certain predisposing factors lowers the threshold for the development of delirium (Table 3.1).

Aetiology

The list of possible causes of delirium is virtually endless. Any factor which disturbs the metabolism of brain sufficiently can cause delirium. The aetiology of delirium demonstrates a *threshold phenomenon*, with a combination of factors adding up to cross a threshold for causing delirium, which appears to be different for each individual.

Table 3.1: Predisposing Factors in Delirium

1. Pre-existing brain damage or dementia
2. Extremes of age (very old or very young)
3. Previous history of delirium
4. Alcohol or drug dependence
5. Generalised or focal cerebral lesion
6. Chronic medical illness
7. Surgical procedure and postoperative period
8. Severe psychological symptoms (such as fear)
9. Treatment with psychotropic medicines
10. Present or past history of head injury
11. Individual susceptibility to delirium

One of the important causes of delirium, namely post-cardiac surgery delirium, is discussed in Chapter 12. The most common causes are listed in Table 3.2.

Management

1. In cases where a cause is not obvious (or other contributory causes are suspected), a battery of investigations should be done which can include complete blood count, urinalysis, blood glucose, blood urea, serum electrolytes, liver and renal function tests, thyroid function tests, serum B_{12} and folate levels, X-ray chest, ECG, CSF examination, urine for porphyrins, drug screens, VDRL, HIV testing, arterial pO_2 and pCO_2, EEG, and brain imaging (such as cranial CT scan or MRI scan).
2. Identification of the cause and its immediate correction, e.g. 50 mg of 50% dextrose IV for hypoglycaemia, O_2 for hypoxia, 100 mg of B_1 IV

Table 3.2: Delirium: Some Important Causes

Metabolic Causes 　i. Hypoxia, Carbon dioxide narcosis 　ii. Hypoglycaemia 　iii. Hepatic encephalopathy, Uremic encephalopathy 　iv. Cardiac failure, Cardiac arrhythmias, Cardiac arrest 　v. Water and electrolyte imbalance (Water, Na^+, K^+, Mg^{++}, Ca^{++}) 　vi. Metabolic acidosis or alkalosis 　vii. Fever, Anaemia, Hypovolemic shock 　viii. Carcinoid syndrome, Porphyria **Endocrine Causes** 　i. Hypo- and Hyperpituitarism 　ii. Hypo- and Hyperthyroidism 　iii. Hypo- and Hyperparathyroidism 　iv. Hypo- and Hyperadrenalism **Drugs (Both ingestion and withdrawal can cause delirium) and Poisons** 　i. Digitalis, Quinidine, Antihypertensives 　ii. Alcohol, Sedatives, Hypnotics (especially barbiturates) 　iii. Tricyclic antidepressants, Antipsychotics, Anticholinergics, Disulfiram	iv. Anticonvulsants, L-dopa, Opiates 　v. Salicylates, Steroids, Penicillin, Insulin 　vi. Methyl alcohol, heavy metals, biocides. **Nutritional Deficiencies** 　i. Thiamine, Niacin, Pyridoxine, Folic acid, B_{12} 　ii. Proteins **Systemic Infections** 　i. Acute and Chronic, e.g. Septicaemia, Pneumonia, Endocarditis **Intracranial Causes** 　i. Epilepsy (including post-ictal states) 　ii. Head injury, Subarachnoid haemorrhage, Subdural haematoma 　iii. Intracranial infections, e.g. Meningitis, Encephalitis, Cerebral malaria 　iv. Migraine 　v. Stroke (acute phase), Hypertensive encephalopathy 　vi. Focal lesions, e.g. right parietal lesions (such as abscess, neoplasm) **Miscellaneous** 　i. Postoperative states (including ICU delirium) 　ii. Sleep deprivation 　iii. Heat, Electricity, Radiation

for thiamine deficiency, and IV fluids for fluid and electrolyte imbalance.

3. *Symptomatic measures:* As many patients are agitated, emergency psychiatric treatment may be needed. Small doses of benzodiazepines(lorazepam or diazepam) or antipsychotics (haloperidol or risperidone) may be given either orally or parenterally. Maintenance treatment can continue till recovery occurs, usually within a week's time. There is an increased risk of stroke in elderly patients with dementia with prescription of atypical antipsychotics such as olanzapine and risperidone.

4. Supportive medical and nursing care.

DEMENTIA

Dementia is a chronic organic mental disorder, characterised by the following main clinical features:

1. Impairment of *intellectual functions*,
2. Impairment of *memory* (predominantly of recent memory, especially in early stages),
3. Deterioration of *personality* with lack of personal care.

Impairment of all these functions occurs *globally*, causing interference with day-to-day activities and interpersonal relationships. There is impairment of judgement and impulse control, and also impairment of abstract thinking. There is however usually no impairment of consciousness (unlike in delirium; Table 3.3). The course of dementia is usually progressive though some forms of dementia can be reversible.

Additional features may also be present. These include:

1. Emotional *lability* (marked variation in emotional expression).
2. *Catastrophic reaction* (when confronted with an assignment which is beyond the residual intellectual capacity, patient may go into a sudden rage).
3. Thought abnormalities, e.g. perseveration, delusions.
4. Urinary and faecal incontinence may develop in later stages.
5. Disorientation in time; disorientation in place and person may also develop in later stages.
6. Neurological signs may or may not be present, depending on the underlying cause.

Table 3.3: A Comparison of Delirium and Dementia

Features	Delirium	Dementia
1. Onset	Usually acute	Usually insidious
2. Course	Usually recover in 1 week; may take up to 1 month	Usually protracted, although may be reversible in some cases
3. Clinical features		
a. Consciousness	Clouded	Usually normal
b. Orientation	Grossly disturbed	Usually normal; disturbed only in late stages
c. Memory	Immediate retention and recall disturbed	Immediate retention and recall normal
	Recent memory disturbed	Recent memory disturbed
		Remote memory disturbed only in late stages
d. Comprehension	Impaired	Impaired only in late stages
e. Sleep-wake cycle	Grossly disturbed	Usually normal
f. Attention and concentration	Grossly disturbed	Usually normal
g. Diurnal variation	Marked; sundowning may be present	Usually absent
h. Perception	Visual illusions and hallucinations very common	Hallucinations may occur
i. Other features	Asterixis; multifocal myoclonus	Catastrophic reaction; perseveration

Diagnosis

Like delirium, the diagnosis of dementia is clinical though ancillary laboratory investigations may help in elucidating the underlying aetiology.

According to ICD-10, the following features are required for diagnosis: evidence of decline in both memory and thinking, sufficient enough to impair personal activities of daily living, memory impairment (typically affecting registration, storage, and retrieval of new information though previously learned material may also be lost particularly in later stages, impaired thinking, presence of clear consciousness (consciousness can be impaired if delirium is also present), and a duration of at least 6 months.

The following conditions must be kept in mind in the *differential diagnosis* of dementia.

1. *Normal aging process:* Although impairment of memory and intellect are commoner in elderly, their mere presence does not justify a diagnosis of dementia. Dementia is diagnosed only when there is demonstrable evidence of memory and other intellectual impairment which is of sufficient severity to interfere with social and/or occupational functioning. The normal memory impairment in old age is called as *benign senescent forgetfulness*.

2. *Delirium*: The syndromes of delirium and dementia may overlap. See Table 3.3 for a comparison of clinical features.

3. *Depressive pseudodementia:* Depression in the elderly patients may mimic dementia clinically. It is called as *depressive pseudodementia* (Table 3.4). Identification of depression is very important as it is far more easily treatable than dementia.

The depressed patients often complain of memory impairment, difficulty in sustaining attention and concentration, and reduced intellectual capacity. In contrast, patients with dementia do not often complain of these disturbances. In fact, when confronted with evidence of memory impairment, they often confabulate. As depression may often be superimposed on dementia, it is at times necessary to undertake a therapeutic trial with antidepressants, if the clinical picture is unclear.

It is useful to differentiate dementia into cortical and subcortical subtypes (Table 3.5).

Aetiology

A large number of conditions can cause dementia (Table 3.6). However, a majority of cases are due to a few common causes such as Alzheimer's disease and multi-infarct dementia. Some clinically important types of dementia are briefly discussed here.

Alzheimer's Dementia

This is the commonest cause of dementia, seen in about 70% of all cases of dementia in USA. It is more commonly seen in women. Earlier, it was differentiated

Table 3.4: Dementia vs Pseudodementia

Dementia	Pseudodementia (Depressive)
1. Patient rarely complains of cognitive impairment	Patient usually always complains about memory impairment
2. Patient often emphasises achievements	Patient often emphasises disability
3. Patient often appears unconcerned	Patient very often communicates distress
4. Usually labile affect	Severe depression on examination
5. Patient makes errors on cognitive examination	'Do not know' answers are more frequent
6. Recent memory impairment found on examination	Recent memory impairment rarely found on examination
7. Confabulation may be present	Confabulation very rare
8. Consistently poor performance on similar tests	Marked variability in performance on similar tests
9. History of depression less common	Past history of manic and/or depressive episodes may be present

Table 3.5: Cortical and Subcortical Dementia

Features	Cortical Dementia	Subcortical Dementia
1. Site of lesion	Cortex (frontal and temporoparieto-occipital association areas, and hippocampus)	Subcortical grey matter (thalamus, basal ganglia, and rostral brain stem)
2. Examples	Alzheimer's disease, Pick's disease	Huntington' chorea, Parkinson's disease, Progressive supranuclear palsy, Wilson's disease
3. Severity	Severe	Mild to moderate
4. Motor system	Usually normal	Dysarthria, flexed/extended posture, tremors, dystonia, chorea, ataxia, rigidity
5. Other features	Simple delusions; depression uncommon; severe aphasia, amnesia, agnosia, apraxia, acalculia, slowed cognitive speed (bradyphrenia)	Complex delusions; depression common; rarely mania
6. Memory deficit (Short-term)	Recall helped very little by cues	Recall partially helped by cues and recognition tasks

Table 3.6: Some Common Causes of Dementia

A. **Parenchymatous brain disease**
   Alzheimer's disease, Pick's disease, Parkinson's disease, Huntington's chorea, Lewy body dementia, Steel Richardson syndrome (Progressive Supra-nuclear Palsy)

B. **Vascular dementia**
   Multi-infarct dementia, subcortical vascular dementia (Binswanger's disease)

C. **Toxic dementias**
   Bromide intoxication, drugs, heavy metals, alcohol, carbon monoxide, analgesics, anticonvulsants, benzodiazepines, psychotropic drugs

D. **Metabolic dementias**
   Chronic hepatic or uraemic encephalopathy, dialysis dementia, Wilson's disease

E. **Endocrine causes**
   Thyroid, parathyroid, pituitary, adrenal dysfunction

F. **Deficiency dementias**
   Pernicious anaemia, pellagra, folic acid deficiency, thiamine deficiency

G. **Dementias due to infections**
   Creutzfeldt-Jacob disease, neurosyphilis, chronic meningitis, viral encephalitis, AIDS dementia, other HIV-related disorders, subacute sclerosing panencephalitis (SSPE)

H. **Neoplastic dementias**
   Neoplasms and other intracranial space-occupying lesions

I. **Traumatic dementias**
   Chronic subdural haematoma, head injury

J. **Hydrocephalic dementia**
   Normal pressure hydrocephalus

into two forms: a presenile form and a senile form. Now it is known that these two forms represent the same disease clinically and pathologically. There is some evidence to suggest that Alzheimer's disease may have a genetic basis.

The diagnosis of Alzheimer's dementia is by exclusion of all other causes of dementia, as there are no distinct diagnostic clinical features or laboratory investigations. Autopsy shows macroscopic changes such as enlarged cerebral ventricles, widened cerebral sulci and shrinkage of cerebral cortex, as well as microscopic changes such as senile plaques, neurofibrillary tangles, cortical nerve cell loss, and granulovacuolar degeneration. However, these changes are only quantitatively, and not qualitatively, different from a normal aged brain. Neurochemically, there is a marked decrease in brain choline acetyltransferase (CAT) with a similar decrease in brain acetylcholinesterase (AchE).

At present, Alzheimer's dementia is not considered a treatable disorder. However, Cholinesterase Inhibitors such as Rivastigmine (1.5 mg twice a day to 6 mg twice a day), Donepezil (5-10 mg/day), and Galantamine (4 mg twice a day to 12 mg twice a day) have been used in the recent past for treatment of moderate dementia with Alzheimer's disease. These elevate acetylcholine (Ach) concentrations in cerebral cortex by slowing the degradation of acetylcholine released by still intact cholinergic neurons in Alzheimer's disease.

Memantine (5-20 mg/day), an N-methyl-D-aspartate (NMDA) antagonist, is also available for the treatment of moderately severe to severe Alzheimer's disease. There are several other drugs (such as ginkgo biloba, piracetam, and vitamin C and E) used for treatment, though their value remains uncertain.

Multi-infarct Dementia

Multi-infarct dementia is the second commonest cause of dementia, seen in 10-15% of all cases, though some studies indicate that multi-infarct dementia is probably far more common in India. It is also one of the important treatable causes of dementia.

Occurrence of multiple cerebral infarctions can lead to a progressive disruption of brain function, leading to dementia. The most typical form of multi-infarct dementia is characterised by the following features:
1. An abrupt onset,
2. Acute exacerbations (due to repeated infarctions),
3. Stepwise clinical deterioration (*step-ladder pattern*),
4. Fluctuating course,
5. Presence of hypertension (most commonly) or any other significant cardiovascular disease, and
6. History of previous stroke or transient ischemic attacks (TIAs).

Focal neurological signs are frequently present. Insight into the illness is usually present in the early part of the course. Emotional lability is common. EEG (showing focal area of slowing) and brain imaging (CT scan or MRI scan of brain showing multiple infarcts) help in diagnosis. The treatment of the underlying cause can prevent further deterioration by preventing further infarctions.

Hypothyroid Dementia

This has been considered one of the most important treatable and reversible causes of dementia, second only to toxic dementias. Although it accounts for less than 1% of dementias, hypothyroidism should be suspected in every patient of dementia.

Since clinical diagnosis of hypothyroid dementia may be difficult, laboratory tests should be used for correct diagnosis. Prompt treatment can reverse the dementing process and can lead to complete recovery if the treatment is started within two years of the onset of dementia.

AIDS Dementia Complex

About 50-70% of patients suffering from AIDS exhibit a triad of cognitive, behavioural and motoric deficits of *subcortical dementia* type and this is known as the AIDS-dementia complex (ADC). Dementia can in fact be an initial presentation in about 25% cases of AIDS.

As the AIDS virus (a lenti-virus, a type of retrovirus) is highly neurotropic and the virus crosses the blood-brain barrier early in the course of the disease cognitive impairment is nearly ubiquitous in AIDS. The diagnosis is established by ELISA (enzyme-linked immuno-sorbent assay) showing anti-HIV antibodies, and the Western Blot test (blotting of antibody specificities to HIV-specific proteins). A Cranial CT scan can show cortical atrophy 1-4 months before the onset of clinical dementia while MRI scan is helpful in detecting the white matter lesions.

Lewy Body Dementia

Lewy body dementia is now believed to be the second most common cause of the degenerative dementias, accounting for about 4% of all dementias. Typically, the clinical features of Lewy body dementia include:

i. Fluctuating cognitive impairment over weeks or months, with involvement of memory and higher cortical functions (such as language, visuo-spatial ability, praxis and reasoning). Lucid intervals can be present in between fluctuations.

ii. Recurrent and detailed visual hallucinations.

iii. Spontaneous extrapyramidal or parkinsonian symptoms such as rigidity and tremors.

iv. *Neuroleptic sensitivity syndrome*, characterised by a marked sensitivity to the effects of typical doses of antipsychotic drugs (resulting in severe extrapyramidal side-effects with use of antipsychotics).

Other clinical features may include repeated falls, autonomic dysfunction (e.g. orthostatic hypotension), urinary incontinence, delusions and depressive features. Although Lewy bodies (intra-cytoplasmic inclusion bodies) are also present in Parkinson's disease, the occurrence of Lewy bodies in Lewy body dementia is more widespread. A PET (Positron Emission Tomography) or SPECT (Single Photon Emission Computerised Tomography) scan of brain may show low dopamine transporter uptake in basal ganglia.

Antipsychotic medication should be avoided (or used with extreme caution and in low doses) in patients with Lewy body dementia.

Management

Basic Investigations

The diagnostic tests are of great importance in finding the cause, or to exclude all other causes before diagnosing Alzheimer's dementia.

The list of investigations could include complete blood count, urinalysis, blood glucose, serum electrolytes, renal function tests, thyroid function tests, serum B_{12} and folate levels, serological tests for syphilis, arterial pO_2 and pCO_2, X-ray chest, ECG, X-ray skull, EEG, lumbar puncture, CT scan/MRI scan of brain, neuropsychological tests, and drug screens.

Treatment of the Underlying Cause, if Treatable

Some underlying causes of dementia are treatable (*reversible dementias*), for example, treatment of hypertension in multi-infarct dementia, thyroxin replacement in hypothyroid dementia, shunting in hydrocephalic dementia, levodopa in parkinsonism, and removal of the toxic agent in toxic dementias. Early treatment can prevent further deterioration of dementia.

Symptomatic Management

1. Environmental manipulation and focus on coping skills to reduce stress in day-to-day activities.

2. Treatment of medical complications, if any.

3. Care of food and hygiene

4. Supportive care for the patient and family/carers.

5. Anxiety symptoms can be treated with low dose of a short-acting benzodiazepine (such as Lorazepam and Oxazepam), though care should be taken to prevent benzodiazepine dependence/misuse.

6. Depression can be treated with low doses of SSRIs such as Citalopram or Sertraline as these antidepressants have low anticholinergic activity and have a safer cardiac profile. Agents with high anticholinergic activity can cause confusion or even frank delirium.

7. Psychotic symptoms and disruptive behaviours can be treated with low doses of antipsychotics. Haloperidol and Risperidone have usually been preferred as they are less sedating and have low cardiac toxicity, though Risperidone can cause postural hypotension. Recently, the use of antipsychotics in treatment of behavioural symptoms in dementia has decreased markedly due to possible association of antipsychotic use with increased mortality. Antipsychotics should also be avoided if Lewy body dementia is suspected.

8. Short-term hospitalisation may be needed for emergent symptoms whilst a longer term hospitalisation or respite placement may be necessary in later stages.

9. Specific drug treatment such as cholinesterase inhibitors (e.g. donepezil, rivastigmine, galantamine) in moderate Alzheimer's disease, or memantine (NMDA antagonist) in moderate to severe Alzheimer's disease, can be helpful.

ORGANIC AMNESTIC SYNDROME

Organic amnestic syndrome is characterised by the following clinical features:

1. Impairment of memory due to an underlying organic cause,
2. No severe disturbance of consciousness and attention (unlike delirium), and
3. No global disturbance of intellectual function, abstract thinking and personality (unlike dementia).

The *impairment of memory* is characterised by a severe impairment of recent memory or short-term memory (inability to learn new material). This is associated with impaired remote memory or long-term memory (inability to recall previously learned material). There is however no impairment of immediate memory (i.e. immediate retention and recall).

Although recent memory is severely disturbed, very remote events are better remembered, especially in the initial stages. Recent memory impairment also leads to disorientation in time and place. To fill in the memory gaps, the patient uses imaginary events in the early phase of illness (*confabulation*). With the progression of the disease, confabulation often disappears.

Diagnosis

According to ICD-10, the following features are required for the diagnosis: recent memory impairment (anterograde and retrograde amnesia), no impairment of immediate retention and recall, attention, consciousness, and global intellectual functioning, and historical or objective evidence of brain disease or injury (occurs particularly with bilateral involvement of diencephalic and medial temporal structures).

Differential Diagnosis

Amnestic syndrome should be differentiated from delirium, dementia, non-organic mental disorders and transient global amnesia. Differentiation from the first three is relatively easy on the basis of the pattern of memory loss.

Transient Global Amnesia

A rare disorder with an abrupt onset, it resembles amnestic syndrome closely. Differentiation is made on the basis of an abrupt onset and patient's severe distress (because of memory loss) in transient global amnesia. This syndrome is probably caused by temporary cerebral ischaemia in the distribution of posterior cerebral circulation.

Aetiology

1. *Thiamine deficiency:* The most common cause of organic amnestic syndrome is chronic alcohol dependence (alcoholism). It is also called as the *Wernicke-Korsakoff syndrome*. Wernicke's encephalopathy is the acute phase of delirium preceding the organic amnestic syndrome, while Korsakoff's syndrome is the chronic phase of amnestic syndrome.
2. *Any other lesion involving bilaterally the inner core of limbic system* (i.e. mammillary bodies, fornix, hippocampus and para-hippocampal structures of medial temporal lobe, posterior hypothalamus and dorsomedial thalamic nuclei), such as:
   i. Head trauma,
   ii. Surgical procedure (e.g. bilateral temporal lobectomy),
   iii. Hypoxia,
   iv. Posterior cerebral artery stroke (bilateral),
   v. Herpes simplex encephalitis, and
   vi. Space occupying lesions in the region of III ventricle (e.g. neoplasms).

Management

1. Treatment of the underlying cause, e.g. thiamine (high doses) in Wernicke-Korsakoff syndrome. However usually the treatment is of not much help, except in prevention of further deterioration and the prognosis is often poor.
2. Supportive care for general condition and treatment of the associated medical illness.

OTHER ORGANIC MENTAL DISORDERS (DUE TO BRAIN DAMAGE AND DYSFUNCTION, AND TO PHYSICAL DISEASES)

This group includes miscellaneous mental disorders which are causally related to brain dysfunction due to primary cerebral disease, systemic disease (secondary), or toxic substances.

According to ICD-10, an evidence of cerebral disease, damage or dysfunction, or of systemic physical disease, known to be associated with one of the listed syndromes is required, with a temporal relationship between development of the underlying disease and the onset of the mental syndrome, with recovery from the mental disorder following removal or improvement of the underlying presumed cause, and an absence of evidence to suggest an alternative cause of the mental syndrome (such as a strong family history or precipitating stress).

If conditions 1 and 2 are present, a provisional diagnosis can be made; if all four are present, the certainty of diagnosis is significantly increased.

The following clinical conditions are known to be associated with an increased risk for these other organic mental disorders:

Primary Cerebral Diseases

Epilepsy, limbic encephalitis, Huntington's disease, head trauma, brain neoplasms, vascular cerebral disease, cerebral malformations.

Systemic Diseases

Extracranial neoplasms (e.g. carcinoma pancreas), collagen diseases (e.g. SLE), endocrine disease (e.g. hypothyroidism, hyperthyroidism, Cushing's disease), metabolic disorders (e.g. hypoglycaemia, porphyria, hypoxia); infectious diseases (e.g. trypanosomiasis).

Drugs

Steroids, propranolol, levodopa, methyldopa, antihypertensives, antimalarials, alcohol and other psychoactive substances.

ORGANIC HALLUCINOSIS

According to ICD-10, presence of persistent or recurrent hallucinations due to an underlying organic cause is required for the diagnosis of organic hallucinosis, in addition to the general guidelines for the diagnosis of other organic mental disorders, described earlier. It is important to rule out any major disturbance of consciousness, intelligence, memory, mood or thought.

These hallucinations can occur in any sensory modality but are usually *visual* (most common) or auditory in nature. In many cases, they depend on the underlying cause. These *hallucinations* can range from very simple and unformed, to very complex and well-organised. Usually the patients realise that the hallucinations are not real but sometimes there may be a delusional elaboration of hallucinations.

Aetiology

1. *Drugs*: Hallucinogens (LSD, psilocybin, mescaline), cocaine, cannabis, phencyclidine (PCP), levodopa, bromocriptine, amantadine, ephedrine, propranolol, pentazocine, methylphenidate, imipramine, anticholinergics, bromide.
2. *Alcohol:* In *alcoholic hallucinosis,* auditory hallucinations are usually more common.
3. *Sensory deprivation.*
4. *'Release' hallucinations* due to sensory pathway disease, e.g. bilateral cataracts, otosclerosis, optic neuritis.
5. *Migraine.*
6. *Epilepsy:* Complex partial seizures.
7. *Intracranial space occupying lesions.*
8. *Temporal arteritis.*
9. *Brain stem lesions* (peduncular hallucinosis).

Management

1. Treatment of the underlying cause, if treatable.
2. Symptomatic treatment with a low dose of an antipsychotic medication (such as Haloperidol, Risperidone and Olanzapine) may be needed.

ORGANIC CATATONIC DISORDER

According to the ICD-10, the following features are required for the diagnosis of organic catatonic disorder, in addition to the general guidelines for the diagnosis of other organic mental disorders, described earlier:

1. *Stupor* (diminution or complete absence of spontaneous movement with partial or complete mutism, negativism, and rigid posturing);
2. *Excitement* (gross hypermotility with or without a tendency to assaultiveness);
3. *Mixed* (shifting rapidly and unpredictably from hypo- to hyperactivity).

The presence of other catatonic symptoms and signs increases the confidence in the diagnosis. The catatonic symptoms and signs are described in detail in Chapter 5.

Aetiology

The aetiology and management of organic catatonic disorder is described in detail in Chapter 19.

Management

1. Treatment of the underlying cause, if amenable to treatment.
2. Symptomatic treatment with low dose of a short-acting benzodiazepine (e.g. Lorazepam), or electroconvulsive therapy (if needed). Antipsychotics should usually be avoided as they can make catatonic features worse; however small doses of atypical antipsychotics such as Risperidone, Olanzapine, Aripiprazole or Quetiapine can be used with care.

ORGANIC DELUSIONAL (SCHIZOPHRENIA-LIKE) DISORDER

According to ICD-10, presence of predominant delusions caused by an underlying organic cause is required for the diagnosis of organic delusional disorder, in addition to the general guidelines for the diagnosis of other organic mental disorders, described

earlier. It is important to rule out any major disturbance of consciousness, orientation, memory, or mood.

The delusions are variable and the type depends on the underlying aetiology. The most common delusions are *persecutory* in nature. Hallucinations (*visual* more often than auditory) may accompany the delusions. Schneiderian first rank symptoms (SFRS) are usually not seen the organic delusional disorder (in contrast to schizophrenia).

Diagnosis

Organic delusional disorder secondary to amphetamine use may be difficult to differentiate from paranoid schizophrenia. The differentiating points are an acute onset, history of amphetamine use prior to the onset, predominant visual hallucinations which may be fleeting, absence of formal thought disorder and a more 'appropriate' affect.

Aetiology

1. *Drugs:* Amphetamines, hallucinogens, cannabis, disulfiram
2. *Complex partial seizures* (e.g. temporal lobe epilepsy)
3. *Huntington's chorea* (initial stages), *Parkinson's disease, Wilson's disease*, and *idiopathic basal ganglia calcification*
4. *Right parietal lobe lesions,* especially vascular lesions
5. Lesions involving limbic system (e.g. tumours)
6. *Spinocerebellar degeneration*
7. *Cerebral malaria*
8. *Herpes simplex encephalitis*
9. *Nutritional deficiencies* (Vitamin B_{12}, iron)
10. *Demyelinating disorders* (such as multiple sclerosis, metachromatic leukodystrophy)

Management

1. Treatment of the underlying cause such as removal of toxic agent in amphetamine psychosis.
2. Symptomatic management with a low dose of an antipsychotic medication (such as Risperidone, Haloperidol, Olanzapine, or Quetiapine) may be needed.

ORGANIC MOOD (AFFECTIVE) DISORDER

According to ICD-10, presence of prominent and persistent mood disturbance caused by an underlying organic cause is required for the diagnosis of organic mood disorder, in addition to the general guidelines for the diagnosis of other organic mental disorders, described earlier. It is important to rule out any major disturbance of consciousness, orientation, or memory.

The *mood disturbance* can be a major depressive episode, a manic episode, or a mixed affective episode. The severity may vary from mild to severe.

Aetiology

Some of the causes of organic mood disorder are listed below:

1. *Drugs:*
   Mania: INH, Levodopa, Bromide, LSD, Corticosteroids (hypomania), Hallucinogens, Tricyclic antidepressants, Cocaine, Baclofen, Amphetamines, Bromocriptine, Cimetidine, Procyclidine
   Depression: Reserpine, Ethanol, Clonidine, Methyldopa, Propranolol, Corticosteroids, Antipsychotics (particularly typical antipsychotics), Cimetidine, Anticancer chemotherapy, Oral contraceptives.
   Any drug a depressed person is taking should be considered a potential factor in the causation of depressive episode.
2. *Endocrine disorders:*
   Mania: Hyperthyroidism
   Depression: Hypothyroidism, Cushing's syndrome, Addison's disease, hyper- and hypoparathyroidism.
3. *CNS disorders:* Parkinsonism, Huntington's chorea, PSP (progressive supranuclear palsy; depression more likely), CVAs (cerebrovascular accidents; left-sided anterior lesions and right-sided posterior lesions cause depression in stroke), cerebral tumours, epilepsy (complex partial seizures), neurosyphilis (GPI), head injury (mania more likely), multiple sclerosis.
4. *Post-viral illnesses:* Influenza, infectious mononucleosis, viral pneumonia, infectious hepatitis.
5. *Deficiencies*: Pellagra, deficiency of thiamine, folate, niacin, folate, B$_{12}$.
6. *Others:* Carcinoma pancreas (depression), SLE, pernicious anaemia, temporal arteritis (depression), carcinoid syndrome (mania).

Management

1. Management of the underlying organic cause, if treatable.
2. Symptomatic management, if the episodes are severe. For example, for a *manic episode*, low dose antipsychotic medication (such as risperidone, haloperidol, olanzapine) and/or a mood stabiliser (such as valproate); and for a *depressive episode*, low dose antidepressants (such as sertraline or mirtazapine). Antipsychotics are not recommended in patients who have suffered from stroke and/or dementia as the risk of mortality is higher.
   Pathological laughter and crying (associated with multiple sclerosis or stroke) can similarly respond to small dose SSRIs or small dose amitriptyline.

ORGANIC ANXIETY DISORDER

According to ICD-10, presence of prominent and persistent generalised anxiety or panic caused by an underlying cause is required for diagnosis of organic anxiety disorder, in addition to the general guidelines for the diagnosis of other organic mental disorders, described earlier. It is important to rule out any major disturbance of consciousness, orientation, memory, personality, thought, perception, or mood.

Aetiology

1. *Drugs and toxins:* Cocaine, caffeine, amphetamines and other sympathomimetics, alcohol and drug withdrawal, heavy metals, penicillin.
2. *Endocrine disorders:* Thyroid, pituitary, parathyroid, or adrenal dysfunction; pheochromocytoma; fasting hypoglycaemia, carcinoid syndrome.

3. *Systemic diseases:* Cardiac arrhythmias, mitral valve prolapse syndrome, chronic obstructive pulmonary disease, coronary artery disease, pulmonary embolism, anaemia, fever, deficiency diseases.

4. *CNS diseases:* Cerebral tumours, epilepsy (especially complex partial seizures of temporal lobe origin), cerebrovascular disease, postconcussional syndrome.

Management

1. Treatment of the underlying organic cause, if treatable.

2. Symptomatic treatment with benzodiazepines, beta-blockers (such as propranolol), cognitive behaviour therapy, and relaxation techniques may be needed.

ORGANIC PERSONALITY DISORDER (PERSONALITY AND BEHAVIOURAL DISORDERS DUE TO BRAIN DISEASE, DAMAGE AND DYSFUNCTION)

The organic personality disorder is characterised by a significant alteration of the premorbid personality caused by an underlying organic cause without major disturbance of consciousness, orientation, memory or perception. The *personality change* may be characterised by poor impulse control, emotional lability, apathy, accentuation of earlier personality traits, or hostility.

According to ICD-10, the following features are required for diagnosis of organic personality disorder, in addition to the general guidelines for the diagnosis of other organic mental disorders, described earlier. In addition to an established history or other evidence of brain disease, damage, or dysfunction, a definitive diagnosis requires the presence of two or more of six features described. These include consistently reduced ability to persevere with goal-directed activities, altered emotional behaviour (emotional lability, euphoria, inappropriate jocularity, irritability or short-lived anger outbursts), expression of needs and impulses without consideration of the consequences, cognitive disturbances (such as suspiciousness, paranoid ideation, and/or excessive preoccupation with a single theme), marked alteration of language production (such as circumstantiality, over-inclusiveness, viscosity, and hypergraphia), and altered sexual behaviour.

Aetiology

1. *Temporal lobe epilepsy* (complex partial seizures) which can be associated with temporal lobe (personality) syndrome (see Table 3.7).

2. *Concussion* (postconcussional syndrome).

3. *Encephalitis* (postencephalitis syndrome).

4. *Multiple sclerosis* (early).

Table 3.7: Organic Personality Disorders

Organic Personality Disorder	*Clinical Features*
1. Frontal lobe syndrome (Types)	
a. Orbito-frontal syndrome (*Pseudo-psychopathic*)	Disinhibition, jocularity, impulsivity, impaired insight and judgement
b. Frontal convexity type (*Pseudo-depressive*)	Apathy, lack of initiative, retardation, perseveration
c. Medial frontal syndrome (*Akinetic*)	Akinesis, incontinence, poor verbal output
2. Temporal lobe syndrome	Egocentricity, explosive affect, perseveration, excessive religiosity, obsessional traits
3. Bilateral temporal lobe or limbic system lesions	Emotional placcidity, hyper-orality, altered sexual behaviour, excessive exploration of environment (hyper-metamorphosis)

5. *Cerebral neoplasms,* especially in frontal lobe (frontal lobe syndromes) and parietal lobe (see Table 3.7).
6. *Cerebrovascular disease.*
7. *Psychoactive drugs* (rarely).

Management

1. Treatment of the underlying cause, if treatable.
2. Symptomatic treatment, with lithium or carbamazepine for aggressive behaviour and impulse dyscontrol, and/or antipsychotics (occasionally) for violent behaviour may be needed.

MISCELLANEOUS ORGANIC MENTAL DISORDERS

Other organic mental disorders described in ICD-10 include organic dissociative disorder, organic emotionally labile (asthenic) disorder, and mild cognitive disorder.

Chapter 4

Psychoactive Substance Use Disorders

A *drug* is defined (by WHO) as any substance that, when taken into the living organism, may modify one or more of its functions. This definition conceptualises 'drug' in a very broad way, including not only the medications but also the other pharmacologically active substances.

The words 'drug addiction' and 'drug addict' were dropped from scientific use due to their derogatory connotation. Instead 'drug abuse', 'drug dependence', 'harmful use', 'misuse', and 'psychoactive substance use disorders' are the terms used in the current nomenclature. A *psychoactive drug* is one that is capable of altering the mental functioning.

There are four important patterns of substance use disorders, which may overlap with each other.
1. Acute intoxication,
2. Withdrawal state,
3. Dependence syndrome, and
4. Harmful use.

Acute Intoxication

According to the ICD-10, acute intoxication is a transient condition following the administration of alcohol or other psychoactive substance, resulting in disturbances in level of consciousness, cognition, perception, affect or behaviour, or other psychophysiological functions and responses. This is usually associated with high blood levels of the drug.

However, in certain cases where the threshold is low (due to a serious medical illness such as chronic renal failure or idiosyncratic sensitivity) even a low dose may lead to intoxication. The intensity of intoxication lessens with time, and effects eventually disappear in the absence of further use of the substance. The recovery is therefore complete, except where tissue damage or another complication has arisen.

The following codes may be used to indicate whether the acute intoxication was associated with any complications:
    i. *uncomplicated* (symptoms of varying severity, usually dose-dependent, particularly at high dose levels);
    ii. *with trauma or other bodily injury;*
    iii. *with other medical complications* (such as haematemesis, inhalation of vomitus);
    iv. *with delirium;*
    v. *with perceptual distortions;*
    vi. *with coma;*
    vii. *with convulsions;* and
    viii. *pathological intoxication* (only for alcohol).

Withdrawal State

A withdrawal state is characterised by a cluster of symptoms, often specific to the drug used, which develop on total or partial withdrawal of a drug, usually after repeated and/or high-dose use. This, too, is a short-lasting syndrome with usual duration of few hours to few days.

Typically, the patient reports that the withdrawal symptoms are relieved by further substance use.

The withdrawal state is further classified as:
i.   *uncomplicated;*
ii. *with convulsions;* and
iii. *with delirium.*

Dependence Syndrome

According to the ICD-10, the dependence syndrome is a cluster of physiological, behavioural, and cognitive phenomena in which the use of a substance or a class of substances takes on a much higher priority for a given individual than other behaviours that once had greater value.

A central descriptive characteristic of the dependence syndrome is the desire (often strong and sometimes overpowering) to take psychoactive substances (which may or may not have been medically prescribed), alcohol, or tobacco. There may be evidence that return to substance use after a period of abstinence leads to a more rapid reappearance of other features of the syndrome than occurs with non-dependent individuals.

A definite diagnosis of dependence should usually be made only if at least three of the following have been experienced or exhibited at sometime during the previous year:

1. A strong *desire* or sense of *compulsion* to take the substance.
2. *Difficulties in controlling* the substance-taking behaviour in terms of its onset, termination, or levels of use.
3. A physiological *withdrawal state* when the substance use has ceased or reduced, as evidenced by the characteristic withdrawal syndrome for the substance; or use of the same (or a closely related) substance with the intention of relieving or avoiding withdrawal symptoms.
4. Evidence of *tolerance*, such that increased doses of the psychoactive substance are required in order to achieve effects originally produced by lower doses (clear examples of this are found in the alcohol- and opiate-dependent individuals who may take daily doses that are sufficient to incapacitate or kill non-tolerant users).

5. Progressive *neglect* of alternative pleasures or interests because of psychoactive substance use, increased amount of time necessary to obtain or take the substance or to recover from its effects.
6. *Persisting* with substance use despite clear evidence of overtly harmful consequences, such as harm to the liver through excessive drinking, depressive mood states consequent to periods of heavy substance use, or drug-related impairment of cognitive functioning; efforts should be made to determine that the user was actually, or could be expected to be, aware of the nature and extent of the harm.

A *narrowing of personal repertoire of patterns* of psychoactive substance use has also been described as a characteristic feature of the dependence syndrome (e.g. a tendency to drink in the same way on weekdays and weekends, regardless of the social constraints that determine appropriate drinking behaviour).

The dependence syndrome can be further coded as (ICD-10):

i.   *currently abstinent;*
ii. *currently abstinent, but in a protected environment* (e.g. in hospital, in a therapeutic community, in prison, etc.);
iii. *currently on a clinically supervised maintenance or replacement regime* (controlled dependence, e.g. with methadone; nicotine gum or nicotine patch);
iv. *currently abstinent, but receiving treatment with aversive or blocking drugs* (e.g. naltrexone or disulfiram);
v.   *currently using the substance* (active dependence);
vi. *continuous use;* and
vii. *episodic use (dipsomania).*

The dependence can be either *psychic*, or *physical*, or both.

Harmful Use

Harmful use is characterised by:
1. Continued drug use, despite the awareness of harmful medical and/or social effect of the drug being used, and/or

2. A pattern of physically hazardous use of drug (e.g. driving during intoxication).

The diagnosis requires that the actual damage should have been caused to the mental or physical health of the user. Harmful use is not diagnosed, if a dependence syndrome is present. DSM-IV-TR uses the term *substance abuse* instead, with minor variations in description.

The other syndromes associated with the psycho-active substance use in ICD-10 include psychotic disorder, amnesic syndrome, and residual and late-onset (delayed onset) psychotic disorder.

Psychoactive Substances

The major dependence producing drugs are:
1. Alcohol
2. Opioids, e.g. opium, heroin
3. Cannabinoids, e.g. cannabis
4. Cocaine
5. Amphetamine and other sympathomimetics

6. Hallucinogens, e.g. LSD, phencyclidine (PCP)
7. Sedatives and hypnotics, e.g. barbiturates
8. Inhalants, e.g. volatile solvents
9. Nicotine, and
10. Other stimulants (e.g. caffeine).

The various psychoactive substances are summarised in Table 4.1.

Aetiology

The various aetiological factors in substance use disorders are briefly summarised in Table 4.2.

ALCOHOL USE DISORDERS

Alcohol dependence was previously called as *alcoholism*. This term much like 'addiction' has been dropped due to its derogatory meaning.

According to Jellinek, there are five 'species' of alcohol dependence (*alcoholism*) on the basis of the patterns of use (and not on the basis of severity).

Table 4.1: Psychoactive Substance Use Disorders

	Drug	Usual Route of Administration	Physical Dependence	Psychic Dependence	Tolerance
1	Alcohol	Oral	+ +	+ +	+
2	Amphetamines	Oral, Parenteral	+ +	+ +	+ + +
3	Barbiturates	Oral, Parenteral	+ +	+ +	+ + +
4	Benzodiazepines	Oral, Parenteral	+	+	+
5	Caffeine	Oral	+	+ +	+
6	Cannabis (Marihuana)	Smoking, Oral	±	+ +	+
7	Cocaine	Inhalation, Oral, Smoking, Parenteral	±	+ +	–
8	Lysergic acid diethylamide (LSD)	Oral	–	+	+
9	Nicotine	Oral, Smoking	+	+ +	+
10	Opioids	Oral, Parenteral, Smoking	+ + +	+ + +	+ + +
11	Phencyclidine (PCP)	Smoking, Inhalation, Parenteral, Oral	±	+	+
12	Volatile solvents	Inhalation	±	+ +	+

– = None; ± = Probable/Little; + = Some/Mild; + + = Moderate; + + + = Severe.

The dependence can be either *psychic*, or *physical*, or both.

Table 4.2: Aetiological Factors in Substance Use Disorders

1. **Biological Factors**
   i. Genetic vulnerability (family history of substance use disorder; for example in type II alcoholism)
   ii. Co-morbid psychiatric disorder or personality disorder
   iii. Co-morbid medical disorders
   iv. Reinforcing effects of drugs (explains continuation of drug use)
   v. Withdrawal effects and craving (explains continuation of drug use)
   vi. Biochemical factors (for example, role of dopamine and norepinephrine in cocaine, ethanol and opioid dependence)
2. **Psychological Factors**
   i. Curiosity; need for novelty seeking
   ii. General rebelliousness and social non-conformity
   iii. Early initiation of alcohol and tobacco
   iv. Poor impulse control
   v. Sensation-seeking (high)
   vi. Low self-esteem (*anomie*)
   vii. Concerns regarding personal autonomy
   viii. Poor stress management skills
   ix. Childhood trauma or loss
   x. Relief from fatigue and/or boredom
   xi. Escape from reality
   xii. Lack of interest in conventional goals
   xiii. Psychological distress
3. **Social Factors**
   i. Peer pressure (often more important than parental factors)
   ii. Modelling (imitating behaviour of important others)
   iii. Ease of availability of alcohol and drugs
   iv. Strictness of drug law enforcement
   v. Intrafamilial conflicts
   vi. Religious reasons
   vii. Poor social/familial support
   viii. 'Perceived distance' within the family
   ix. Permissive social attitudes
   x. Rapid urbanisation.

A. Alpha (α)
i. Excessive and inappropriate drinking to relieve physical and/or emotional pain.
ii. No loss of control.
iii. Ability to abstain present.

B. Beta (β)
i. Excessive and inappropriate drinking.
ii. Physical complications (e.g. cirrhosis, gastritis and neuritis) due to cultural drinking patterns and poor nutrition.
iii. No dependence.

C. Gamma (γ); also called as *malignant alcoholism*
i. Progressive course.
ii. Physical dependence with tolerance and withdrawal symptoms.
iii. Psychological dependence, with inability to control drinking.

D. Delta (δ)
i. Inability to abstain.
ii. Tolerance.
iii. Withdrawal symptoms.
iv. The amount of alcohol consumed can be controlled.
v. Social disruption is minimal.

E. Epsilon (ε)
i. *Dipsomania* (compulsive-drinking).
ii. Spree-drinking.

Earlier, it was believed that γ-alcoholism was more common in America, while δ-alcoholism was commoner in the wine-drinking countries such as France. At present the existence of this pattern of distribution is doubted and its inclusion in this book is mainly for historical reasons.

Cloninger has classified alcoholism into two types, on the basis of the relative importance of genetic and environmental factors (Table 4.3).

Alcohol dependence is more common in males, and has an onset in late second or early third decade. The course is usually insidious. There is often an associated abuse or dependence of other drugs. If the onset occurs late in life, especially after 40 years of age, an underlying mood disorder should be looked for.

Table 4.3: Classification of Alcoholism

Factors	Type I	Type II
Synonym	Milieu-limited	Male-limited
Gender	Both sexes	Mostly in males
Age of onset	> 25 years	< 25 years
Aetiological factors	Genetic factors important; strong *environmental influences* are contributory	*Heritable*; environmental influences are limited
Family history	May be positive	Parental alcoholism and antisocial behaviour usually present
Loss of control	Present	No loss of control
Other features	Psychological dependence; and guilt present	Drinking followed by aggressive behaviour; spontaneous alcohol seeking
Pre-morbid personality traits	Harm avoidance; high reward dependence	Novelty-seeking

Certain laboratory markers of alcohol dependence have been suggested. These include:

i. *GGT* (γ-glutyl-transferase) is raised to about 40 IU/L in about 80% of the alcohol dependent individuals. GGT returns to normal rapidly (i.e. within 48 hours) on abstinence from alcohol. An increase of GGT of more than 50% in an abstinent individual signifies a resumption of heavy drinking or an abnormality of liver function.

ii. *MCV* (mean corpuscular volume) is more than 92 fl (normal = 80-90 fl) in about 60% of the alcohol dependent individuals. MCV takes several weeks to return to normal values after abstinence.

iii. *Other lab markers* include alkaline phosphatase, AST, ALT, uric acid, blood triglycerides and CK.

GGT and MCV together can usually identify three out of four problem drinkers. In addition, BAC (blood alcohol concentration) and breath analyser can be used for the purpose of identification.

For detection of the problem drinkers in the community, several screening instruments are available. MAST (Michigan Alcoholism Screening Test) is frequently used for this purpose whilst CAGE questionnaire (Table 4.5) is the easiest to be administered (it takes only about 1-2 minutes).

Acute Intoxication

After a brief period of excitation, there is a generalised central nervous system depression with alcohol use. With increasing intoxication, there is increased reaction time, slowed thinking, distractibility and poor motor control. Later, dysarthria, ataxia and incoordination can occur. There is progressive loss of self-control with frank disinhibited behaviour.

The duration of intoxication depends on the amount and the rapidity of ingestion of alcohol. Usually the signs of intoxication are obvious with blood levels of 150-200 mg%. With blood alcohol levels of 300-450 mg%, increasing drowsiness followed by coma and respiratory depression develop. Death occurs with blood alcohol levels between 400 to 800 mg% (Table 4.6).

Occasionally a small dose of alcohol may produce acute intoxication in some persons. This is known as *pathological intoxication*. Another feature, sometimes seen in acute intoxication, is the development of amnesia or *blackouts*.

Withdrawal Syndrome

The most common withdrawal syndrome is a *hangover* on the next morning. Mild tremors, nausea, vomiting, weakness, irritability, insomnia and anxiety are the other common withdrawal symptoms. Sometimes the withdrawal syndrome may be more severe, characterised by one of the following three disturbances: delirium tremens, alcoholic seizures and alcoholic hallucinosis. It is important to remember that alcohol withdrawal syndrome can be associated with marked morbidity as well as significant mortality, and it is important to treat it correctly.

1. Delirium tremens

Delirium tremens (DT) is the most severe alcohol withdrawal syndrome. It occurs usually within 2-4 days of complete or significant abstinence from heavy alcohol drinking in about 5% of patients, as compared to acute tremulousness which occurs in about 34% of patients.

The course is short, with recovery occurring within 3-7 days. This is an acute organic brain syndrome (delirium) with characteristic features of:

i.   Clouding of consciousness with disorientation in time and place.
ii. Poor attention span and distractibility.
iii. Visual (and also auditory) hallucinations and illusions, which are often vivid and very frightening. Tactile hallucinations of insects crawling over the body may occur.
iv. Marked autonomic disturbance with tachycardia, fever, hypertension, sweating and pupillary dilatation.
v.   Psychomotor agitation and ataxia.
vi. Insomnia, with a reversal of sleep-wake pattern.
vii. Dehydration with electrolyte imbalance.

Death can occur in 5-10% of patients with delirium tremens and is often due to cardiovascular collapse, infection, hyperthermia or self-inflicted injury. At times, intercurrent medical illnesses such as pneumonia, fractures, liver disease or pulmonary tuberculosis may complicate the clinical picture.

2. Alcoholic seizures ('rum fits')

Generalised tonic clonic seizures occur in about 10% of alcohol dependence patients, usually 12-48 hours after a heavy bout of drinking. Often these patients have been drinking alcohol in large amounts on a regular basis for many years.

Multiple seizures (2-6 at one time) are more common than single seizures. Sometimes, status epilepticus may be precipitated. In about 30% of the cases, delirium tremens follows.

3. Alcoholic hallucinosis

Alcoholic hallucinosis is characterised by the presence of hallucinations (usually auditory) during partial or complete abstinence, following regular alcohol intake. It occurs in about 2% of patients.

These hallucinations persist after the withdrawal syndrome is over, and classically occur in clear consciousness. Usually recovery occurs within one month and the duration is very rarely more than six months.

Complications of Chronic Alcohol Use

Alcohol dependence is often associated with several complications; both medical and social (Table 4.4). Some withdrawal and intoxication related complications have described above whilst the neuropsychiatric complications are discussed below.

Wernicke's encephalopathy

This is an acute reaction to a severe deficiency of thiamine, the commonest cause being chronic alcohol use. Characteristically, the onset occurs after a period of persistent vomiting. The important clinical signs are:

i.   *Ocular signs:* Coarse nystagmus and ophthalmoplegia, with bilateral external rectus paralysis occurring early. In addition, pupillary irregularities, retinal haemorrhages and papilloedema can occur, causing an impairment of vision
ii. *Higher mental function disturbance:* Disorientation, confusion, recent memory disturbances, poor attention span and distractibility are quite common. Other early symptoms are apathy and ataxia.

Peripheral neuropathy and serious malnutrition are often co-existent. Neuropathologically, neuronal degeneration and haemorrhage are seen in thalamus, hypothalamus, mammillary bodies and midbrain.

Korsakoff's psychosis

As Korsakoff's psychosis often follows Wernicke's encephalopathy; these are together referred to as Wernicke-Korsakoff syndrome.

Table 4.4: Some Complications of Alcohol Dependence

I. Medical Complications

A. *Gastrointestinal System*

   i. Fatty liver, cirrhosis of liver, hepatitis, liver cell carcinoma, liver failure

   ii. Gastritis, reflux oesophagitis, oesophageal varices, Mallory-Weiss syndrome, achlorhydria, peptic ulcer, carcinoma stomach and oesophagus

   iii. Malabsorption syndrome, protein-losing enteropathy

   iv. Pancreatitis: acute, chronic, and relapsing

B. *Central Nervous System*

   i. Peripheral neuropathy

   ii. Delirium tremens

   iii. *Rum fits* (Alcohol withdrawal seizures)

   iv. Alcoholic hallucinosis

   v. Alcoholic jealousy

   vi. Wernicke-Korsakoff psychosis

   vii. Marchiafava-Bignami disease

   viii. Alcoholic dementia

   ix. Suicide

   x. Cerebellar degeneration

   xi. Central pontine myelinosis

   xii. Head injury and fractures.

C. *Miscellaneous*

   i. Acne rosacea, palmar erythema, rhinophyma, spider naevi, ascitis, parotid enlargement

   ii. Foetal alcohol syndrome (craniofacial anomalies, growth retardation, major organ system malformations)

   iii. Alcoholic hypoglycaemia and ketoacidosis

   iv. Cardiomyopathy, cardiac beri-beri

   v. Alcoholic myopathy

   vi. Anaemia, thrombocytopenia, Vitamin K factor deficiency, haemolytic anaemia

   vii. Accidental hypothermia

   viii. Pseudo-Cushing's syndrome, hypogonadism, gynaecomastia (in men), amenorrhoea, infertility, decreased testosterone and increased LH levels

   ix. Risk for coronary artery disease

   x. Malnutrition, pellagra

   xi. Decreased immune function and proneness to infections such as tuberculosis

   xii. Sexual dysfunction

II. Social Complications

   i. Accidents

   ii. Marital disharmony

   iii. Divorce

   iv. Occupational problems, with loss of productive man-hours

   v. Increased incidence of drug dependence

   vi. Criminality

   vii. Financial difficulties.

Table 4.5: CAGE Questionnaire

The CAGE questionnaire basically consists of four questions:

   i. Have you ever had to **C**ut down on alcohol (amount)?

   ii. Have you ever been **A**nnoyed by people's criticism of alcoholism?

   iii. Have you ever felt **G**uilty about drinking?

   iv. Have you ever needed an **E**ye opener drink (early morning drink)?

A score of 2 or more identifies problem drinkers.

Clinically, Korsakoff's psychosis presents as an *organic amnestic syndrome*, characterised by gross memory disturbances, with confabulation. Insight is often impaired. The neuropathological lesion is usually wide-spread, but the most consistent changes are seen in bilateral dorsomedial nuclei of thalamus

Table 4.6: Body Fluid Alcohol Levels

BAC* (mg%)	Behavioural Correlates
25-100	Excitement
80	Legal limit for driving (in UK)**
100-200	Serious intoxication, slurred speech, incoordination, nystagmus
200-300	Dangerous
300-350	Hypothermia, dysarthria, cold sweats
350-400	Coma, respiratory depression
>400	Death may occur

Urinary Alcohol (mg%)	Diagnostic Use	Equivalent BAC (mg%)
>120	Suggestive	80
>200	Diagnostic	150

*BAC - Blood Alcohol Concentration

**30 mg/100 ml in India (Section 185 of the Motor Vehicle Act, 1988)

and mammillary bodies. The changes are also seen in periventricular and periaqueductal grey matter, cerebellum and parts of brain stem.

The underlying cause is believed to be usually severe untreated thiamine deficiency secondary to chronic alcohol use.

Marchiafava-Bignami disease

This is a rare disorder characterised by disorientation, epilepsy, ataxia, dysarthria, hallucinations, spastic limb paralysis, and deterioration of personality and intellectual functioning. There is a widespread demyelination of corpus callosum, optic tracts and cerebellar peduncles. The cause is probably an alcohol-related nutritional deficiency.

Other Complications

These include:

i.   Alcoholic dementia.
ii. Cerebellar degeneration.
iii. Peripheral neuropathy.
iv. Central pontine myelinosis.

Treatment

Before starting any treatment, it is important to follow these steps:

i.   Ruling out (or diagnosing) any physical disorder.
ii. Ruling out (or diagnosing) any psychiatric disorder and/or co-morbid substance use disorder.
iii. Assessment of motivation for treatment.
iv. Assessment of social support system.
v.   Assessment of personality characteristics of the patient.
vi. Assessment of current and past social, interpersonal and occupational functioning.

The treatment can be broadly divided into two categories which are often interlinked. These are detoxification and treatment of alcohol dependence.

Detoxification

Detoxification is the treatment of alcohol withdrawal symptoms, i.e. symptoms produced by the removal of the 'toxin' (alcohol). The best way to stop alcohol (or any other drug of dependence) is to stop it suddenly unless the risks of acute discontinuation are felt to be high by the treating team. This decision is often based on several factors including chronicity of alcohol dependence, daily amount consumed, past history of alcohol withdrawal complications, level of general health and the patient's wishes.

The usual duration of uncomplicated withdrawal syndrome is 7-14 days. The aim of detoxification is symptomatic management of emergent withdrawal symptoms.

The drugs of choice for detoxification are usually *benzodiazepines*. Chlordiazepoxide (80-200 mg/day in divided doses) and diazepam (40-80 mg/day in divided doses) are the most frequently used benzodiazepines. The higher limit of the normal dose range is used in delirium tremens.

A typical dose of Chlordiazepoxide in moderate alcohol dependence is 20 mg QID (four times a day) on day 1, 15 mg QID on day 2, 10 mg QID on day 3, 5 mg QID on day 4, 5 mg BD on day 5 and none on day 6. However, in more severe dependence, higher doses are needed for longer periods (up to 10 days). These drugs are used in a standardised protocol, with the dosage steadily decreasing everyday before being stopped, usually on the tenth day. Clormethiazole (1-2 g/day) and carbamazepine (600-1600 mg/day) are experimental drugs and should not be used routinely for detoxification.

In addition, vitamins should also be administered. In patients suffering from (or likely to suffer from) delirium tremens, peripheral neuropathy, Wernicke-Korsakoff syndrome, and/or with other signs of vitamin B deficiency (especially thiamine and nicotinic acid), a preparation of vitamin B containing 100 mg of thiamine (vitamin B_1) should be administered parenterally, twice everyday for 3-5 days. This should be followed by oral administration of vitamin B_1 for at least 6 months.

Care of *hydration* is another important step; it is extremely important not to administer 5% dextrose (or any carbohydrate) in delirium tremens (or even in uncomplicated alcohol withdrawal syndrome) *without* thiamine.

Although detoxification can be achieved on an outpatient (OPD) basis, some patients do require hospitalisation. These patients may present with:

i. Signs of impending delirium tremens (tremor, autonomic hyperactivity, disorientation, or perceptual abnormalities), or

ii. Psychiatric symptoms (psychotic disorder, mood disorder, suicidal ideation or attempts, alcohol-induced neuropsychiatric disorders), or

iii. Physical illness (caused by chronic alcohol use or incidentally present), or

iv. Inability to stop alcohol in the home setting.

Detoxification is the first step in the treatment of alcohol dependence.

Treatment of Alcohol Dependence

After the step of detoxification is over, there are several methods to choose from, for further management. Some of these important methods include:

i. Behaviour therapy

The most commonly used behaviour therapy in the past has been *aversion therapy*, using either a sub-threshold electric shock or an emetic such as apomorphine. Many other methods (*covert sensitisation*, relaxation techniques, assertiveness training, self-control skills, and positive reinforcement) have been used alone or in combination with aversion therapy. Currently, in most settings, it is considered unethical to use aversion therapy for the treatment of alcohol dependence.

ii. Psychotherapy

Both group and individual psychotherapy have been used. The patient should be educated about the risks of continuing alcohol use, asked to resume personal responsibility for change and be given a choice of options for change. Motivational enhancement therapy with or without cognitive behaviour therapy and life-style modification is often useful, if available.

iii. Group therapy

Of particular importance is the voluntary self-help group known as AA (Alcoholics Anonymous), with branches all over the world and a membership in hundreds of thousands. Although the approach is partly religious in nature, many patients derive benefits from the group meetings which are non-professional in nature.

iv. Deterrent agents

The deterrent agents are also known as *alcohol sensitising drugs*.

Disulfiram (tetraethyl thiuram disulfide) was discovered in 1930s, when it was observed that workers in the rubber industry developed unpleasant reactions to alcohol intake, due to accidental absorption of antioxidant disulfiram. The mechanism of action of disulfiram is summarised in Figure 4.1.

When alcohol is ingested by a person who is on disulfiram, alcohol-derived acetaldehyde cannot be oxidised to acetate and this leads to an accumulation of acetaldehyde in blood. This causes the important *disulfiram-ethanol reaction* (DER) characterised by flushing, tachycardia, hypotension, tachypnoea, palpitations, headache, sweating, nausea, vomiting, giddiness and a sense of impending doom associated with severe anxiety.

The onset of the reaction occurs within 30 minutes, becomes full blown within 1 hour, and subsides usually within 2 hours of ingestion of alcohol. In sensitive patients or in those who have ingested a large amount of alcohol, DER can be very severe and life threatening due to one or more of the following: shock, myocardial infarction, convulsions, hypoxia, confusion and coma.

Therefore, treatment with disulfiram is usually begun in an inpatient hospital setting, usually after a *challenge test* with alcohol to demonstrate that unpleasant and dangerous side-effects occur, if either alcohol or alcohol-containing eatable/drink is consumed whilst treatment is continued with disulfiram.

The usual dose of disulfiram is 250-500 mg/day (taken before bedtime to avoid drowsiness in daytime) in the first week and 250 mg/day subsequently for the maintenance treatment. The effect begins within 12 hours of first dose and remains for 7-10 days after the last dose. The patient should carry a *warning card* detailing the forbidden alcohol-containing articles, the possible effects and their emergency treatment, along with patient identification details.

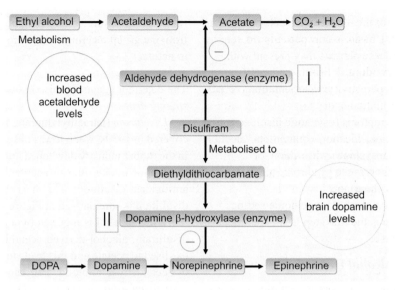

Fig. 4.1: Disulfiram: Mode of Action

The *contraindications* of disulfiram use are first trimester of pregnancy, coronary artery disease, liver failure, chronic renal failure, peripheral neuropathy, muscle disease and psychotic symptoms presently or in the past.

In selected patients (such as an older age group, good motivation, good social support, absent underlying psychopathology and good treatment concordance), the response can be dramatic. In addition to oral preparations, subcutaneous disulfiram implants are also now available. However, they provide unpredictable blood levels of disulfiram.

Other deterrent agents

1. Citrated calcium carbimide (CCC): The mechanism of action is similar to disulfiram but onset of action occurs within 1 hour and is reversible. The usual dosage is 100 mg/d in two divided doses.
2. Metronidazole.
3. Animal charcoal, a fungus (*Coprinus atramentarius*), sulfonylureas and certain cephalosporins also cause a disulfiram like action.

v. Anti-craving agents

Acamprosate, naltrexone and SSRIs (such as fluoxetine) are among the medications tried as anti-craving agents in alcohol dependence.

Acamprosate (the Ca^{++} salt of N-acetyl-homotaurinate) interacts with NMDA receptor-mediated glutamatergic neurotransmission in the various brain regions and reduces Ca^{++} fluxes through voltage-operated channels.

Naltrexone (oral opioid receptor antagonist) probably interferes with alcohol-induced reinforcement by blocking opioid receptors. *Fluoxetine* (and other SSRIs) have been occasionally used as anti-craving agents in their usual antidepressant doses.

vi. Other medications

A variety of other medicines such as benzodiazepines, antidepressants, antipsychotics, lithium, carbamazepine, and even narcotics have been tried. These should be used only if there is a special indication for their use (for example, antidepressants for underlying depression).

vii. Psychosocial rehabilitation

Rehabilitation is an integral part of the multi-modal treatment of alcohol dependence.

OPIOID USE DISORDERS

Dried exudate obtained from unripe seed capsules of *Papaver somniferum* has been used and abused for centuries. The natural alkaloids of opium and their synthetic preparations are highly dependence producing. These are listed in Table 4.7.

In the last few decades, use of opioids has increased markedly all over the world. India, surrounded on both sides by the infamous routes of illicit transport, namely the *Golden Triangle* (Burma-Thailand-Laos) and the *Golden Crescent* (Iran-Afghanistan-Pakistan) has been particularly severely affected.

The most important dependence producing derivatives are morphine and heroin. They both like majority of dependence producing opioids bind to μ (mu) opioid receptors. The other opioid receptors are k (kappa, e.g. for pentazocine), δ (delta, e.g. for a type of enkephalin), σ (sigma, e.g. for phencyclidine), ϵ (epsilon) and λ (lambda).

Heroin or di-acetyl-morphine is about two times more potent than morphine in injectable form. Apart from the parenteral mode of administration, heroin can also be smoked or 'chased' (*chasing the dragon*), often in an impure form (called *'smack'* or *'brown sugar'* in India). Heroin is more addicting than morphine and can cause dependence even after a short period of exposure. Tolerance to heroin occurs rapidly and can be increased to up to more than 100 times the first dose needed to produce an effect.

Acute Intoxication

Intoxication is characterised by apathy, bradycardia, hypotension, respiratory depression, subnormal core body temperature, and pin-point pupils. Later, delayed reflexes, thready pulse and coma may occur in case of a large overdose. In severe intoxication, mydriasis may occur due to hypoxia.

Withdrawal Syndrome

The onset of withdrawal symptoms occurs typically within 12-24 hours, peaks within 24-72 hours, and symptoms usually subside within 7-10 days of the last dose of opioid.

The characteristic symptoms include lacrimation, rhinorrhoea, pupillary dilation, sweating, diarrhoea,

Table 4.7: Opioid Derivatives

A. **Natural Alkaloids of Opium**
   1. Morphine
   2. Codeine
   3. Thebaine
   4. Noscapine
   5. Papaverine

B. **Synthetic Compounds**
   1. Heroin
   2. Nalorphine
   3. Hydromorphone
   4. Methadone
   5. Dextropropoxyphene
   6. Meperidine (Pethidine)
   7. Cyclazocine
   8. Levallorphan
   9. Diphenoxylate

yawning, tachycardia, mild hypertension, insomnia, raised body temperature, muscle cramps, generalised bodyache, severe anxiety, piloerection, nausea, vomiting and anorexia.

There are marked individual differences in presentation of withdrawal symptoms. Heroin withdrawal syndrome is far more severe than the withdrawal syndrome seen with morphine.

Complications

The important complications of chronic opioid use may include one or more of the following:

1. Complications due to illicit drug (contaminants): Parkinsonism, degeneration of globus pallidus, peripheral neuropathy, amblyopia, transverse myelitis.

2. Complications due to intravenous use: AIDS, skin infection(s), thrombophlebitis, pulmonary embolism, septicaemia, viral hepatitis, tetanus, endocarditis.

3. Drug peddling and involvement in criminal activities (social complication).

Treatment

Before treatment, a correct diagnosis must be made on the basis of history, examination (pin-point pupils during intoxication or withdrawal symptoms) and/or laboratory tests. These tests are:

1. *Naloxone challenge test* (to precipitate withdrawal symptoms).
2. Urinary opioids testing: With radioimmunoassay (RIA), free radical assay technique (FRAT), thin layer chromatography (TLC), gas-liquid chromatography (GLC), high pressure liquid chromatography (HPLC) or enzyme-multiplied immunoassay technique (EMIT).

The treatment can be divided into three main types:

1. Treatment of overdose.
2. Detoxification.
3. Maintenance therapy.

Treatment of Opioid Overdose

An overdose of opioid can be treated with *narcotic antagonists* (such as naloxone, naltrexone). Usually an intravenous injection of 2 mg naloxone, followed by a repeat injection in 5-10 minutes, can cause reversal of overdose. But as naloxone has a short half-life repeated doses may be needed every 1-2 hours. This should be combined with general care and supportive treatment.

Detoxification

This is a mode of treatment in which the dependent person is 'taken off' opioids. This is usually done abruptly, followed by management of emergent withdrawal symptoms. It is highly recommended that detoxification is conducted in a safe manner under expert guidance of a specialist.

The withdrawal symptoms can be managed by one of the following methods:

1. *Use of substitution drugs* such as methadone (not available in India at present) to ameliorate the withdrawal symptoms.

   The aim is to gradually taper off the patient from methadone (which is less addicting, has a longer half-life, decreases possible criminal behaviour, and has a much milder withdrawal syndrome). However, relapses are common and its opponents argue that one type of dependence is often replaced by another (methadone).

2. *Clonidine* is an α_2 agonist that acts by inhibiting norepinephrine release at presynaptic α_2 receptors. The usual dose is 0.3-1.2 mg/day, and drug is tapered off in 10-14 days. It can be started after stoppage of either the opioid itself or the substitution drug (methadone). The important side effects of clonidine are excessive sedation and postural hypotension. Clonidine treatment is usually started in an inpatient psychiatric or specialist alcohol and drug treatment centre setting.

3. *Naltrexone with Clonidine:* Naltrexone is an orally available narcotic antagonist which, when given to an opioid dependent individual, causes withdrawal symptoms. These symptoms are managed with the addition of clonidine for 10-14 days after which clonidine is withdrawn and the patient is continued on naltrexone alone. Now if the person takes an opioid, there are no pleasurable experiences, as the opioid receptors are blocked by naltrexone. Therefore, this method is a combination of detoxification and maintenance treatment. The usual dose of naltrexone is 100 mg orally, administered on alternate days. Once again treatment is usually started in an inpatient psychiatric or specialist alcohol and drug treatment centre setting.

4. *Other Drugs:* The other detoxification agents include LAAM (levo-alpha-acetyl-methadol), propoxyphene, diphenoxylate, buprenorphine (long acting synthetic partial μ-agonist which can be administered sublingually), and lofexidine (α_2 agonist, similar to clonidine).

   In particular, Buprenorphine has recently been used widely for detoxification as well as for maintenance treatment in many parts of the World. Care must be exercised as there is potential for misuse with buprenorphine.

Maintenance Therapy

After the detoxification phase is over, the patient is maintained on one of the following regimens:

1. *Methadone maintenance*
   (Agonist substitution therapy)

This a very popular method used widely in the Western World. 20-50 mg/day of methadone is given to the patients to 'shift' them from 'hard' drugs, thus decreasing IV use and criminal behaviour. Its use in India has not been recommended by an expert committee for de-addiction services.

Other drugs such as LAAM and buprenorphine can be used for maintenance treatment.

2. *Opioid antagonists*

Opioid antagonists have been in use for a long time but they were either partial antagonists (such as nalorphine) or had to be administered parenterally (such as naloxone). Now with the availability of orally effective and very potent antagonists, such as naltrexone, the use of opioid antagonists in routine practice has been simplified. The usual maintenance dose is 100 mg on Mondays and Wednesdays, and 150 mg on Fridays. Naltrexone combined with clonidine, as described above, is a very effective method for detoxification as well as for maintenance treatment.

3. *Other methods*

These include individual psychotherapy, behaviour therapy, interpersonal therapy, cognitive behaviour therapy (CBT), motivational enhancement therapy, self-control strategies, psychotropic drugs for associated psychopathology, family therapy, and group therapy (e.g. in therapeutic communities such as *Synanon,* self-help groups such as *Narcotic Anonymous or NA*). These methods have to be tailored for use in an individual patient.

4. *Psychosocial rehabilitation*

This is a very important step in the post-detoxification phase, in the absence of which relapse rates can be very high. Rehabilitation should be at both occupational and social levels.

CANNABIS USE DISORDER

Cannabis is derived from the hemp plant, *Cannabis sativa*, which has several varieties named after the region in which it is found (e.g. *sativa indica* in India and Pakistan, and *americana* in America).

Cannabis (street names: *grass*, *hash* or *hashish*, *marihuana*) produces more than 400 identifiable chemicals of which about 50 are cannabinoids, the most active being Δ-9-tetrahydrocannabinol (Δ^9-THC). The pistillate form of the female plant is more important in cannabis production (Table 4.8).

Recently, a G_i-protein (inhibitory G-protein) linked cannabinoid receptor has been found (in basal ganglia, hippocampus and cerebellum) which inhibits the adenylate cyclase activity in a dose-dependent manner.

Cannabis produces a very mild physical dependence, with a relatively mild withdrawal syndrome, which is characterised by fine tremors, irritability, restlessness, nervousness, insomnia, decreased appetite and craving. This syndrome begins within few hours of stopping cannabis use and lasts for 4 to 5 days. However, some health professionals feel that there is no true physical dependence with cannabis.

Table 4.8: Cannabis Preparations

	Cannabis Preparation	Portion of Plant	THC Content (%)	Potency (as compared to 'Bhang')
1	Hashish/Charas	Resinous exudate from the flowering tops of cultivated plantsh	8-14	10
2	Ganja	Small leaves and brackets of inflorescence of highly cultivated plants	1-2	2
3	Bhang	Dried leaves, flowering shoots and cut tops of uncultivated plants	1	1
4	Hash oil	Lipid soluble plant extract	15-40	25

On the other hand, psychological dependence ranges from mild (occasional 'trips') to marked (compulsive use). All the active ingredients are called as *marijuana* or *marihuana*. Cannabis can be detected in urine for up to 3 weeks after chronic heavy use.

Acute Intoxication

Mild cannabis intoxication is characterised by mild impairment of consciousness and orientation, light-headedness, tachycardia, a sense of floating in the air, a euphoric dream-like state, alternation (either an increase or decrease) in psychomotor activity and tremors, in addition to photophobia, lacrimation, tachycardia, reddening of conjunctiva, dry mouth and increased appetite. There is often a curious splitting of consciousness, in which the user seems to observe his own intoxication as a non-participant observer, along with a feeling that time is slowed down.

Perceptual disturbances are common and can include depersonalisation, derealisation, *synaesthesias* (sensation in one sensory modality caused by a sensation in another sensory modality, e.g. 'seeing' the music) and increased sensitivity to sound. However, hallucinations are seen only in marked to severe intoxication. These are often visual, ranging from elementary flashes of lights and geometrical figures to complex human faces and pictures.

Mild cannabis intoxication releases inhibitions, which is expressed in words and emotions rather than in actions. 'Flashback phenomenon' has been described, and is characterised by a recurrence of cannabis use experience in the absence of current cannabis use.

Complications

The complications of cannabis use can include:

1. *Transient or short-lasting psychiatric disorders:* Acute anxiety, paranoid psychosis, hysterical fugue-like states, suicidal ideation, hypomania, schizophrenia-like state (which is characterised by persecutory delusions, hallucinations and at times catatonic symptoms), acute organic psychosis and, very rarely, depression.

2. *Amotivational syndrome:* Chronic cannabis use is postulated to cause lethargy, apathy, loss of interest, anergia, reduced drive and lack of ambition. The aetiological role of cannabis in this disorder is however far from proven.

3. *'Hemp insanity' or cannabis psychosis: Indian hemp insanity* was first described by Dhunjibhoy in 1930. Thereafter, several reports appeared in literature from India, Egypt, Morocco and Nigeria. It was described as being similar to an acute schizophreniform disorder with disorientation and confusion, and with a good prognosis. The validity of this specific disorder is currently doubted.

4. *Other complications:* Chronic cannabis use sometimes leads to memory impairment, worsening or relapse in schizophrenia or mood disorder, chronic obstructive airway disease, pulmonary malignancies, alteration in both the humoral and cell-mediated immunity, decreased testosterone levels, anovulatory cycles, reversible inhibition of spermatogenesis, blockade of gonadotropin releasing hormone, and increased risk for the developing foetus (if taken during pregnancy).

Treatment

As the withdrawal syndrome is usually very mild, the management consists of supportive and symptomatic treatment, if the patient comes to medical attention. The psychiatric symptoms may require appropriate psychotropic medication and sometimes hospitalisation. Psychotherapy and psychoeducation are very important in the management of psychic dependence.

COCAINE USE DISORDER

Cocaine is an alkaloid derived from the coca bush, *Erythroxylum coca*, found in Bolivia and Peru. It was isolated by Albert Neimann in 1860 and was used by Karl Koller (a friend of Freud) in 1884 as the first effective local anesthetic agent.

Cocaine (common street name: *Crack*) can be administered orally, intranasally, by smoking *(free basing)* or parenterally, depending on the preparation available (Fig. 4.2). Cocaine HCl is the commonest form used, followed by the free base alkaloid. Both intravenous use and free base inhalation produce a 'rush' of pleasurable sensations.

Cocaine is a central stimulant which inhibits the reuptake of dopamine, along with the reuptake of norepinephrine and serotonin. In animals, cocaine is the most powerful reinforcer of the drug-taking behaviour. A typical pattern of cocaine use is cocaine 'runs' (binges), followed by the cocaine 'crashes' (interruption of use). Cocaine is sometimes used in combination with opiates like heroin ('speed ball') or at times amphetamines. Previously uncommon, cocaine misuse appears to be recently a growing problem in the metros of India.

Acute Intoxication

Acute cocaine intoxication is characterised by pupillary dilatation, tachycardia, hypertension, sweating, and nausea or vomiting. A hypomanic picture with increased psychomotor activity, grandiosity, elation of mood, hypervigilance and increased speech output may be present. Later, judgement is impaired and there is impairment of social or occupational functioning.

Withdrawal Syndrome

Cocaine use produces a very mild physical, but a very strong psychological, dependence. A triphasic withdrawal syndrome usually follows an abrupt discontinuation of chronic cocaine use (Table 4.9).

Complications

The complications of chronic cocaine use include acute anxiety reaction, uncontrolled compulsive behaviour, psychotic episodes (with persecutory delusions, and tactile and other hallucinations), delirium and delusional disorder. High doses of cocaine can often lead to seizures, respiratory depression, cardiac arrhythmias, coronary artery occlusion, myocardial infarction, lung damage, gastrointestinal necrosis, foetal anoxia and perforation of nasal septum.

Treatment

Before starting treatment, it is essential to diagnose (or rule out) co-existent psychiatric and/or physical disorder, and assess the motivation for treatment.

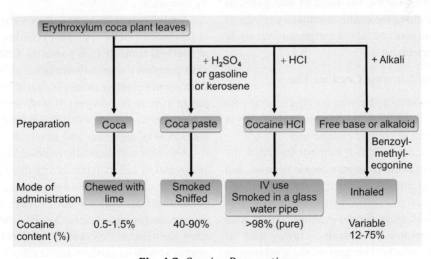

Fig. 4.2: Cocaine Preparations

Table 4.9: Phases in Cocaine Withdrawal Syndrome

Phase	Sub-stage	Duration	Clinical Features
I (Crash phase)	i	9 hours to	Agitation, depression, anorexia, craving + + +
	ii	4 days	Fatigue, depression, sleepiness, craving +
	iii	after discontinuation	Exhaustion, hypersomnia with intermittent awakening, hyperphagia, craving ±
II	i	4 to 7 days after discontinuation	Normal sleep, improved mood, craving ±
	ii		Anxiety, anergia, anhedonia, craving + +
III (Extinction phase)		After 7-10 days of discontinuation	No withdrawal symptoms, increased vulnerability to relapse

Cocaine use disorder is commonly associated with mood disorder, particularly major depression and cyclothymia.

Treatment of Cocaine Overdose

The treatment of overdose consists of oxygenation, muscle relaxants, and IV thiopentone and/or IV diazepam (for seizures and severe anxiety).

IV propranolol, a specific antagonist of cocaine-induced sympathomimetic effects, can be helpful, administered by a specialist. Haloperidol (or pimozide) can be used for the treatment of psychosis, as well as for blocking the cardio-stimulatory effects of cocaine. These must be administered very carefully by an expert specialist.

Treatment of Chronic Cocaine Use

The management of underlying (or co-existent) psychopathology is probably the most important step in the management of chronic cocaine use.

The pharmacological treatment includes the use of bromocriptine (a dopaminergic agonist) and amantadine (an antiparkinsonian) in reducing cocaine craving.

Other useful drugs are desipramine, imipramine and trazodone (both for reducing craving and for antidepressant effect). The goal of the treatment is total abstinence from cocaine use.

The psychosocial management techniques, such as supportive psychotherapy and contingent behaviour therapy, are useful in the post-withdrawal treatment and in the prevention of relapse.

AMPHETAMINE USE DISORDER

Though synthesised by Edleano in 1887, it was introduced in Medicine in 1932 as benzedrine inhaler, for the treatment of coryza, rhinitis and asthma. Later, it was recommended for a variety of conditions such as narcolepsy, postencephalitic parkinsonism, obesity, depression, and even to heighten energy and capacity to work.

Amphetamine refers to a unique chemical which is basically phenyl-iso-propylamine or methyl-phenethylamine. It is a powerful CNS stimulant, with peripheral sympathomimetic effects too. The dextro-amphetamine isomer is nearly 3-4 times more potent than the levo-isomer. It acts primarily on norepinephrine release in brain, along with an action on the release of dopamine and serotonin.

Although still clinically indicated for narcolepsy and attention deficit hyperactivity disorder (and very rarely for obesity and mild depression), one of the commonest patterns of 'use' is seen amongst the students and sports-persons to overcome the need for sleep and fatigue. Tolerance usually develops to the central as well as cardiovascular effects of amphetamines.

Recently, there has been a resurgence of amphetamine use in USA and Europe, with the availability of 'designer' amphetamines, such as MDMA (3,4-methy-lenedioxy-amphetamine; street name: *ecstasy* or *XTC*).

Intoxication and Complications

The signs and symptoms of acute amphetamine intoxication are primarily cardiovascular (tachycardia, hypertension, haemorrhage, cardiac failure and cardiovascular shock) and central (seizures, hyperpyrexia, tremors, ataxia, euphoria, pupillary dilatation, tetany and coma). The neuropsychiatric manifestations include anxiety, panic, insomnia, restlessness, irritability, hostility and bruxism.

Acute intoxication may present as a paranoid hallucinatory syndrome which closely mimics paranoid schizophrenia. The distinguishing features include rapidity of onset, prominence of visual hallucinations, absence of thought disorder, appropriateness of affect, fearful emotional reaction, and presence of confusion. However, a confident diagnosis requires an estimation of the recent urinary amphetamine levels. Amphetamine-induced psychosis usually resolves within seven days of urinary clearance of amphetamines.

Chronic amphetamine intoxication leads to severe and compulsive craving for the drug. A high degree of tolerance is characteristic, with the dependent individual needing up to 15-20 times the initial dose, in order to obtain the pleasurable effects. A common pattern of chronic use is a cycle of *runs* (heavy use for several days) followed by *crashes* (stopping the drug use).

Tactile hallucinations, in clear consciousness, may sometimes occur in chronic amphetamine intoxication.

Withdrawal Syndrome

The withdrawal syndrome is typically seen on an abrupt discontinuation of amphetamines after a period of chronic use. The syndrome is characterised by depression (may present with suicidal ideation), marked asthenia, apathy, fatigue, hypersomnia alternating with insomnia, agitation and hyperphagia.

Treatment

Treatment of Intoxication

Acute intoxication is treated by symptomatic measures, e.g. hyperpyrexia (cold sponging, parenteral antipyretics), seizures (parenteral diazepam), psychotic symptoms (antipsychotics), and hypertension (antihypertensives). Acidification of urine (with oral NH_4Cl; 500 mg every 4 hours) facilitates the elimination of amphetamines.

Treatment of Withdrawal Symptoms

The presence of severe suicidal depression may necessitate hospitalisation. The treatment includes symptomatic management, use of antidepressants and supportive psychotherapy. The management of withdrawal syndrome is usually the first step towards successful management of amphetamine dependence.

LSD USE DISORDER

Lysergic acid diethylamide, first synthesised by Albert Hoffman in 1938 and popularly known as 'acid', is a powerful hallucinogen. It is related to the psychedelic compounds found in the 'morning glory' seeds, the lysergic acid amides. As little as 100 µg of LSD is sufficient to produce behavioural effects in man. LSD presumably produces its effects by an action on the 5-HT levels in brain.

Although tolerance as well as psychological dependence can occur with LSD use, no physical dependence or withdrawal syndrome is reported. A common pattern of LSD use is a *trip* (occasional use followed by a long period of abstinence).

Intoxication

The characteristic features of acute LSD intoxication are perceptual changes occurring in a clear consciousness. These perceptual changes include depersonalisation, derealisation, intensification of perceptions, synaesthesias (for example, colours are heard, and sounds are felt), illusions, and hallucinations.

In addition, features suggestive of autonomic hyperactivity, such as pupillary dilatation, tachycardia, sweating, tremors, incoordination, palpitations, raised temperature, piloerection and giddiness, can also be present.

These changes are usually associated with marked anxiety and/or depression, though euphoria is more common in small doses. Persecutory and referential ideation may also occur.

Sometimes, acute LSD intoxication presents with an acute panic reaction, known as a *bad trip*, in which the individual experiences a loss of control over his self. The recovery usually occurs within 8-12 hours of the last dose. Rarely, the intoxication is severe enough to produce an acute psychotic episode resembling a schizophreniform psychosis.

Withdrawal Syndrome

No withdrawal syndrome has been described with LSD use.

However, sometimes, there is a spontaneous recurrence of the LSD use experience in a drug free state. Described as a *flashback*, it usually occurs weeks to months after the last experience. Such episodes are often induced by stress, fatigue, alcohol intake, severe physical illness or marihuana intoxication.

Complications

Long-term LSD use is not a common phenomenon. The complications of chronic LSD use include psychiatric symptoms (anxiety, depression, psychosis or visual hallucinosis) and occasionally foetal abnormalities.

Treatment

The treatment of acute LSD intoxication consists of symptomatic management with antianxiety, antidepressant or antipsychotic medication, along with supportive psychotherapy.

BARBITURATE USE DISORDER

Barbiturate use disorder is now subsumed under sedative, hypnotic and anxiolytic use disorders. However, it has been described separately as it has some distinctive features.

Since their introduction in 1903, barbiturates have been used as sedatives, hypnotics, anticonvulsants, anaesthetics and tranquilisers. The commonly abused barbiturates are secobarbital, pentobarbital and amobarbital. Their use has recently decreased markedly as benzodiazepines have replaced barbiturates in the majority of their clinical uses.

Barbiturates produce marked physical and psychological dependence. Tolerance (both central and metabolic) develops rapidly and is usually marked. There is also a cross tolerance with alcohol.

Intoxication and Complications

Acute intoxication, typically occurring as an episodic phenomenon, is characterised by irritability, increased productivity of speech, lability of mood, disinhibited behaviour, slurring of speech, incoordination, attentional and memory impairment, and ataxia. Mild barbiturate intoxication resembles alcohol intoxication; severe forms may present with diplopia, nystagmus, hypotonia, positive Romberg's sign and suicidal ideation. Drug automatism may sometimes lead to lethal accidents.

Intravenous use can lead to skin abscesses, cellulitis, infections, embolism and hypersensitivity reactions.

Withdrawal Syndrome

The barbiturate withdrawal syndrome can be very severe. It usually occurs in individuals who are taking more than 600-800 mg/day of secobarbital equivalent for more than one month.

It is usually characterised by marked restlessness, tremors, hypertension, seizures, and in severe cases, a psychosis resembling delirium tremens. The withdrawal syndrome is at its worst about 72 hours after the last dose. Coma, followed by death, can occur in some cases.

Treatment

The barbiturate intoxication should be treated symptomatically. If patient is conscious induction of vomiting and use of activated charcoal can reduce drug absorption. If coma ensues, intensive care measures should be employed on an emergency basis.

The treatment of withdrawal syndrome is usually conservative. However, pentobarbital substitution therapy has been suggested for treatment of withdrawal from short-acting barbiturates. After detoxification phase is over, follow-up supportive treatment and treatment of associated psychiatric disorder, usually depression, are important steps to prevent relapses.

BENZODIAZEPINES AND OTHER SEDATIVE-HYPNOTIC USE DISORDER

Since the discovery of chlordiazepoxide in 1957 by Sternbach, benzodiazepines have replaced other sedative-hypnotics in treatment of insomnia and anxiety. These are currently one of the most often prescribed drugs. Benzodiazepines produce their effects by acting on the benzodiazepine receptors (GABA-benzodiazepine receptor complex), thereby indirectly increasing the action of GABA, the chief inhibitory neurotransmitter in the human brain.

Benzodiazepine (or sedative-hypnotic) use disorder can be either iatrogenic or originating with illicit drug use. Dependence, both physical and psychological, can occur and tolerance is usually moderate.

Intoxication and Complications

Acute intoxication resembles alcohol intoxication whilst chronic intoxication causes tolerance, especially to the sedative and anticonvulsant actions of benzodiazepines. Excessive doses can lead to respiratory depression, coma and death while chronic use has been reported to cause amnestic syndrome.

Some of the other complications of benzodiazepines, particularly with high dose and chronic use, include behavioural disinhibition, impulsivity, blackouts, memory loss, worsening of depression and interactions with other prescribed medications.

Withdrawal Syndrome

A typical withdrawal syndrome, after cessation of prolonged use (more than 4-6 weeks) of moderate to heavy doses (more than 60-80 mg per day of diazepam), is characterised by marked anxiety, irritability, tremors, insomnia, vomiting, weakness, autonomic hyperactivity with postural hypotension, and seizures.

Depression, transient psychotic episodes, suicidal ideation, perceptual disturbances and rarely delirium have also been reported in withdrawal period.

Treatment

The treatment of benzodiazepine intoxication is usually symptomatic. However, in cases of coma caused by benzodiazepine overdose, flumazenil (a benzodiazepine receptor antagonist) can be used in a dose of 0.3-1.0 mg IV, administered over 1-2 minutes.

The treatment of low dose dependence syndrome (~15 mg/day of diazepam) is abrupt withdrawal and symptomatic management of withdrawal symptoms. However, moderate to high dose dependence is best managed by gradual withdrawal in a step-wise manner (a reduction of ~10% of the dose every day). Sometimes a slower withdrawal is clinically indicated (see Ashton Manual in Suggested Further Reading List).

The best treatment is probably prevention by limiting benzodiazepine use to no more than 2-4 weeks of prescription at most.

After the detoxification phase, an adequate follow-up and supportive treatment is essential to prevent relapses.

INHALANTS OR VOLATILE SOLVENT USE DISORDER

The commonly used volatile solvents include gasoline (petrol), glues, aerosols (spray paints), thinners, varnish remover and industrial solvents. The active ingredients usually include toluene, benzene, acetone and halogenated hydrocarbons.

Volatile solvent misuse is more common in early adolescence as a group activity, particularly in low socioeconomic status groups (e.g. rag-pickers in Mumbai and Delhi).

Intoxication and Complications

Inhalation of a volatile solvent leads to euphoria, excitement, belligerence, dizziness, slurring of speech, apathy, impaired judgement, and neurological signs (such as decreased reflexes, ataxia, nystagmus, incoordination and coma). Death can occur due to respiratory depression, cardiac arrhythmias, or asphyxia.

The complications include irreversible damage to liver and kidneys, peripheral neuropathy, perceptual disturbances and brain damage.

There appears to be no specific treatment of the inhalant use disorder. There is often an associated psychiatric disorder (usually schizophrenia or personality disorder, particularly in solitary sniffers), or there is a history of criminal background. The prognosis is usually guarded.

PHENCYCLIDINE USE DISORDER

Phencyclidine (PCP) was introduced as a dissociative anaesthetic agent (similar to ketamine) in 1950s. However, its use was soon restricted to veterinary anaesthesia as some human subjects developed delirium while emerging from anaesthesia. Classified as an atypical hallucinogen (street names: *Peace pill; angel dust*), PCP selectively antagonises the neuronal action of NMDA (N-methyl-D-aspartate).

PCP is usually taken either occasionally or in binges (called as *runs*); however, some individuals do take PCP in a regular manner. It can be administered orally, intravenously or by snorting.

Intoxication and Complications

Acute PCP intoxication produces euphoria in small doses; higher doses produce dysphoria. Other features may include impulsiveness, agitation, impaired social judgement, assaultativeness, feeling of numbness and inability to move. PCP intoxication can sometimes present with psychiatric syndromes (catatonic syndrome, delirium, stupor, paranoid hallucinatory psychosis, mania or depression) and/or neurological symptoms (nystagmus, ataxia, dysarthria, rigidity, seizures or coma).

Withdrawal Syndrome

Although no clear-cut withdrawal syndrome has been described, craving, social withdrawal, anxiety,

depression and impairment in cognitive functions have been reported.

Treatment

The treatment of PCP intoxication is symptomatic and usually involves gastric lavage, isolation, and use of anticonvulsants (for seizures) and antipsychotics (for PCP induced psychosis).

There is no specific treatment for phencyclidine withdrawal syndrome.

OTHER USE DISORDERS

Caffeine and nicotine are among the most widely used substances, as they are both legally available. Both of these can cause intoxication, dependence, tolerance, and withdrawal syndrome.

Nicotine use (often in the form of smoking) is more common in schizophrenia and depression. Smoking predisposes to increased risk of cardiovascular disease, respiratory disease and cancer, and can affect metabolism of several psychotropic drugs. Smoking also decreases serum levels of clozapine (and other drugs such as olanzapine, duloxetine, fluphenazine) by up to 50%. Clozapine levels can therefore rise significantly after smoking cessation even whilst the patient is on nicotine replacement therapy. This is due to induction of liver enzymes CYP1A2 (cytochrome P450 1A2) by hydrocarbons in tobacco smoke rather than nicotine.

Nicotine withdrawal can occur 12-14 hours after last smoke and can present with anxiety, restlessness, poor concentration, decreased sleep, increased appetite and exacerbation of psychiatric symptoms in those with pre-existing psychiatric disorder(s).

Nicotine replacement therapy is widely used despite equivocal evidence, delivered in a variety of preparations such as a sublingual tablet (2 mg), lozenge (1, 2 or 4 mg), chewing gum (2 or 4 mg), nasal spray (0.5 mg), inhalator (10 mg), and patches (7, 14 or 21 mg).

In addition, bupropion (also called as amfebutamone; a norepinephrine and dopamine reuptake inhibitor – NDRI antidepressant) and varenicline (a partial α4β2 nicotinic acetylcholine receptor partial agonist) are pharmacological agents recently used in promoting smoking cessation as adjuncts to behavioural or cognitive behavioural treatment(s). These should only be initiated after a discussion of possible adverse effects with the patient.

Similarly, caffeine is widely used in general population as well as in patients with psychiatric disorders. DSM-IV-TR defines *caffeinism* (caffeine intoxication) as a recent consumption of caffeine, usually in excess of 250 mg per day, along with five or more of the following: restlessness, nervousness, excitement, insomnia, flushed face, diuresis, GI (gastrointestinal) disturbance, muscle twitching, rambling flow of thought and speech, tachycardia or cardiac arrhythmia, periods of inexhaustibility and psychomotor agitation.

These symptoms should be accompanied by clinically significant distress or impairment in social, occupational or other areas of functioning, and the symptoms should not be better accounted by a general medical condition or another mental disorder.

The typical content of caffeine in the commonly used drinks is usually as follows: tea (45 mg/cup), instant coffee (60 mg/cup), brewed coffee (100 mg/cup), and cola drinks (25-50 mg/can). Caffeine is also present in chocolate. Caffeine can affect metabolism of several psychotropic drugs, most importantly clozapine. It can elevate the levels of clozapine (and other drugs) by inhibiting CYP1A2.

Chapter 5

Schizophrenia

Schizophrenia has puzzled physicians, philosophers, and general public for centuries. The systematic study of schizophrenia, however, is but a century old. A clinical syndrome with a profound influence on public health, schizophrenia has been called "arguably the worst disease affecting mankind, even AIDS not excepted" (Nature 1988).

To understand what schizophrenia is, it is important to have a brief look at the history of evolution of the concept of schizophrenia.

HISTORICAL BACKGROUND

Although earlier descriptions of schizophrenia-like illness are recorded in literature (such as in Ayurveda; Morel's description of demence precoce; Kahlbaum's description of catatonia; Hecker's description of hebephrenia), the scientific study of the disorder began with the description of dementia praecox by Emil Kraepelin.

Emil Kraepelin

In 1896, Emil Kraepelin differentiated the major psychiatric illnesses into two clinical types: Dementia praecox, and Manic depressive illness.

Under dementia praecox, he brought together the various psychiatric illnesses (such as paranoia, catatonia and hebephrenia), which were earlier thought to be distinct illnesses. The emphasis in diagnosis of dementia praecox was on an early onset and a poor outcome (*dementia*: deterioration; *praecox*: early onset).

He recognised the characteristic features of dementia praecox, such as delusions, hallucinations, disturbances of affect and motor disturbances.

Eugen Bleuler

Eugen Bleuler (1911), while renaming dementia praecox as schizophrenia (meaning mental splitting), recognised that this disorder did not always have a poor prognosis as described by Kraepelin. He also recognised that schizophrenia consisted of a group of disorders rather than being a distinct entity. Therefore, he used the term, *a group of schizophrenias*.

Bleuler described the characteristic symptoms (fundamental symptoms) which were then thought to be diagnostic of schizophrenia (Table 5.1). He also described accessory symptoms of schizophrenia (thought to be secondary to fundamental symptoms). These accessory symptoms included delusions, hallucinations and negativism.

Kurt Schneider

Kurt Schneider (1959) described symptoms which, though not specific of schizophrenia, were of great help in making a clinical diagnosis of schizophrenia. These are popularly called as *Schneider's first rank symptoms of schizophrenia* (FRS or SFRS) (Table 5.2). He also described the second rank symptoms of schizophrenia (which were considered by him as less

Table 5.1: Eugen Bleuler's Fundamental Symptoms of Schizophrenia (Also called as 4 A's of Bleuler)

1. *Ambivalence*: Marked inability to decide for or against
2. *Autism*: Withdrawal into self
3. *Affect disturbances*: Disturbances of affect such as inappropriate affect
4. *Association disturbances*: Loosening of associations; thought disorder

Table 5.2: First Rank Symptoms (SFRS) of Schizophrenia

1. *Audible thoughts*: Voices speaking out thoughts aloud or '*thought echo*'.
2. *Voices heard arguing*: Two or more hallucinatory voices discussing the subject in third person.
3. *Voices commenting on one's action*.
4. *Thought withdrawal*: Thoughts cease and subject experiences them as removed by an external force.
5. *Thought insertion*: Experience of thoughts imposed by some external force on person's passive mind.
6. *Thought diffusion or broadcasting*: Experience of thoughts escaping the confines of self and as being experienced by others around.
7. '*Made' feelings or affect*.
8. '*Made' impulses*.
9. '*Made' volition or acts*: In 'made' affect, impulses and volitions, the person experiences feelings, impulses or acts which are imposed by some external force. In 'made' volition, for example, one's own acts are experienced as being under the control of some external force.
10. *Somatic passivity*: Bodily sensations, especially sensory symptoms, are experienced as imposed on body by some external force.
11. *Delusional perception*: Normal perception has a private and illogical meaning.

important for diagnosis of schizophrenia), such as other forms of hallucinations, perplexity, and affect disturbances.

These symptoms (SFRS) have been described in some detail here as they have very often been used for diagnosis of schizophrenia and have significantly influenced the diagnostic criteria and classification of schizophrenia and other related psychotic disorders. As mentioned earlier, SFRS are not specific for schizophrenia and may be seen in other psychiatric disorders such as mood disorders and organic psychiatric disorders.

EPIDEMIOLOGY

According to the World (Mental) Health Report 2001, about 24 million people worldwide suffer from schizophrenia. The point prevalence of schizophrenia is about 0.5-1%. Schizophrenia is prevalent across racial, sociocultural and national boundaries, with a few exceptions in the prevalence rates in some isolated communities.

The incidence of schizophrenia is believed to be about 0.5 per 1000. The onset of schizophrenia occurs usually later in women and often runs a relatively more benign course, as compared to men.

CLINICAL FEATURES

Schizophrenia is characterised by disturbances in thought and verbal behaviour, perception, affect, motor behaviour and relationship to the external world. The diagnosis is entirely clinical and is based on the following clinical features, none of which are pathognomonic if present alone.

Thought and Speech Disorders

Autistic thinking is one of the most classical features of schizophrenia. Here thinking is governed by private and illogical rules. The patient may consider two things identical because they have identical predicates or properties (*von Domarus Law*); for example, Lord Hanuman was celibate, I am celibate too; So, I am Lord Hanuman.

Loosening of associations is a pattern of spontaneous speech in which things said in juxtaposition lack a meaningful relationship or there is idiosyncratic shifting from one frame of reference to another. The speech is often described as being 'disjointed'. If the loosening becomes very severe, speech becomes virtually incomprehensible. This is then known as *incoherence*.

Thought blocking is a characteristic feature of schizophrenia, although it can also be seen in complex partial seizures (temporal lobe epilepsy). There is a sudden interruption of stream of speech before the thought is completed. After a pause, the subject cannot recall what he had meant to say. This may at times be associated with *thought withdrawal*.

Neologisms are newly formed words or phrases whose derivation cannot be understood. These are created to express a concept for which the subject has no dictionary word. Sometimes, normal words are used in an unconventional or distorted way but the derivation can be understood, even if bizarre. These are called *word approximations* or *paraphasias*; for example, describing stomach as a 'food vessel'.

A patient with schizophrenia may show complete *mutism* (with no speech production), *poverty of speech* (decreased speech production), *poverty of ideation* (speech amount is adequate but content conveys little information), *echolalia* (repetition or echoing by the patient of the words or phrases of examiner), *perseveration* (persistent repetition of words beyond their relevance), or *verbigeration* (senseless repetition of same words or phrases over and over again). These are disorders of verbal behaviour or speech.

Delusions are false unshakable beliefs which are not in keeping with patient's socio-cultural and educational background. These are of two types: primary and secondary.

1. *Primary delusions* arise *de novo* and cannot be explained on the basis of other experiences or perceptions. Also known as *autochthonous delusions*, these are though to characteristic of schizophrenia and are usually seen in early stages.
2. *Secondary delusions* are the commonest type of delusions seen in clinical practice and are not diagnostic of schizophrenia as these can also be seen in other psychoses. Secondary delusions can be explained as arising from other abnormal experiences.

The commonly seen delusions in schizophrenia include:
1. Delusions of persecution (being persecuted against, e.g. 'people are against me').
2. Delusions of reference (being referred to by others; e.g. 'people are talking about me').
3. Delusions of grandeur (exaggerated self-importance; e.g. 'I am God almighty').
4. Delusions of control (being controlled by an external force, known or unknown; e.g. 'My neighbour is controlling me").
5. Somatic (or hypochondriacal) delusions (e.g. 'there are insects crawling in my scalp').

The other clinical features of schizophrenic thought disorder include: *overinclusion* (tending to include irrelevant items in speech), *impaired abstraction* (loss of ability to generalise), *concreteness* (due to impaired abstraction), *perplexity* and *ambivalence*.

Schneider's first rank symptoms (such as thought insertion, thought withdrawal, thought broadcasting, 'made' feeling, 'made' impulses and 'made' volitions), which have already been discussed earlier (Table 5.2), may also be present.

Disorders of Perception

Hallucinations (perceptions without stimuli) are common in schizophrenia. Auditory hallucinations are by far the most frequent. These can be:
i.   Elementary auditory hallucinations (i.e. hearing simple sounds rather than voices)
ii. 'Thought echo' ('audible thoughts')
iii. 'Third person hallucinations' ('voices heard arguing', discussing the patient in third person)
iv. 'Voices commenting on one's action'.

Only the 'third person hallucinations' are believed to be characteristic of schizophrenia. Visual hallucinations can also occur, usually along with auditory hallucinations. The tactile, gustatory and olfactory types are less common.

Disorders of Affect

The disorders of affect include apathy, emotional blunting, emotional shallowness, *anhedonia* (inability to experience pleasure) and inappropriate emotional response (emotional response inappropriate to thought).

The difficulty of a patient with schizophrenia in establishing emotional contact with other individuals can lead to *lack of rapport* with the physician.

Disorders of Motor Behaviour

There can be either a decrease (decreased spontaneity, inertia, stupor) or an increase in psychomotor activity (excitement, aggressiveness, restlessness, agitation).

Mannerisms, grimacing, stereotypies (repetitive strange behaviour), decreased self-care, and poor grooming are common features. Catatonic features are commonly seen in the catatonic subtype of schizophrenia (and are discussed in detail under that heading).

Negative Symptoms

The prominent negative symptoms of schizophrenia include *affective flattening* or *blunting*, *attentional impairment*, *avolition-apathy* (lack of initiative associated with psychomotor slowing), *anhedonia*, *asociality* (social withdrawal), and *alogia* (lack of speech output). There is poor verbal as well as non-verbal communication with poor facial expression, decreased eye contact, with usually poor self-care and social interaction.

Other Features

1. Decreased functioning in work, social relations and self-care, as compared to the earlier levels achieved by the individual.
2. *Loss of ego boundaries* (feeling of blurring of boundaries of self with the environment; uncertainty and perplexity regarding own identity and meaning of existence).
3. Multiple somatic symptoms, especially in the early stages of illness.
4. Insight (into the illness) is absent and social judgement is usually poor.
5. There is usually no clinically significant disturbance of consciousness, orientation, attention, memory and intelligence.

6. There is usually *variability* in symptomatology over time which in some cases can be marked.
7. There is no obvious underlying organic cause that can explain the causation of the symptoms.
8. There is no prominent mood disorder of depressive or manic type.

Suicide in Schizophrenia

Suicide can occur in schizophrenia due to several reasons. Some of the common reasons can include the presence of co-morbid depressive symptoms, command hallucinations commanding the patient to commit suicide, impulsive behaviour, presence of anhedonia, and/or return of insight in the illness (with the painful awareness that one has suffered from schizophrenia or psychosis).

It is important to be aware of possibility of suicide whilst treating a patient with schizophrenia so that the various risk factors can be addressed in management.

DIAGNOSIS

According to ICD-10, for the diagnosis of schizophrenia, a minimum of 1 very clear symptom (and usually 2 or more if less clear cut) belonging to any one of the groups referred to as (a) to (d) or symptoms from at least 2 of the groups referred to as (e) to (h), should have been clearly present for most of the time during a period of 1 month or more (DSM-IV-TR on the other hand requires a minimum period of 6 months).

If the duration of illness is less than 1 month, then a diagnosis of acute schizophrenia-like psychotic disorder should be made. These symptoms include (ICD-10):

Thought echo/insertion/withdrawal/broadcasting; delusions of control/influence/passivity; delusional perception; hallucinatory voices commenting or discussing the patient, or other voices coming from some part of body; and/or persistent culturally inappropriate delusions are included in groups (a) to (d) mentioned above.

Persistent hallucinations in any modality, or by persistent overvalued ideas; incoherence or irrelevant speech; neologisms; catatonic behaviour; negative symptoms not due to depression or antipsychotics are included in groups (a) to (d) mentioned above.

This is associated with a significant and consistent change in personal behaviour, manifest as loss of interest, aimlessness, or social withdrawal.

If the patient also meets the criteria for manic episode or depressive episode, the guidelines mentioned above must have been met before the disturbance of mood developed. The disorder is not diagnosed in the presence of overt brain disease, or alcohol- or drug-related intoxication, dependence, or withdrawal.

CLINICAL TYPES

Schizophrenia can be classified into several subtypes (Table 5.3). The catatonic and hebephrenic subtypes of schizophrenia together have been called as *nuclear schizophrenia*, as they present with typical symptomatology of schizophrenia and can most frequently result in personality deterioration over time (especially if chronic).

Paranoid Schizophrenia

Paranoid schizophrenia is characterised by the following clinical features, in addition to the general guidelines of schizophrenia described earlier:
1. Delusions of persecution, reference, grandeur (or 'grandiosity'), control, or infidelity (or 'jealousy'). The delusions are usually well-systematised (i.e. thematically well connected with each other)
2. The hallucinations usually have a persecutory or grandiose content.

Table 5.3: Clinical Types of Schizophrenia

1. Paranoid schizophrenia
2. Hebephrenic schizophrenia
3. Catatonic schizophrenia
4. Residual schizophrenia
5. Undifferentiated schizophrenia
6. Simple schizophrenia
7. Post-schizophrenic depression
8. Others

3. No prominent disturbances of affect, volition, speech, and/or motor behaviour.

Personality deterioration in the paranoid subtype is much less than that seen in other types of schizophrenias. The patient may be quite apprehensive (due to delusions and hallucinations) and anxious, and appear evasive and guarded on mental status examination.

The onset of paranoid schizophrenia is usually insidious, occurs later in life (i.e. late 3rd and early 4th decade) as compared to the other subtypes of schizophrenia. The course is usually progressive and complete recovery usually does not occur. There may be frequent remissions and relapses. At other times, the functional capability may be only slightly impaired. The differential diagnosis is usually from delusional (or paranoid) disorders and paranoid personality disorders.

Disorganised (or Hebephrenic) Schizophrenia

Disorganised schizophrenia is characterised by the following features, in addition to the general guidelines of schizophrenia described earlier:
1. Marked thought disorder, incoherence and severe loosening of associations. Delusions and hallucinations are fragmentary and changeable.
2. Emotional disturbances (inappropriate affect, blunted affect, or senseless giggling), mannerisms, 'mirror-gazing' (for long periods of time), disinhibited behaviour, poor self-care and hygiene, markedly impaired social and occupational functioning, extreme social withdrawal and other oddities of behaviour.

ICD-10 recommends a period of 2 or 3 months of continuous observation for a confident diagnosis of disorganised (or hebephrenic) schizophrenia to be made.

The onset is insidious, usually in the early 2nd decade. The course is progressive and downhill. The recovery from the episode is classically poor. Severe deterioration, without any significant remissions, usually occurs over time. Hebephrenic schizophrenia has one of the worst prognoses among the various subtypes of schizophrenia.

Catatonic Schizophrenia

Catatonic schizophrenia (*Cata*: disturbed, *tonic*: tone) is characterised by a marked disturbance of motor behaviour, in addition to the general guidelines of schizophrenia described earlier.

It can present in three clinical forms: excited catatonia, stuporous catatonia, and catatonia alternating between excitement and stupor.

Excited Catatonia

This is characterised by the following features:
1. Increase in psychomotor activity, ranging from restlessness, agitation, excitement, aggressiveness to, at times, violent behaviour (furore).
2. Increase in speech production, with increased spontaneity, pressure of speech, loosening of associations and frank incoherence.

The excitement has no apparent relationship with the external environment; instead inner stimuli (e.g. thought and impulses) influence the excited behaviour. So, the excitement is not goal-directed.

Sometimes the excitement can become very severe, and is accompanied by rigidity, hyperthermia and dehydration, finally culminating in death. It is then known as *acute lethal catatonia* or *pernicious catatonia*. Fortunately, with the availability of new treatment choices, and early diagnosis and treatment, lethal catatonia has become increasingly rare in most parts of the world.

Stuporous (or Retarded) Catatonia

This is characterised by extreme retardation of psychomotor function. The characteristic catatonic signs (Table 5.4) are usually observed. Delusions and hallucinations may be present but are usually not prominent. Not all the features are present at the same time.

Catatonia Alternating between Excitement and Stupor

This clinical picture is very common with features of both excited catatonia and stuporous catatonia alternatingly present.

Table 5.4: Some Important Clinical Features of Retarded Catatonia

1. *Mutism*: Complete absence of speech
2. *Rigidity*: Maintenance of a rigid posture against efforts to be moved
3. *Negativism*: An apparently motiveless resistance to all commands and attempts to be moved, or doing just the opposite
4. *Posturing*: Voluntary assumption of an inappropriate and often bizarre posture for long periods of time
5. *Stupor*: Akinesis (no movement) with mutism but with evidence of relative preservation of conscious awareness
6. *Echolalia*: Repetition, echo or mimicking of phrases or words heard
7. *Echopraxia*: Repetition, echo or mimicking of actions observed
8. *Waxy flexibility*: Parts of body can be placed in positions that will be maintained for long periods of time, even if very uncomfortable; flexible like wax
9. *Ambitendency*: Due to ambivalence, conflicting impulses and tentative actions are made, but no goal directed action occurs, e.g. on asking to take out tongue, tongue is slightly protruded but taken back again
10. Other signs such as *mannerisms*, *stereotypies* (verbal and behavioural), *automatic obedience* (commands are followed automatically, irrespective of their nature) and *verbigeration* (incomprehensible speech).

The onset of catatonic schizophrenia is usually acute, usually in the late 2nd and early 3rd decade. The course is often episodic and recovery from the episode is usually complete. However, residual features are present after two or more episodes. Differential diagnosis is from other causes of stupor and catatonia. (This is discussed in further detail in Chapter 19).

Residual and Latent Schizophrenia

Residual schizophrenia is similar to latent schizophrenia and symptoms are similar to prodromal symptoms of schizophrenia. The only difference is that residual schizophrenia is diagnosed after at least one episode has occurred.

There are prominent negative symptoms described above, with absence or marked reduction of florid psychotic symptoms such as delusions and hallucinations. It is important to rule out antipsychotic-induced negative symptoms as well as negative symptoms secondary to associated depression, organic brain disease or institutionalisation.

Undifferentiated Schizophrenia

This is a very common type of schizophrenia and is diagnosed either:
1. When features of no subtype are fully present, or
2. When features of more than one subtype are exhibited, and the general criteria for diagnosis of schizophrenia are met.

Simple Schizophrenia

Although called simple, it is one of the subtypes which is the most difficult to diagnose. It is characterised by an early onset (early 2nd decade), very insidious and progressive course, presence of characteristic 'negative symptoms' of residual schizophrenia (such as marked social withdrawal, shallow emotional response, with loss of initiative and drive), vague hypochondriacal features, a drift down the social ladder, and living shabbily and wandering aimlessly. Delusions and hallucinations are usually absent, and if present they are short lasting and poorly systematised.

The prognosis is usually very poor.

Post-Schizophrenic Depression

Some schizophrenic patients develop depressive features within 12 months of an acute episode of schizophrenia. The depressive features develop in the presence of residual or active features of schizophrenia and are associated with an increased risk of suicide. The depressive features can occur due to side-effect of antipsychotics, regaining insight after recovery, or just be an integral part of schizophrenia.

It is important to distinguish the depressive features from negative symptoms of schizophrenia and extrapyramidal side-effects of antipsychotic medication.

Other Subtypes

Historically, there have been many other subtypes of schizophrenia described, but a majority of them would easily fit in one of the above-mentioned seven subtypes. A few are briefly mentioned due to their historical interest and their popular names; though others are important in their own right.

Pseudoneurotic Schizophrenia

Pseudoneurotic schizophrenia was first described by Hoch and Polatin. In initial phases, there are predominant neurotic symptoms that last for years and show a poor response to treatment.

The three classical features described are pananxiety (diffuse, free-floating anxiety which hardly ever subsides), pan-neurosis (almost all neurotic symptoms may be present) and pansexuality (constant preoccupation with sexual problems).

Nowadays, this subtype is subsumed under borderline personality disorder.

Schizophreniform Disorder

This is a diagnostic category in DSM-IV-TR with features of schizophrenia as diagnostic criteria. The only difference is that the duration is less than 6 months and prognosis is usually better than that of schizophrenia. This term was originally introduced by Langfeldt (1961) to designate good prognosis cases, distinct from "true" schizophrenia. A similar condition in ICD-10 is called acute schizophrenia-like psychotic disorder (see Chapter 7 for details).

Oneiroid Schizophrenia

Described first by Mayer-Gross, this is a subtype of schizophrenia with an acute onset, clouding of consciousness, disorientation, dream-like states (oneiroid means 'dream'), and perceptual disturbances with rapid shifting.

Classically, the episode is usually brief.

Van Gogh Syndrome

Dramatic self-mutilation occurring in schizophrenia has been also called as Van Gogh syndrome, after the name of the famous painter Vincent Van Gogh who had cut his ear during the active phase of illness.

Late Paraphrenia

Described by Sir Martin Roth, this is a disorder which occurs late in life, usually in the sixth decade. It is more common in women, especially unmarried or widowed women. Delusions of persecution are seen, with bizarre and fantastic content (for example, being raped or gassed or strangers entering their rooms and interfering with them).

Hallucinations of all kinds (visual, auditory, tactile, gustatory and olfactory) can be present. Intelligence and social judgement outside the arena of persecutory delusions are usually normal. Approximately 25-40% of the patients have some defect of sight or hearing.

At present, this syndrome is placed under paranoid schizophrenia, late onset type.

Pfropf Schizophrenia

This is a syndrome of schizophrenia occurring in the presence of mental retardation. It differs from schizophrenia in only that there is often a poverty of ideation and delusions are not usually very well-systematised. Therefore, behavioural disturbances are much more prominent than delusions and hallucinations. However, both ICD-10 and DSM-IV-TR do not suggest a separate category and it is best to diagnose both schizophrenia and mental retardation, when present together.

Type I and Type II Schizophrenia

TJ Crow had divided schizophrenia into two subtypes, namely Type I and II schizophrenias. The Type I syndrome is characterised by positive symptoms while the Type II syndrome is predominantly characterised by presence of negative symptoms.

Type I syndrome is supposed to have an acute presentation, good response to medication and a good outcome, while Type II is theorised to be chronic in course, have a poor response to medication and a poor outcome. Crow also described dilated ventricles on CT Scan of Brain in Type II syndrome.

Although a useful concept theoretically, it has not been found to be valid in the recent research studies. Very few patients have a pure Type I or Type II syndrome, and admixtures are far more common.

Table 5.5 summarises symptom clusters in schizophrenia with enumeration of positive, negative and disorganised symptoms.

DIFFERENTIAL DIAGNOSIS

The first step in the differential diagnosis is to exclude psychoses with known organic causes, such as complex partial seizures, drug-induced psychoses (such as amphetamine-induced psychoses), metabolic disturbances, or cerebral space occupying lesions. There would often be clinical features suggestive of underlying disorders in these conditions.

The second step is to rule out a possibility of mood disorder (such as mania, depression, or mixed affective disorder) or schizo-affective disorder.

The third step is to exclude the possibility of other nonorganic psychoses such as delusional disorders, or acute and transient psychotic disorders (ATPD).

In addition to the main diagnosis, it is also important to look for co-morbid medical (such as diabetes, hypertension) and/or psychiatric disorders (such as depression, anxiety, alcohol or drug misuse, or personality disorder) on a multi-axial diagnostic system (see Table 1.4).

PROGNOSIS

The important prognostic factors in schizophrenia are summarised in Table 5.6.

COURSE AND OUTCOME

Since the time of Kraepelin, when the disorder was conceptualised as dementia paecox, schizophrenia has been associated with a progressive downhill course, with a large number of patients hospitalised in mental asylums.

However, the longitudinal studies of schizophrenia suggest that this pattern occurs in only a minority of

Table 5.5: Symptom Clusters in Schizophrenia

Positive Symptoms	Negative Symptoms	Disorganised Symptoms
Delusions	Affective flattening	Inappropriate affect
Hallucinations	Alogia (poverty of speech)	Disorganised behaviour
	Anhedonia—asociality	Thought disorder
	Avolition—apathy	Loosening of associations
	Attentional impairment	

Table 5.6: Prognostic Factors in Schizophrenia

	Good Prognostic Factors	Poor Prognostic Factors
1.	Acute or abrupt onset	Insidious onset
2.	Onset >35 years of age (late onset)	Onset <20 years of age (early onset)
3.	Presence of precipitating stressor	Absence of stressor
4.	Good premorbid adjustment	Poor premorbid adjustment
5.	Catatonic subtype (paranoid subtype has an intermediate prognosis)	Disorganised, simple, undifferentiated, or chronic catatonic subtypes
6.	Short duration (< 6 months)	Chronic course (> 2 years)
7.	Presence of depression	Absence of depression
8.	Predominance of positive symptoms	Predominance of negative symptoms
9.	Family history of mood disorder	Family history of schizophrenia
10.	First episode	Past history of schizophrenia
11.	Pyknic (fat) physique	Asthenic (thin) physique
12.	Female sex	Male sex
13.	Good social support	Poor social support or unmarried
14.	Presence of confusion, perplexity, or disorientation in the acute phase	Flat or blunted affect
15.	Proper treatment, good treatment concordance, and good response to treatment	Absence of proper treatment or poor response to treatment
16.	Outpatient treatment	Institutionalisation (long-term hospitalisation)
17.	Normal cranial CT scan	Evidence of ventricular enlargement on cranial CT scan

patients. According to a major study (Luc Ciompi 1980), where 5661 cases were followed up for an average of 36.9 years, the outcome was as follows:

- Complete remission (27%)
- Remission with minor residual deficit (22%)
- Intermediate outcome (24%)
- Severe disability (18%)
- Unstable or uncertain outcome (9%).

So, almost 50% patients reached complete or near complete recovery, and only 18% were left with severe disability, with only 9% needing institutionalisation.

A Study of Factors Associated with Course and Outcome of Schizophrenia (SOFACOS) was conducted by ICMR (Indian Council of Medical Research) at three centres (Vellore, Madras and Lucknow) in India. A total of 386 patients were followed up for a period of 5 years (1981 to 1986), at the end of which the outcome was as follows:

- Very favourable outcome (27%)
- Favourable outcome (40%)
- Intermediate outcome (31%)
- Unfavourable outcome (2%).

So, about two-thirds (67%) of the patients had a favourable outcome as compared to 50% in Luc Ciompi's study.

The International Pilot Study on Schizophrenia (IPSS), conducted on 811 schizophrenic patients selected in 1968-1969 (patients selected from 9 countries, namely USA, Columbia, UK, Czechoslovakia, USSR, India, Nigeria, Denmark and China), found interesting outcome results. It was apparent that the course and prognosis of schizophrenia was better in the developing countries such as Nigeria and India, as compared to the developed countries (Fig. 5.1).

In ICD-10, the course of schizophrenia is specified under the categories of:

i. Continuous;
ii. Episodic with progressive deficit;
iii. Episodic with stable deficit;
iv. Episodic remittent;
v. Incomplete remission; and
vi. Complete remission.

If the period of observation is less than one year, the course is not specified.

Some studies have suggested that longer the DUP (duration of untreated psychosis), worse is the outcome, underlining the importance of early diagnosis and treatment of schizophrenia. There is an increased mortality in patients with schizophrenia by almost one and half times. The most important cause of death is suicide, the life-time risk of which is about 5-10 times higher in schizophrenia as compared to normal population.

There is also a higher prevalence of *metabolic syndrome* (characterised by abdominal obesity, atherogenic dyslipidaemia, hypertension, raised fasting blood glucose, and insulin resistance) in schizophrenia which can be worsened by administration of antipsychotic medication. Patients with schizophrenia can die 10-15 years prematurely as compared to general population. There are several factors responsible for this increased morbidity and mortality, including high prevalence of smoking, caffeine, alcohol and drug misuse, obesity, poor treatment concordance, poor help-seeking behaviour, decreased activity levels, higher incidence of suicide, and metabolic syndrome.

AETIOLOGY

The aetiology of schizophrenia is currently unknown. However, several theories have been propounded; these include the following:

Biological Theories

Genetic Hypothesis

About 8-10% of first degree relatives (and 3% of second degree relatives and 2% of third degree relatives) of patients with schizophrenia can present with schizophrenia, as compared with the 0.5-1% prevalence rate in general population.

The concordance rate for monozygotic twins is 46% and for dizygotic twins is 14%. If one parent has schizophrenia, the chances of the child developing schizophrenia are 10-12%. However, if both parents have schizophrenia, chances of the child developing schizophrenia increase to about 40%.

Therefore, genetic factors are very important in making an individual vulnerable to schizophrenia. However, environmental factors and stress are probably also important in precipitating an episode in several individuals.

Biochemical Theories

Schizophrenia is presently thought to be probably due to a functional increase of dopamine at the postsyn-

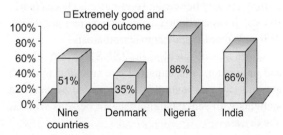

Fig. 5.1: IPSS Outcome

aptic receptor, though other neurotransmitters such as serotonin (especially 5-HT$_2$ receptors), GABA and acetylcholine are also presumably involved.

Brain Imaging

Cranial CT Scan, MRI Scan, and postmortem studies show enlarged ventricles (not amounting to hydrocephalus) and mild cortical atrophy (with an overall reduction in brain volume and cortical grey matter by 5-10%) in some patients of schizophrenia.

PET (positron emission tomography) scan shows hypofrontality and decreased glucose utilisation in the dominant temporal lobe. Attempts are being made to localise symptoms of schizophrenia (such as auditory hallucinations, negative symptoms) to the various brain regions by PET studies.

At present brain imaging does not have a role in confirming a diagnosis of schizophrenia though it can be used to rule out an organic basis of psychotic symptoms where clinically appropriate.

Other Theories

The following findings also point towards a biological basis of schizophrenia. Antipsychotics, which act by blocking the dopamine (D$_2$) receptor, cause significant improvement in schizophrenia and relapse usually occurs on stopping antipsychotic medication. The newer, atypical antipsychotics (such as risperidone, olanzapine, quetiapine) are D$_2$-5-HT$_2$ antagonists.

Drugs such as amphetamines and mescaline can cause schizophrenia-like symptoms in normal subjects. Organic mental disorders with schizophrenia-like symptoms may be seen in Huntington's chorea (early stages), homocystinuria, acute intermittent porphyria, Wilson's disease and haemachromatosis.

Soft neurological signs (SNS), minor physical anomalies, and impaired eye tracking (smooth pursuit eye movements) are more often seen in patients with schizophrenia than in persons without the disease.

Viral and autoimmune factors have also been implicated by some, while others (e.g. Weinberger) have suggested a neurodevelopmental hypothesis for schizophrenia.

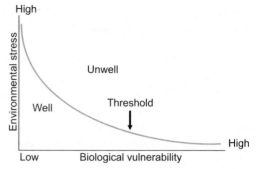

Fig. 5.2: Stress Vulnerability Hypothesis in Schizophrenia.
Ref: Zubin and Spring (1977)

Psychological Theories

Stress

Increased number of stressful life events before the onset or relapse probably has a triggering effect on the onset of schizophrenia, in a genetically vulnerable person (*Stress-Vulnerability Hypothesis*) (Fig. 5.2). According to this hypothesis, higher the genetic vulnerability in a person, lesser the environmental stress needed to precipitate a relapse.

Increased expressed emotions (EE; such as hostility, critical comments, emotional over-involvement) of 'significant others' in the family can lead to an early relapse. Figure 5.3 depicts the 9-month relapse rates in patients with schizophrenia in the study conducted by Vaughn and Leff in 1976. In this study, patients who were without any antipsychotic medication and were exposed to more than 35 hours contact per week with a 'significant other' with expressed emotions, were particularly likely to relapse (92%). The comparable rate in patients who received antipsychotic medication and faced less expressed emotions was 12%. In the research conducted in the last 30 years, these findings have been replicated all over the globe, though the period of 35 hours/weeks has not been found to be significant.

Family Theories

Several theories have been propounded in the past but are currently of doubtful value. These include

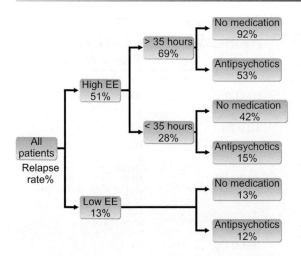

9 months relapse rate in 128 patients with schizophrenia (Vaughn and Leff 1976)

Fig. 5.3: Expressed Emotions (EE) in Schizophrenia

'schizophrenogenic mothers', lack of 'real' parents, dependency on mother, anxious mother, parental marital schism or skew, double-bind theory, communication deviance, and pseudomutuality.

Some of these theories were unfortunately responsible for arousing a sense of unnecessary guilt in parents for causation of schizophrenia in their children.

Information Processing Hypothesis

Disturbances in attention, inability to maintain a set, and inability to assimilate and integrate percepts are common findings in schizophrenia. Patients with schizophrenia may at first be overly attentive to stimuli but later may reduce or exclude attention to stimuli. There is possibly a breakdown in the internal representation of mental events.

Psychoanalytical Theories

According to Freud, there is regression to the preoral (and oral) stage of psychosexual development, with the use of defense mechanisms of *denial*, *projection*, and *reaction formation* (see Table 17.1). There is a

loss of ego-boundaries (described by Federn), with a loss of touch with reality.

Sociocultural Theories

Although the prevalence of schizophrenia is quite uniform across cultures, it was found to be more common in lower socioeconomic status in some studies. This has now been explained due to a 'downward social drift', which is a result of having developed schizophrenia rather than causing it.

Higher rates of schizophrenia have been found among some migrants, not only among the first generation migrants but also among the second generation.

MANAGEMENT

The treatment of schizophrenia can be discussed under the following major headings:
1. Somatic treatment
   a. Pharmacological treatment
   b. Electro-convulsive therapy (ECT)
   c. Miscellaneous treatments.
2. Psychosocial treatment and rehabilitation.

Pharmacological Treatment

The first drug to be used with beneficial effect in schizophrenia was probably reserpine (Rauwolfia serpentina extract), in India by Sen and Bose (1931). Reserpine is no longer used for the treatment of schizophrenia for a variety of reasons, including its propensity to cause severe and suicidal depression.

Antipsychotics were formally discovered by Delay and Deniker in 1952. Since their introduction, they have changed the outcome of schizophrenia significantly. These are discussed in some detail in Chapter 15. Only some relevant clinical points are briefly mentioned here. A list of commonly used antipsychotics with their routinely used doses is available in Table 5.7.

Atypical (or the second generation) antipsychotic drugs, such as risperidone, olanzapine, quetiapine,

Table 5.7: Antipsychotic Dose in Schizophrenia

Drug	Oral Dose Range (mg/day)	Parenteral Dose (mg/day)	Equivalent Oral Dose* (Equal to 100 mg CPZ)
A. Typical/Traditional/First Generation Antipsychotics			
1. Chlorpromazine (CPZ)	300-1000	50-100 IM	100
2. Flupentixol	3-18	—	2
3. Haloperidol	5-30	5-10 IM	2-3
4. Loxapine	25-250	—	10
5. Pimozide	4-12	—	2
6. Prochlorperazine	45-150	40-80 IM	15
7. Sulpiride	400-2400	—	200
8. Thioridazine	300-600	—	100
9. Trifluoperazine	15-50	1-5 IM	5
10. Triflupromazine	100-400	30-60 IM	25
11. Zuclopenthixol	25-150	50-100 IM	25
B. Atypical/Second Generation Antipsychotics			
12. Amisulpride	400-1200	—	—
13. Aripiprazole	5-30	5.25-15 IM	—
14. Clozapine	50-900	—	50
15. Olanzapine	5-20	2.5-10 IM	2-3
16. Paliperidone	3-12	—	—
17. Quetiapine	150-800	—	50-100
18. Risperidone	2-16	—	0.5-1.0
19. Ziprasidone	40-160	—	20
20. Zotepine	75-300	—	—

*Equivalent doses are at best approximations only. The dose in a particular patient should be chosen on an individualised basis by the treating professional.

aripiprazole, and ziprasidone, are more commonly used than the older typical (or first generation) antipsychotics such as trifluoperazine and haloperidol, in acute stages. Atypical antipsychotics are also more useful when negative symptoms are prominent, e.g. in chronic schizophrenia.

Clozapine, another atypical antipsychotic, is available in the Indian market. The clinical trials have shown that clozapine is effective in about 30% of patients who had no beneficial response to traditional (typical and atypical) antipsychotics. It is an effective drug; however, as it can cause agranulocytosis and seizures as side-effects, it should be used with caution, with regular WBC and neutrophil counts as advised by the Summary of Product Characteristics (SPC).

Drug treatment is usually administered in the outpatient setting as:
1. There are very few number of psychiatric beds in India,
2. Majorities of families are willing to care for the patients at home, and
3. Majority of patients do not require hospitalisation.

However, hospitalisation is indicated if there is:
1. Neglect of food and water intake,
2. Danger to self or others,
3. Poor treatment adherence,
4. Significant neglect of self-care, or
5. Lack of social support with evidence of above-mentioned risks.

In the presence of acute excitement, haloperidol 5 mg IV or IM, with/without 10 mg diazepam or 50 mg of promethazine can be administered. Given IM, chlorpromazine can cause painful injection abscess at the injection site. It should never be given IV, as severe hypotension can occur. It is really important to exercise care in administering parenteral antipsychotics to any patient, but particularly one who is treatment (antipsychotic) naïve. Oral antipsychotics are preferable to parenteral antipsychotic in routine clinical practice.

A majority of patients require maintenance treatment with antipsychotics to prevent relapse. Generally, the treatment is continued for 6 months to 1 year for the first episode, for 1-2 years for the subsequent episodes, and for indefinite period for repeated episodes or persistent symptoms. However, the decision regarding the duration of treatment in a particular case has to be assessed individually by the treating psychiatrist in consultation with the patient and family (if appropriate), in view of past history and possible risks.

To ensure drug concordance, depot antipsychotic preparations with long duration of action can be used. (See Table 15.5 for some common preparations of depot antipsychotics).

Many patients require adjuvant antiparkinsonian medication to prevent extrapyramidal side-effects; for example, trihexiphenidyl 6 mg/day, orphenadrine 150 mg/day, procyclidine 7.5-15 mg/day. This is particularly true if the patient is receiving an older, typical antipsychotic (such as haloperidol). However, at times atypical antipsychotics such as risperidone can also cause extrapyramidal symptoms, particularly in higher doses.

Ideally speaking, during hospitalisation, no patient should receive anticholinergic antiparkinsonian medication till extrapyramidal side-effects appear. Anticholinergics can worsen cognitive function, have an abuse potential, can cause delirium (especially in elderly), can worsen or contribute to negative symptoms in schizophrenia, and may increase the risk of tardive dyskinesia. But, in routine clinical practice, often a majority of patients do receive anticholinergics in addition to traditional antipsychotics.

Antipsychotics probably act by blocking the post-synaptic dopamine (D_2) receptors in the mesolimbic system. Other receptors such as 5-HT, muscarinic receptors and GABA are also probably important. Atypical antipsychotics are also called as Serotonin-Dopamine Antagonists (SDAs) due of their action on both dopamine and 5-HT.

Electroconvulsive Therapy (ECT)

Schizophrenia is not a primary indication for ECT. The indications for ECT in schizophrenia include:
1. Catatonic stupor.
2. Uncontrolled catatonic excitement.
3. Acute exacerbation not controlled with drugs.
4. Severe side-effect with drugs, in presence of untreated schizophrenia.

Usually 8-12 ECTs are needed (although up to 18 have been given in poor responders), administered two or three times a week.

Miscellaneous Treatments

Psychosurgery is not routinely indicated in the treatment of schizophrenia. It is a treatment which is extremely rarely used in clinical practice. When used, the treatment of choice is limbic leucotomy (a small subcaudate lesion with a cingulate lesion) in some cases with severe and very prominent depression, anxiety or obsessional symptoms.

Severely deteriorated patients are unlikely to benefit. The maximum benefit would be in acute episodes, but antipsychotics are far better obviously both in efficacy and safety.

Many other methods such as megavitamin therapy, dialysis, malaria therapy, high dose propranolol and insulin coma therapy have been used in past but are no longer used in clinical practice due to either poor evidence for efficacy and/or risks to the patient.

Psychosocial Treatment

Psychosocial treatment is an extremely important component of comprehensive management of schizophrenia. It can be divided in following steps:
1. *Psychoeducation* of the patient and especially the family/carers (with patient's consent) regarding

the nature of illness, and its course and treatment. Psychoeducation helps in establishing a good therapeutic relationship with the patient (and the family). Psychoeducation also involves explaining the stress-vulnerability model of schizophrenia to the patient and carer(s).

2. *Group psychotherapy* is particularly aimed at teaching problem solving and communication skills. This can be conducted in a form which is known as the '*social skills training package*'.

3. *Family therapy*: Apart from psychoeducation, family members are also provided social skills training to enhance communication and help decrease intrafamilial 'tensions'. Attempts are also made to decrease the 'expressed emotions' (EE) of 'significant others' in the family. The family members' awareness is raised regarding decreasing expectations and avoiding *critical remarks*, *emotional over-involvement*, and *hostility*.

4. *Milieu therapy* (or *therapeutic community*) includes treatment in a living, learning or working environment ranging from inpatient psychiatric unit to day-care hospitals and half-way homes.

5. *Individual psychotherapy* is usually supportive in nature. Rarely, psychoanalytically oriented psychodynamic psychotherapy is used. However, the current consensus does not recommend the use of psychoanalytic psychotherapy in routine treatment of schizophrenia.

Several centres (and guidelines) recommend the use of *cognitive behaviour therapy* (CBT) in the treatment of schizophrenia [e.g. NICE (National Institute of Clinical Excellence, UK) Guidelines for Schizophrenia 2009]. Delivery of CBT in schizophrenia needs specialised training and is often conducted as an adjunct to psychopharmacological therapy.

6. Psychosocial rehabilitation is used, usually along with milieu therapy. This includes activity therapy, to develop the work habit, training in a new vocation or retraining in a previous skill, vocational guidance, independent job placement, sheltered employment or self-employment, and occupational therapy.

However, antipsychotic drug treatment in the acute stages, as well as for maintenance treatment, is the mainstay of management of schizophrenia.

Psychosocial treatment is an important adjunct to drug treatment which enhances its efficacy and leads to a more complete recovery and rehabilitation. However, it is unlikely that psychosocial treatment, in the absence of drug treatment, will be able to treat schizophrenia effectively.

Chapter 6

Mood Disorders

Broadly speaking, the *emotions* can be described as two main types:

1. *Affect,* which is a *short-lived* emotional response to an idea or an event, and
2. *Mood,* which is a *sustained and pervasive* emotional response which colours the whole psychic life.

So according to these definitions, depression and mania are *mood disorders* and not 'affective disorders' as they have been called so frequently in the past. Throughout this chapter (and this book), the more correct word *mood disorder* will be used (as indeed in DSM-IV-TR and ICD-10).

Mood disorders have been known to man since antiquity. The Old Testament describes King Saul as suffering from severe depressive episodes and responding slightly to David's soothing music. While Hippocrates coined the words mania and melancholia, it was Aretaeus who first described mania and depression occurring in the same individual. Emil Kraepelin, borrowing from the work of Kahlbaum, Falret and Baillarger, described the manic-depressive illness as separate from dementia praecox on the basis of course, clinical symptoms and outcome.

Recently, the World Health Report 2001 has identified *unipolar depression* as the 4th cause of Disability-Adjusted Life Years (DALYs) in all ages, and the 2nd cause in the age group of 15-44 years. Unipolar depression is also the 1st cause of YLD (Years of Life Lived with Disability) in all ages. The comparison was with all medical disorders, and not only psychiatric disorders. The World Health Report 2001 estimates that there are 121 million people worldwide suffering from depression.

CLASSIFICATION

The classification of mood disorders is an area which is fraught with multiple controversies. According to the ICD-10, the mood disorders are classified as follows:

1. Manic episode
2. Depressive episode
3. Bipolar mood (affective) disorder
4. Recurrent depressive disorder
5. Persistent mood disorder (including cyclothymia and dysthymia)
6. Other mood disorders (including mixed affective episode and recurrent brief depressive disorder).

CLINICAL FEATURES AND DIAGNOSIS

Manic Episode

The life-time risk of manic episode is about 0.8-1%. This disorder tends to occur in episodes lasting usually 3-4 months, followed by complete clinical recovery. The future episodes can be manic, depressive or mixed.

A manic episode is typically characterised by the following features (which should last for at least one week and cause disruption in occupational and social activities).

Elevated, Expansive or Irritable Mood

The elevated mood can pass through following four stages, depending on the severity of manic episode:

a. *Euphoria* (mild elevation of mood): An increased sense of psychological well-being and happiness, not in keeping with ongoing events. This is usually seen in hypomania (Stage I).

b. *Elation* (moderate elevation of mood): A feeling of confidence and enjoyment, along with an increased psychomotor activity. Elation is classically seen in mania (Stage II).

c. *Exaltation* (severe elevation of mood): Intense elation with delusions of grandeur; seen in severe mania (Stage III).

d. *Ecstasy* (very severe elevation of mood): Intense sense of rapture or blissfulness; typically seen in delirious or stuporous mania (Stage IV).

Along with these variations in elevation of mood, expansive mood may also be present, which is an unceasing and unselective enthusiasm for interacting with people and surrounding environment. At times, elevated mood may not be apparent and instead an irritable mood may be predominant, especially when the person is stopped from doing what he wants. There may be rapid, short lasting shifts from euphoria to depression or irritability.

Psychomotor Activity

There is an increased psychomotor activity, ranging from overactiveness and restlessness, to manic excitement where the person is 'on-the-toe-on-the-go', (i.e. involved in ceaseless activity). The activity is usually goal-oriented and is based on external environmental cues. Rarely, a manic patient can go in to a stuporous state (*manic stupor*).

Speech and Thought

The person is more talkative than usual; describes thoughts racing in his mind; develops pressure of speech; uses playful language with punning, rhyming, joking and teasing; and speaks loudly.

Later, there is *'flight of ideas'* (rapidly produced speech with abrupt shifts from topic to topic, using external environmental cues. Typically the connections between the shifts are apparent). When the 'flight' becomes severe, incoherence may occur. A less severe and a more ordered 'flight', in the absence of pressure of speech, is called *'prolixity'*.

There can be delusions (or ideas) of grandeur (grandiosity), with markedly inflated self-esteem. Delusions of persecution may sometimes develop secondary to the delusions of grandeur (e.g. I am so great that people are against me). Hallucinations (both auditory and visual), often with religious content, can occur (e.g. God appeared before me and spoke to me). Since these psychotic symptoms are in keeping with the elevated mood state, these are called *mood-congruent psychotic features*.

Distractibility is a common feature and results in rapid changes in speech and activity, in response to even irrelevant external stimuli.

Goal-directed Activity

The person is unusually alert, trying to do many things at one time.

In hypomania, the ability to function becomes much better and there is a marked increase in productivity and creativity. Many artists and writers have contributed significantly in such periods. As past history of hypomania and mild forms of mania is often difficult to elicit, it is really important to take additional historical information from reliable informants (e.g. family members).

In mania, there is marked increase in activity with excessive planning and, at times, execution of multiple activities. Due to being involved in so many activities and distractibility, there is often a decrease in the functioning ability in later stages. There is marked increase in sociability even with previously unknown people. Gradually this sociability leads to an interfering behaviour though the person does not recognise it as abnormal at that time. The person becomes impulsive and disinhibited, with sexual indiscretions, and can later become hypersexual and promiscuous.

Due to grandiose ideation, increased sociability, overactivity and poor judgement, the manic person is often involved in the high-risk activities such as buying sprees, reckless driving, foolish business investments, and distributing money and/or personal articles to unknown persons. He is usually dressed up in gaudy and flamboyant clothes, although in severe mania there may be poor self-care.

Other Features

Sleep is usually reduced with a *decreased need for sleep*. Appetite may be increased but later there is usually decreased food intake, due to marked over-activity. Insight into the illness is absent, especially in severe mania.

Psychotic features such as delusions, hallucinations which are not understandable in the context of mood disorder (called *mood incongruent psychotic features*), e.g. delusions of control, may be present in some cases.

Absence of Underlying Organic Cause

If manic episode is secondary to an organic cause, a diagnosis of organic mood disorder should be made.

Depressive Episode

The life-time risk of depression in males is 8-12% and in females is 20-26%. However, the life-time risk of major depression (or depressive episode) is about 8%.

The typical depressive episode is characterised by the following features (which should last for at least two weeks for a diagnosis to be made):

Depressed Mood

The most important feature is the sadness of mood or loss of interest and/or pleasure in almost all activities (*pervasive sadness*), present throughout the day (*persistent sadness*). This sadness of mood is quantitatively as well as qualitatively different from the sadness encountered in 'normal' sadness or grief. The depressed mood varies little from day to day and is often not responsive to the environmental stimuli.

The loss of interest in daily activities results in social withdrawal, decreased ability to function in occupational and interpersonal areas and decreased involvement in previously pleasurable activities. In severe depression, there may be complete *anhedonia* (inability to experience pleasure).

Depressive Ideation/Cognition

Sadness of mood is usually associated with pessimism, which can result in three common types of depressive ideas. These are:

a. Hopelessness (there is no hope in the future).
b. Helplessness (no help is possible now).
c. Worthlessness (feeling of inadequacy and inferiority).

The ideas of worthlessness can lead to self-reproach and guilt-feelings. The other features are difficulty in thinking, difficulty in concentration, indecisiveness, slowed thinking, subjective poor memory, lack of initiative and energy. Often there are ruminations (repetitive, intrusive thoughts) with pessimistic ideas. Thoughts of death and preoccupation with death are not uncommon.

Suicidal ideas may be present. In severe cases, delusions of nihilism (e.g. 'world is coming to an end', 'my brain is completely dead', 'my intestines have rotted away') may occur.

Psychomotor Activity

In younger patients (< 40 year old), retardation is more common and is characterised by slowed thinking and activity, decreased energy and monotonous voice. In a severe form, the patient can become stuporous (*depressive stupor*).

In the older patients (e.g. post-menopausal women), agitation is commoner. It often presents with marked anxiety, restlessness (inability to sit still, hand-wriggling, picking at body parts or other objects) and a subjective feeling of unease.

Anxiety is a frequent accompaniment of depression. Irritability may present as easy annoyance and frustration in day-to-day activities, e.g. unusual anger at the noise made by children in the house.

Physical Symptoms

Multiple physical symptoms (such as heaviness of head, vague body aches) are particularly common in the elderly depressives and depressed patients from the developing countries (such as India).

However, the recent literature has shown that multiple physical symptoms (called *general aches and pains*) are present in most patients even in the Western world and they can be elicited only if physicians routinely ask the patients for their presence.

Hypochondriacal features may be present in up to a quarter of depressives presenting for treatment. These physical symptoms are almost always present in severe depressive episode.

Another common symptom is the complaints of reduced energy and easy fatigability. The patients, therefore, not surprisingly attribute their symptoms to physical cause(s) and consult a physician instead of a psychiatrist.

Biological Functions

Disturbance of biological functions is common, with *insomnia* (or sometimes increased sleep), *loss of appetite and weight* (or sometimes hyperphagia and weight gain), and loss of sexual drive.

When the disturbance is severe, it is called as melancholia (*somatic syndrome* in ICD-10-DCR; Diagnostic Criteria for Research). The somatic syndrome of depression is described in Table 6.1.

The presence of somatic syndrome in depressive disorder signifies higher severity and more biological nature of the disturbance. It often also implies a good response to somatic methods of treatment (e.g. pharmacotherapy, ECT).

Psychotic Features

About 15-20% of depressed patients have psychotic symptoms such as delusions, hallucinations, grossly inappropriate behaviour or stupor. The psychotic features can be either mood-congruent (e.g. nihilistic delusions, delusions of guilt, delusions of poverty, stupor) which are understandable in the light of depressed mood, or can be mood-incongruent (e.g. delusions of control) which are not directly related to depressive mood.

Suicide

Suicidal ideas in depression should always be taken very seriously. Although there is a risk of suicide in every depressed patient with suicidal ideation, presence of certain factors increases the risk of suicide (Table 6.2).

Absence of Underlying Organic Cause

If depressive episode is secondary to an organic cause, a diagnosis of *organic mood disorder* should be made.

In ICD-10, the severity of depressive episode is defined as mild, moderate or severe, depending primarily on the number of the symptoms, but also on the severity of symptoms and the degree of impairment.

Table 6.1: Somatic Syndrome in Depression (ICD-10)

The somatic syndrome is characterised by:
a. Significant decrease in appetite or weight
b. Early morning awakening, at least 2 (or more) hours before the usual time of awakening
c. Diurnal variation, with depression being worst in the morning
d. Pervasive loss of interest and loss of reactivity to pleasurable stimuli
e. Psychomotor agitation or retardation.

Table 6.2: Suicidal Risk: Some Important Factors

Suicidal risk is much more in the presence of following factors:
a. Presence of marked hopelessness
b. Males; age > 40; unmarried, divorced/widowed
c. Written/verbal communication of suicidal intent and/or plan
d. Early stages of depression
e. Recovering from depression (At the peak of depression, the patient is usually either too depressed or too retarded to commit suicide)
f. Period of 3 months from recovery.

Bipolar Mood (or Affective) Disorder

This disorder, earlier known as manic depressive psychosis (MDP), is characterised by recurrent episodes of mania and depression in the same patient at different times (Fig. 6.1).

These episodes can occur in any sequence. The patients with recurrent episodes of mania (unipolar mania) are also classified here as they are rare and often resemble the bipolar patients in their clinical features.

The current episode in bipolar mood disorder is specified as one of the following (ICD-10):
   i. hypomanic,
   ii. manic without psychotic symptoms,
   iii. manic with psychotic symptoms,
   iv. mild or moderate depression,
   v. severe depression, without psychotic symptoms,
   vi. severe depression, with psychotic symptoms,
   vii. mixed, or
   viii. in remission.

Bipolar mood disorder is further classified in to bipolar I and bipolar II disorders (Table 6.3).

Recurrent Depressive Disorder

This disorder is characterised by recurrent (at least two) depressive episodes (unipolar depression).

The current episode in recurrent depressive disorder is specified as one of the following:
i.   mild,
ii. moderate,
iii. severe, without psychotic symptoms,
iv. severe, with psychotic symptoms,
v.   in remission.

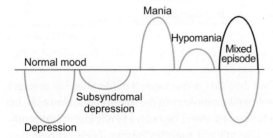

Fig. 6.1: Bipolar Disorder: Clinical Picture

Persistent Mood Disorder

These disorders are characterised by persistent mood symptoms which last for more than 2 years (1 year in children and adolescents) but are not severe enough to be labelled as even hypomanic or mild depressive episode.

If the symptoms consist of persistent mild depression, the disorder is called as *dysthymia*; and if symptoms consist of persistent instability of mood between mild depression and mild elation, the disorder is called as *cyclothymia*.

Other Mood Disorders

This category includes the diagnosis of mixed affective episode. This is a frequently missed diagnosis clinically. In this type, the full clinical picture of depression and mania is present either at the same time intermixed (Fig. 6.1), or alternates rapidly with each other (*rapid cycling*), without a normal intervening period of euthymia.

COURSE AND PROGNOSIS

Bipolar mood disorder has an earlier age of onset (third decade) than recurrent depressive (unipolar) disorder. Unipolar depression, on the other hand, is common in two age groups: late third decade and fifth to sixth decades.

An average manic episode lasts for 3-4 months while a depressive episode lasts from 4-6 months. Unipolar depression usually lasts longer than bipolar depression. With rapid institution of treatment, the major symptoms of mania are controlled within 2 weeks and of depression within 6-8 weeks.

Table 6.3: Subtypes of Bipolar Disorder

1. Bipolar I   Characterised by episodes of severe mania and severe depression
2. Bipolar II   Characterised by episodes of hypomania (not requiring hospitalisation) and severe depression

Nearly 40% of depressives with episodic course improve in 3 months, 60% in 6 months and 80% improve within a period of one year. 15-20% of patients develop a chronic course of illness, which may last for two or more years.

Chronic depression is usually characterised by less intense depression, hypochondriacal symptoms, presence of co-morbid disorders (such as dysthymic disorder, alcohol dependence, personality disorders and medical disorders), presence of ongoing stressors and unfavourable early environment. As the age advances, the intervals between two episodes shorten and, the duration of the episodes and their frequency tends to increase. Although not all patients have relapses, it has been estimated that up to 75% of patients have a second episode within 5 years.

Some patients with bipolar mood disorder have more than 4 episodes per year; they are known as *rapid cyclers* (Figure 6.2). About 70-80% of all rapid cyclers are women. When phases of mania and depression alternate very rapidly (e.g. in matter of hours or days), the condition is known as *ultra-rapid cycling*. Some of the factors associated with rapid cycling include the use of antidepressants (especially tricyclic antidepressants), low thyroxin levels, female gender, bipolar II pattern of illness, and the presence of neurological disease.

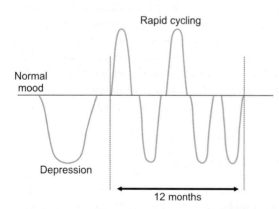

Fig. 6.2: Bipolar Disorder: Rapid Cycling Clinical Picture

There is an increased mortality in patients with mood disorders by almost two times the general population. The most important cause of death is suicide, the life-time risk of which is 10-15 times higher in depression. Patients with depression also have higher mortality rates from cardiovascular diseases and co-morbid alcohol and drug use disorders. Patients with depression also exhibit a variety of disturbances in immune function.

PROGNOSIS

Classically, the prognosis in mood disorders is generally described as better than in schizophrenia. Some of the good (and poor) prognostic factors in mood disorders are described in Table 6.4.

Table 6.4: Some Prognostic Factors in Mood Disorders

Good Prognostic Factors
1. Acute or abrupt onset
2. Typical clinical features
3. Severe depression
4. Well-adjusted premorbid personality
5. Good response to treatment.

Poor Prognostic Factors
1. Co-morbid medical disorder, personality disorder or alcohol dependence
2. Double depression (acute depressive episode superimposed on chronic depression or dysthymia)
3. Catastrophic stress or chronic ongoing stress
4. Unfavourable early environment
5. Marked hypochondriacal features, or mood-incongruent psychotic features
6. Poor drug compliance.

AETIOLOGY

Over the years, a vast amount of literature has emerged probing the aetiology of mood disorders. However, the aetiology of mood disorders is not known currently, despite several theories having been propounded. Some of these include:

Biological Theories

The following findings (and theories) point towards a biological basis of mood disorders.

Genetic Hypothesis

The life-time risk for the first degree relatives of bipolar mood disorder patients is 25%, and of recurrent depressive disorder patients is 20%.

The life-time risk for the children of one parent with bipolar mood disorder is 27% and of both parents with bipolar mood disorder is 74%.

The concordance rate in *bipolar disorders* for monozygotic twins is 65% and for dizygotic twins is 20%; the concordance rate in *unipolar depression* for monozygotic twins is 46% and for dizygotic twins is 20%.

Therefore, genetic factors are very important in making an individual vulnerable to mood disorders, particularly so in bipolar mood disorders. However, environmental factors are also probably important.

Biochemical Theories

There are several biochemical hypotheses for the causation of mood disorders. The monoamine hypothesis suggests an abnormality in the monoamine [catecholamine (norepinephrine and dopamine) and serotonin] system in the central nervous system at one or more sites. Acetylcholine and GABA are also presumably involved.

The earlier models of a functional increase (in mania) or decrease (in depression) of amines at the synaptic cleft now appear simplistic, though urinary and CSF levels of amine metabolites indicate decreased norepinephrine and/or 5-HT function in depression, and increased norepinephrine in mania.

The postsynaptic events involving the second messenger system, and alterations in the receptor number and function, are also important in addition to the synaptic and presynaptic events.

The effects of antidepressants and mood stabilisers in mood disorders also provide additional evidence to the biochemical hypothesis of mood disorders.

Patients suffering from severe depression with suicidal intent/attempt appear to have a marked decrease in the serotonergic function, evidenced by decreased urinary and plasma 5-HIAA levels and the postmortem studies.

Neuroendocrine Theories

Mood symptoms are prominently present in many endocrine disorders, such as hypothyroidism, Cushing's disease, and Addison's disease.

Endocrine function is often disturbed in depression, with cortisol hypersecretion, non-suppression with dexamethasone challenge (Dexamethasone suppression test or DST), blunted TSH response to TRH, and blunted growth hormone (GH) production during sleep.

The neuroendocrine and biochemical mechanisms are closely inter-related.

Sleep Studies

Sleep abnormalities are common in mood disorders (e.g. decreased need for sleep in mania; insomnia and frequent awakenings in depression).

In depression, the commonly observed abnormalities include decreased REM latency (i.e. the time between falling asleep and the first REM period is decreased), increased duration of the first REM period, and delayed sleep onset.

Brain Imaging

In mood disorders, brain imaging studies (CT scan/ MRI scan of brain, PET scan, and SPECT) have yielded inconsistent, yet suggestive findings.

These findings include ventricular dilatation, white matter hyper-intensities, and changes in the blood flow and metabolism in several parts of brain (such as prefrontal cortex, anterior cingulate cortex, and caudate).

Psychosocial Theories

Psychoanalytic Theories

In depression, loss of a libidinal object, *introjection* of the lost object, fixation in the oral sadistic phase of development, and intense craving for narcissism or self-love are some of the postulates of different psychodynamic theories.

Mania represents a *reaction formation* (Table 17.1) to depression according to the psychodynamic theory.

Stress

Increased number of stressful life events before the onset or relapse has a *formative* rather than a precipitating effect in depression though they can serve a precipitant role in mania. Increased stressors in the early period of development are probably more important in depression.

Cognitive and Behavioural Theories

The mechanisms of causation of depression, according to these theories, include depressive negative cognition (cognitive theory), learned helplessness (animal model), and anger directed inwards. These concepts are useful in the psychological treatment of mild (to moderate) depression.

Several other theories have also been propounded but are currently considered to be of doubtful value as theories of causation of depression.

DIFFERENTIAL DIAGNOSIS

The first step in the differential diagnosis of any mood disorder is to exclude a disorder with known organic cause, e.g. *organic* (especially drug-induced) *mood disorders* and *dementia* (differential diagnosis from depressive pseudodementia).

The second step is to rule out a possibility of *acute and transient psychotic disorders, schizo-affective disorder*, and *schizophrenia*.

The third step is to exclude the possibility of other non-organic psychoses such as *delusional disorders*.

The fourth step is to exclude the possibility of *adjustment disorder with depressed mood, generalised anxiety disorder, normal grief reaction*, and *obsessive compulsive disorder* (with or without secondary depression).

In addition to the main diagnosis, it is also important to look for co-morbid medical (such as diabetes, hypertension) and/or psychiatric disorders (such as

Table 6.5: Some Commonly used Antidepressants

	Generic Name	Usual Therapeutic Range (mg/day)
1.	Agomelatin	25-50
2.	Amitriptyline	75-300
3.	Amoxapine	150-300
4.	Bupropion	150-450
5.	Citalopram	10-40
6.	Clomipramine	75-250
7.	Doxepine	75-300
8.	Dosulepin/Dotheipin	75-150
9.	Duloxetine	30-120
10.	Escitalopram	10-20
11.	Fluoxetine	20-60
12.	Fluvoxamine	50-200
13.	Imipramine	75-300
14.	Lofepramine	140-210
15.	Mianserin	30-120
16.	Mirtazapine	15-45
17.	Moclobemide	300-600
18.	Nortriptyline	150-300
19.	Paroxetine	10-40
20.	Reboxetine	10-12
21.	Sertraline	50-200
22.	Tianeptin	37.5
23.	Trazodone	300-600
24.	Venlafaxine	75-375

anxiety, panic, alcohol or drug misuse, or personality disorder) on a multi-axial diagnostic system (Table 1,4).

MANAGEMENT

Somatic Treatment

Antidepressants

Antidepressants are the treatment of choice for a vast majority of depressive episodes. Some of the commonly used antidepressants with their usual range of therapeutic dosage are listed in Table 6.5. (Antidepressants are discussed in more detail in Chapter 15).

The usual starting dose is about 75-150 mg of imipramine equivalent. The clinical improvement is assessed after about two weeks. In case of non-improvement, the dose can usually be increased up to 300 mg of imipramine equivalent.

It should be remembered that it may take up to 3 weeks before any appreciable response may be noticed. Before stopping or changing a drug, the particular drug should be given in a therapeutically adequate dose for at least 6 weeks.

A variety of antidepressants are now available in the market. Since almost all antidepressants are equal in antidepressant efficacy and there is no single antidepressant effective for all depressed patients, the choice of antidepressant is often dictated by other factors. These factors include cost and ease of availability of the drug, the side-effect profile of the drug, past history of response and (any) co-morbid medical or psychiatric disorders. An individualised choice has to be made in each patient, keeping these various factors in mind.

Imipramine, amitriptyline and other related drugs are called *tricyclic antidepressants (TCAs)*. The newer antidepressants such as *selective serotonin reuptake inhibitors (SSRIs)* (e.g. fluoxetine, sertraline, citalopram), mirtazapine, and *serotonin norepine-phrine reuptake inhibitors (SNRIs)* (e.g. venlafaxine, duloxetine) have very little anticholinergic side effects and, hence, are generally safer drugs to use in elderly patients with benign hypertrophy of prostate. However, both venlafaxine and duloxetine have been associated with hypertension and should be used with care in those with a history of cardiac illness.

The antidepressant dosage is monitored on the basis of clinical improvement. Routine monitoring of blood levels is not usually indicated.

For the first, uncomplicated, depressive episode, the patient should receive full therapeutic dose of the chosen antidepressant for a period of 6-9 months, after achieving full remission. It is wise to taper the antidepressant medication, when the treatment is to be stopped after the continuation phase.

There are three main phases of treatment:
i. *Acute treatment* (till remission occurs),
ii. *Continuation treatment* (from remission till end of treatment), and
iii. *Maintenance treatment* (to prevent further recurrences).

Maintenance treatment may be indicated in the following patients:
i. Partial response to acute treatment.
ii. Poor symptom control during the continuation treatment.
iii. More than 3 episodes (90% chances of recurrence).
iv. More than 2 episodes with early age of onset, or recurrence within 2 years of stopping antidepressants, or severe and/or life-threatening depression, or family history of mood disorder.
v. Chronic depression (> 2 years) or double depression.

About 20-35% of depressed patients are *refractory* to antidepressant medication. The management of a treatment refractory depressed patient is best done by a psychiatrist, often at a tertiary care centre. These patients may require one of the following alternatives:
i. A change of antidepressant (*Switch*),
ii. Combination of two types of antidepressants,
iii. Augmentation with lithium,
iv. Augmentation with T_3 or T_4,
v. Augmentation with antipsychotics,
vi. Electroconvulsive therapy, or
vii. Use of newer and experimental techniques.

One type of depression, namely delusional depression (depression with *psychotic* features), is usually refractory to antidepressants alone. The treatments of choice in this condition include:
i. An antidepressant with ECT, or
ii. An antidepressant with antipsychotics, or
iii. An antidepressant with lithium.

Electroconvulsive Therapy (ECT)

The indications for ECT in depression include:
i. Severe depression with suicidal risk.

ii.   Severe depression with stupor, severe psycho-motor retardation, or somatic syndrome.
iii. Severe treatment refractory depression.
iv.   Delusional depression (psychotic features).
v.   Presence of significant antidepressant side-effects or intolerance to drugs.

Severe depression with suicidal risk is the first and foremost indication for use of ECT. The prompt use of ECT can be life-saving in such a situation.

The response is usually rapid, resulting in a marked improvement. In most clinical situations, usually 6-8 ECTs are needed, given three times a week. When six ECTs are administered, the usual pattern is three ECTs in the first week, two in the second week and one in the third week.

However, improvement is not sustained after stopping the ECTs. Therefore, antidepressants are often needed along with ECTs, in order to maintain the improvement achieved. The safety of the ECT procedure has now been well-established.

ECT can also be used for acute manic excitement, if it is not adequately responding to antipsychotics and mood stabilisers.

Lithium (Li)

Lithium has traditionally been the drug of choice for the treatment of manic episode (acute phase) as well as for prevention of further episodes in bipolar mood disorder. It has also been used in treatment of depression with less success. (Lithium is discussed in detail in Chapter 15).

There is usually a 1-2 week lag period before any appreciable response is observed. So, for treatment of acute manic episode, antipsychotics are usually administered along with lithium, in order to provide cover for the first few weeks.

The usual therapeutic dose range is 900-1500 mg of lithium carbonate per day. Lithium treatment needs to be closely monitored by repeated blood levels, as the difference between the therapeutic and lethal blood levels is not very wide (*narrow therapeutic index*).

Therapeutic blood lithium = 0.8-1.2 mEq/L
Prophylactic blood lithium = 0.6-1.2 mEq/L

A blood lithium level of >2.0 mEq/L is often associated with toxicity, while a level of more than 2.5-3.0 mEq/L may be lethal.

Although lithium is indicated for therapeutic use in all manic episodes, the preventive use is best in usually those patients with bipolar disorder, in whom the frequency of episodes is 1-3 per year or 2-5 per two years.

The common acute toxic symptoms of lithium are neurological while the common chronic side-effects are nephrological and endocrinal (usually hypothyroidism).

The important investigations before starting lithium therapy include a complete general physical examination, full blood counts, ECG, urine routine examination (with/without 24 hour urine volume), renal function tests and thyroid function tests.

Antipsychotics

Antipsychotics are an important adjunct in the treatment of mood disorder. The commonly used drugs include risperidone, olanzapine, quetiapine, haloperidol, and aripiprazole. It is customary to use the atypical antipsychotics first, before considering the older typical antipsychotics.

Some of the indications include:

1. Acute manic episode
•   Along with mood stabilisers for the first few weeks, before the effect of mood stabilisers becomes apparent.
•   Where mood stabilisers are not effective, not indicated, or have significant side-effects.
•   Given parenterally (IM or IV) for emergency treatment of mania.
•   Recently, there has been some early evidence that atypical antipsychotics (e.g. olanzapine) might have some mood stabilising properties.

2. Delusional depression
As stated above, antipsychotics are important adjuncts in the treatment of delusional depression. Once again, it is customary to use atypical antipsychotics such as olanzapine, quetiapine, risperidone, and ziprasidone first, although any antipsychotic can be used.

iii. Bipolar depression

There is recent evidence that quetiapine has antidepressant efficacy in bipolar depression.

iv. Maintenance or prophylactic treatment in bipolar
disorder

Recent evidence shows that several atypical antipsychotics such as olanzapine, quetiapine and aripiprazole can be successfully used in the maintenance treatment of bipolar disorder.

Other Mood Stabilisers

The other mood stabilisers which are used in the treatment of bipolar mood disorders include:

1. Sodium valproate

- For acute treatment of mania and prevention of bipolar mood disorder.
- Particularly useful in those patients who are refractory to lithium.
- The dose range is usually 1000-3000 mg/day (the therapeutic blood levels are 50-125 mg/ml).
- It has a faster onset of action than lithium, therefore, it can be used in acute treatment of mania effectively.

2. Carbamazepine and Oxcarbazepine

- For acute treatment of mania and prevention of bipolar mood disorder.
- Particularly useful in those patients who are refractory to lithium and valproate.
- Particularly effective when EEG is abnormal (although this is not necessary for the use of carbamazepine).
- The dose range of carbamazepine is 600-1600 mg/day (the therapeutic blood levels are 4-12 mg/ml).
- The use of carbamazepine in treatment of bipolar disorder has recently declined, partly due to its potential for drug interactions.
- Oxcarbazepine has a narrow evidence base and its use in bipolar disorder is quite recent.

3. Benzodiazepines

Lorazepam (IV and orally) and *clonazepam* are used for the treatment of manic episode alone rarely; however, they have been used more often as adjuvants to antipsychotics.

4. *Lamotrigine* is particularly effective for bipolar depression and is recommended by several guidelines.

5. T_3 and T_4 as adjuncts for the treatment of rapid cycling mood disorder and resistant depression.

Other Treatments

Psychosurgery is an extremely rarely used method of treatment and is resorted to only in exceptional circumstances.

In depressive episode, which is either chronic or persistently recurrent with a limited or absent response to other modes of treatment, one of the following procedures may very rarely be performed:

   i. Stereotactic subcaudate tractotomy, or

   ii. Stereotactic limbic leucotomy.

In carefully selected patients, the results are reported to be satisfactory. However, in the current day and age, psychosurgery is hardly ever considered in routine clinical practice.

Psychosocial Treatment

Although somatic treatment appears to be the primary mode of management in major mood disorders, psychosocial treatment is often helpful. These indications include:

   i. As an adjunct to somatic treatment.

   ii. In mild to moderate cases of depression.

   iii. Certain selected cases.

These methods include (see Chapter 18 for details):

Cognitive Behaviour Therapy

Cognitive behaviour therapy (CBT) aims at correcting depressive negative cognitions (ideations) such as hopelessness, worthlessness, helplessness and pessimistic ideas, and replacing them by new cognitive and behavioural responses.

CBT is useful in mild to moderate, non-bipolar depression and can be used with or without somatic treatment.

Interpersonal Therapy

Interpersonal therapy (IPT) attempts to recognise and explore interpersonal stressors, role disputes and transitions, social isolation, or social skills deficits, which act as precipitants for depression.

It is useful in the treatment of mild to moderate unipolar depression, with or without antidepressants.

Psychoanalytic Psychotherapy

The short-term psychoanalytic psychotherapies aim at changing the personality itself rather than just ameliorating the symptoms.

Their usefulness is uncertain, particularly in florid depressive or manic episode. These techniques are however helpful in the treatment of selected patients (such as dysthymic disorder, depression co-morbid with personality disorders, or depression with history of childhood loss/child abuse).

Behaviour Therapy

This includes the various short-term modalities such as social skills training; problem solving techniques, assertiveness training, self-control therapy, activity scheduling and decision-making techniques.

It can be useful in mild cases of depression or as an adjunct to antidepressants in moderate depression.

Group Therapy

Group psychotherapy can be useful in mild cases of depression. It is a very useful method of psychoeducation in both recurrent depressive disorder and bipolar disorder.

Family and Marital Therapy

Apart from educating the family about the nature of illness and the usefulness of somatic treatment, family therapy has not been found very useful in treatment of mood disorders per se.

These therapies can however help decrease the intrafamilial and interpersonal difficulties, and to reduce or modify stressors, which may help in a faster and more complete recovery. Their most common use in clinical practice is to ensure continuity of treatment (such as lithium prevention in patients with bipolar disorder) and adequate drug concordance.

OTHER SYNDROMES OF DEPRESSION AND MANIA

Involutional Melancholia

Described by Kraepelin, this is a form of severe depression which occurs in the involutional period of life (i.e. 40-65 years of age).

It is typically characterised by marked agitation, presence of psychotic features (such as delusions of persecution, tactile and auditory hallucinations) and multiple somatic symptoms (or hypochondriacal delusions). Presently, it is no longer thought of as an independent entity but the term is used to describe the severity of a depressive episode.

Mixed Anxiety Depressive Disorder

This disorder is characterised by the presence of depressive and anxiety symptoms which result in significant distress or disability in the person. The symptoms should not meet the criteria of either an anxiety disorder or a mood disorder.

This disorder is apparently seen more frequently in the medical outpatient departments and primary care centres. Several cases probably exist untreated in the general population, but rarely come to medical attention.

In clinical practice, it is important to consider a diagnosis of either a mood disorder or an anxiety disorder, before attempting a diagnosis of mixed anxiety-depressive disorder.

Masked Depression

In masked depression, the depressive mood is not easily apparent and is usually hidden behind the somatic symptoms. This is especially common in the elderly, where the somatic symptoms range from chronic pain, insomnia, atypical facial pain, and paraesthesias. The depressive symptoms can also be masked by drug and/or alcohol misuse. However, a more detailed examination will bring out the tell-tale symptomatology of depression.

The treatment is similar to a depressive episode.

Depressive Equivalents

These are certain conditions which, though not a part of the depressive syndrome, are still thought be comparable to depression (*affective spectrum disorders*). Some of these show clinical response to antidepressant treatment whilst others appear related to depression due to multiple complex reasons.

These disorders include agoraphobia, chronic pain, paraesthesias, panic attacks, alcoholism, drug abuse, hysteria, obsessive compulsive disorder and eating disorders (anorexia nervosa and bulimia nervosa).

This term presently has an uncertain nosological status.

Atypical Depression(s)

These are depressive syndromes which do not present with classical or typical features of depression. These include:

1. *Depression with predominant anxiety:* The anxiety here is far more subjective, in contrast to the objective restlessness seen in agitated depression. The treatment is usually by antidepressants.
2. *Phobic-anxiety-depersonalisation syndrome (PAD syndrome):* Described by Roth, this syndrome is commoner in women aged 20-40 years. It is characterised by diffuse anxiety and panic attacks, multiple phobias (such as agoraphobia and claustrophobia), depersonalisation, derealisation and depressive features. The treatment is usually by antidepressants. It is recognised that ECTs may make the condition worse.
3. *Non-endogenous depression:* Atypical depression of the non-endogenous type is characterised by absence of neurotic traits and significant stressful life events. This differentiates it from neurotic or reactive depression.
4. *Hysteroid-dysphoric depression:* In this type, there are marked fluctuations of mood, ranging from near normal to severe depression. Any stress leads to an abrupt onset of depression, with marked anxiety, pallor and changes in physical appearance. The person usually has histrionic personality traits or disorder.

Atypical depression usually has an onset in the teens and runs a chronic course. Hypersomnia, hyperphagia, reactive nature of symptoms, *rejection sensitivity* and lethargy (*leaden paralysis*) are some of the characteristic features.

The importance of diagnosing atypical depression lies in the fact that many of these patients respond better to MAOIs (monoamine oxidase inhibitors), although SSRIs (Selective Serotonin Reuptake Inhibitors) and TCAs (Tricyclic Antidepressants) should be tried first.

Double Depression

This is a major depressive episode (usually acute), superimposed on an underlying dysthymia or neurotic depression (usually chronic). The response to treatment is usually poor.

Agitated Depression

This is a type of severe depression with marked motor restlessness or agitation. It is either seen alone or along with involutional melancholia. It is more common after the age of 40 years.

The treatment of agitated depression usually requires addition of antipsychotics or benzodiazepines to the antidepressant therapy.

Seasonal Mood Disorder

This is either a bipolar mood disorder or recurrent depressive episode which tends to occur in the same season on each occasion. It is usually more commonly seen in women.

For example, in a bipolar seasonal mood disorder, depression would tend to occur in the same months every time (usually winter months), while mania would occur in the months of some other season every episode (usually summer months).

This is thought to be due to changes in the length of the day (and light) and its effect on hypothalamus. The characteristic symptoms of winter depression are dysphoria, decreased activity and atypical depressive symptoms (increased fatigue, increased sleep, increased appetite and weight, and carbohydrate craving).

The prevalence of winter seasonal mood disorder increases with increasing latitude.

The treatment, in addition to the usual modes of management, also includes *phototherapy*, which consists of increasing the number of hours of day-light (using artificial, full-spectrum, white light of 2,500-10,000 lux intensity, in the early morning, with eyes open) for the treatment of depression. The recent NICE guidelines for treatment of depression cast some doubt on efficacy of light therapy.

Secondary Depression and Secondary Mania

Both depressive and manic episodes can occur secondary to certain physical diseases and drugs. These have been discussed under organic mood disorders (Chapter 3).

Neurotic Depression

Neurotic depression is usually characterised by the following clinical features:
1. Presence of mild to moderate depression.
2. Depressive symptoms usually occur in response to a stressful situation but are often quite disproportionate to the severity of stress.
3. Other 'neurotic' symptoms such as anxiety, obsessive symptoms, phobic symptoms, and multiple somatic symptoms, are often present.
4. Preoccupation with the stressful condition is common.

The typical course of neurotic depression is chronic, with fluctuations. Delusions, hallucinations and other psychotic features are characteristically absent. The other common features include:
1. The reactivity of mood is preserved, i.e. the patient is able to emotionally react to the events occurring in his surroundings.
2. There may be insomnia or hypersomnia. There is usually difficulty in initiating sleep and sometimes difficulty in awakening in the morning.
3. The mood may be worse in the evening, at the end of the day. The mood may also become better in social gatherings and whilst engaged in recreational activities.

4. Suicidal threats and gestures are more common than completed suicide. However, as suicide may be completed accidentally, all such threats should be taken seriously.

An episode of major depression may become superimposed on an underlying neurotic depression. This is then known as *double depression.*

Neurotic depression has been renamed as *dysthymia* or *dysthymic disorder* in DSM-IV-TR and ICD-10. This category does not require the presence of stress as a precipitating factor, and does not put emphasis on the presence of other neurotic symptoms or traits. Dysthymia is defined as any mild depression which is not severe enough to be called a depressive episode, and lasts for two years or more. This is more common in females, with an average age of onset in late third decade.

A large number of psychotherapies have been advocated for neurotic depression. The choice of therapy mainly rests on the therapist's expertise in a particular mode of therapy. Two important issues which often need to be addressed in the therapeutic relationship are:
   i. Dependency needs of the patient, and
   ii. Manipulative behaviour.

Supportive psychotherapy is an important adjunct to the treatment.

When depression is significant and/or is not responding to psychotherapy, *antidepressants* should be used. As mixed depression and anxiety are very common, addition of small doses of benzodiazepines to antidepressants may be needed for the first one or two weeks. However, one must be careful as benzodiazepines tend to get abused if prescribed for more than four weeks at one time.

For non-responders to TCAs and SSRIs, and/or when other neurotic symptoms (such as hypochondriacal symptoms or depersonalisation) are prominent, MAOIs are the drugs of choice. Occasionally, amphetamines (such as methylphenidate) may be useful in mild depression; however, there is a significant risk of dependence.

Chapter 7 — Other Psychotic Disorders

The major nonorganic psychotic disorders are schizophrenia and mood disorders. In addition to these two, there are other nonorganic psychoses some of which have been sometimes labelled as the *third psychoses* or *other psychotic disorders* (psychosis is defined in Table 7.1). These conditions are discussed in this chapter.

PERSISTENT DELUSIONAL DISORDERS

This category in ICD-10 includes all disorders in which persistent delusions are the prominent and most important clinical features.

Delusional Disorder

This disorder, also previously called as *paranoid disorder*, is characterised by the following clinical features in ICD-10. Persistent delusions must be present for at least 3 months and these can include delusions of persecution (being persecuted against), delusions of grandeur (inflated self-esteem and self image), delusions of jealousy (infidelity), somatic (hypochondriacal) delusions, erotomanic delusions (delusions of love), and/or other non-bizarre delusions. It is important to note absence of prominent hallucinations, organic mental disorders, schizophrenia and mood disorders.

The common aetiology appears to be an abrupt change in the environment, for example, in prison inmates, and in immigrants (to a different culture),

Table 7.1: Definition of Psychosis

The term *psychosis* is defined as:

1. Gross impairment in reality-testing ('not in contact' with reality).
2. Marked disturbance in personality, with impairment in social, interpersonal and occupational functioning.
3. Marked impairment in judgement and absent understanding of the current symptoms and behaviour (loss of insight).
4. Presence of the characteristic symptoms, like delusions and hallucinations.

though stressors are not always evident in several other cases. The aetiology of delusional disorders, similar to several other psychiatric disorders, appears to be multifactorial.

It is a disorder with usually a relatively stable and chronic course. It is characterised by presence of well-systematised delusions of nonbizarre type (cf. bizarre delusions can occur in schizophrenia). The emotional response and behaviour is often understandable in the light of their delusional beliefs, with behaviour outside the 'limits' of delusions usually almost normal. Very often, these individuals are able to carry on a near normal social and occupational life without arousing suspicion regarding their delusional disorder. It is only when the area of delusions is probed or confronted that the dysfunction becomes evident.

When the content of delusions is predominantly persecutory (as is often the case), it is important to

Table 7.2: Differential Diagnosis of Delusional Disorders

	Features	Paranoid Schizophrenia	Delusional Disorder (Paranoid disorder)	Paranoid Personality Disorder
1.	General behaviour	Eccentricities, mannerisms, stereotypies, decreased self-care, social withdrawal, guarded and evasive	Eccentricities, decreased social interaction	Restrained social inter-action
2.	Personality	Disorganised (although deterioration is much less than in other types of schizophrenia	Disturbed in delusional area, near normal in other areas	No deterioration
3.	Thought disorder	Delusions, Schneiderian FRS, loosening of associations, formal thought disorder; delusions may be bizarre	Nonbizarre delusions which are well-systematised, no other thought disorder	No thought disorder
4.	Hallucinations	Auditory hallucinations common	Uncommon. If present, are not persistent	Absent
5.	Contact with reality	Markedly disturbed	Disturbed in area of delusional belief	Intact
6.	Insight	Absent	Absent	Present
7.	Affect/mood in relation to thought	Often inappropriate	Usually appropriate	Usually appropriate

differentiate delusional disorder from paranoid schizophrenia and paranoid personality disorder (Table 7.2).

When the content of delusions is predominantly jealousy (infidelity) involving the spouse, it is called as *Othello syndrome* or *conjugal paranoia*.

A syndrome of *late paraphrenia* has also been described in the elderly. Although it was earlier considered a subtype of delusional disorders, it is presently diagnosed under paranoid schizophrenia.

When the content of delusions is predominantly characterised by presence of hypochondriacal delusions, it is called as *monosymptomatic hypochondriacal psychosis* (MHP), *delusional parasitosis*, or *hypochondriacal paranoia*. The common delusions include infestations by worms or foreign bodies, emitting a foul odour (*delusional halitosis*), body (or its parts) being ugly or misshapen (*delusional dysmorphophobia*).

When content of delusions is erotic (erotomanic) the condition is known as *Clerambault's syndrome* or *erotomania*. Occurring most often in women, there is an erotic conviction that a person with (usually a) higher status is in love with the patient.

When the content of delusions is predominantly grandiose, then the patient usually has delusions with religious or political content and may believe self to be a leader with 'higher' aims of spreading peace, making war or spreading a message in the world.

Other Persistent Delusional Disorders

This is a residual category in ICD-10 for other persistent delusional disorders, which do not fulfil the criteria for delusional disorders. The examples of disorders included here are:
1. Delusions associated with persistent hallucinatory voices (but a diagnosis of schizophrenia cannot be made).
2. Delusional disorders with duration of less than 3 months.

Differential Diagnosis

The conditions from which delusional disorders should be differentiated include paranoid schizophrenia, mania, depression, paranoid personality disorder and organic delusional disorder (see Table 7.2).

Treatment

1. Antipsychotics are used to control agitation and treat the psychotic features. For MHP (monosymptomatic hypochondriacal psychosis) or delusional disorder with somatic (hypochondriacal) delusions, pimozide has classically been the drug of choice, though other antipsychotics with or without antidepressants have been used as effectively. Recently, the use of pimozide has declined sharply due to concerns regarding its cardiac adverse effects.
2. Supportive psychotherapy.
3. Antidepressants (such as fluoxetine) and/or ECT may be needed for secondary depression.

INDUCED DELUSIONAL DISORDER

This is an uncommon delusional disorder characterised by a sharing of delusions between usually two (folie à deux) or occasionally more persons (folie à trios, folie à quatre, folie à famille), who usually have a closely knit emotional bond. Only one person usually has authentic delusions due to an underlying psychiatric disorder, most often schizophrenia or delusional disorder.

On separation of the two, the dependent individual may give up his/her delusions and the patient with the primary delusions should then be treated appropriately.

ACUTE AND TRANSIENT PSYCHOTIC DISORDERS

A large number of psychiatrists, especially from the developing countries such as India and Africa, reported that many patients developed an acute psychotic disorder that neither followed the classical course of schizophrenia nor resembled mood disorders in clinical picture, and usually had a better prognosis than schizophrenia.

In a study conducted by the Indian Council of Medical Research (ICMR) on acute psychoses (1989), the following findings were apparent:

1. 85% of these patients exhibited full recovery.
2. Recovery occurred in several cases even in the absence of treatment.
3. 50% of patients had a psychological stressor and 20% of patients had a somatic stressor before the onset of illness.
4. The onset occurred in less than 48 hours in 50% of cases.

ICD-10 has included a new category of 'acute and transient psychotic disorders' (ATPD) in the section on 'schizophrenia, schizotypal and delusional disorders'.

According to ICD-10, these disorders have an abrupt (less than 48 hours) or acute (less than 2 weeks) onset. The onset is often associated with an easily identifiable acute stress (though not necessarily always so) that would be regarded as stressful to most people in similar circumstances, within the culture of the person concerned. The typical events would include bereavement, unexpected loss of partner or job, marriage, or the psychological trauma of combat, terrorism, and torture. Longstanding difficulties or problems are not included here as stressful.

Acute onset is probably associated with a good outcome, and it seems that more abrupt the onset, the better is the outcome. A complete recovery usually occurs within 2-3 months, often even much earlier.

These disorders should not satisfy the criteria for organic mental disorders, psychoactive substance use disorders, schizophrenia, or mood disorders.

The subtypes of acute and transient psychotic disorders include the following:

1. Acute polymorphic psychotic disorder without symptoms of schizophrenia.
2. Acute polymorphic psychotic disorder with symptoms of schizophrenia.
3. Acute schizophrenia-like psychotic disorder.
4. Other acute predominantly delusional psychotic disorders.

The various subtypes of acute and transient psychotic disorders are further classified as:
  i. without associated acute stress, and
  ii. with associated acute stress.

Acute Polymorphic Psychotic Disorder without Symptoms of Schizophrenia

According to ICD-10, this disorder is characterised by an acute onset (from a nonpsychotic state to a clearly psychotic state within 2 weeks) and *polymorphic* picture (unstable and markedly variable clinical picture that changes from day to day or even from hour to hour).

There are several types of hallucinations and/or delusions, changing in both type and intensity from day to day or within the same day. Marked emotional turmoil, which ranges from intense feelings of happiness and ecstasy to anxiety and irritability, is also frequently present.

This disorder is particularly likely to have an abrupt onset (within 48 hours) and a rapid resolution of symptoms; in a large proportion of cases there is no obvious precipitating stress. If the symptoms persist for more than 3 months, the diagnosis should be changed. In spite of the variety of symptoms, none should be present with sufficient consistency to fulfil the criteria for schizophrenia or mood disorder.

Acute Polymorphic Psychotic Disorder with Symptoms of Schizophrenia

According to ICD-10, this disorder meets the descriptive criteria for acute polymorphic psychotic disorder but in which typically schizophrenic symptoms are also consistently present.

If the schizophrenic symptoms persist for more than 1 month, the diagnosis should be changed to schizophrenia.

Acute Schizophrenia-like Psychotic Disorder

According to ICD-10, this disorder is characterised by an acute onset of a psychotic disorder in which the psychotic symptoms are comparatively stable (and *not*

polymorphic) and fulfil the criteria for schizophrenia but have lasted for less than 1 month.

Some degree of emotional variability or instability may be present, but not to the extent described in the acute polymorphic psychotic disorder. The criteria for acute polymorphic psychotic disorder should not be fulfilled.

If the schizophrenic symptoms persist for more than 1 month, the diagnosis should be changed to schizophrenia.

Other Acute Predominantly Delusional Psychotic Disorders

According to ICD-10, this disorder is characterised by an acute onset of a psychotic disorder in which comparatively stable delusions or hallucinations are the main clinical features, but do not fulfil the criteria for schizophrenia.

Delusions of persecution or reference are common, and hallucinations are usually auditory (voices talking directly to the patient). The criteria for acute polymorphic psychotic disorder or schizophrenia should not be fulfilled.

If delusions persist for more than 3 months, the diagnosis should be changed to persistent delusional disorder. If only hallucinations persist for more than 3 months, the diagnosis should then be changed to other nonorganic psychotic disorder.

Differential Diagnosis

The conditions from which acute and transient psychotic disorders should be differentiated include organic mental disorders, psychoactive substance use disorders, schizophrenia, mood disorders, and delusional disorders.

Prognosis

The good prognostic factors in acute and transient psychotic disorders are as follows:
1. Well adjusted premorbid personality.
2. Absence of family history of schizophrenia.
3. Presence of severe precipitating stressor before the onset.

4. Sudden onset of symptoms.
5. Presence of affective symptoms, confusion, perplexity and/or disorientation in clinical picture.
6. Short duration of symptoms.
7. First episode.

Treatment

1. Antipsychotics are the mainstay of treatment, and are used to control agitation and psychotic features. Usually lower doses of antipsychotics are needed.

   However, in the initial stages the patient may not take oral medication. In such cases, parenteral administration of antipsychotics (with or without benzodiazepines such as lorazepam or diazepam) may be needed.

   The first use of parenteral antipsychotics in an antipsychotic-naive patient should be carefully considered, as there is a higher risk of neuroleptic malignant syndrome (NMS) in these patients. Long-term use of antipsychotics should be preferably avoided in these patients (see Chapter 15 for further details).

2. ECT may be needed in cases with marked agitation and emotional turmoil, as well as in cases where there is a danger to self and/or others.

3. Antidepressants may be rarely needed as adjuvants in some cases with associated depression.

4. Psychotherapy and other psychological interventions may be needed in cases with associated stress, as well as for psychoeducation for the patient and family. Engagement with psychological treatment is usually after the acute episode is under control and the patient can communicate his/her fears and anxieties.

SCHIZOAFFECTIVE DISORDER

This is a disorder which lies on the borderland between schizophrenia and mood disorders. In this disorder, the symptoms of schizophrenia and mood disorders are prominently present within the same episode. The symptoms of both disorders may be present simultaneously or may follow within few days of each other.

There are three types described:
1. Schizoaffective disorder, manic (or bipolar) type.
2. Schizoaffective disorder, depressed type.
3. Schizoaffective disorder, mixed type.

The course is usually episodic (particularly in manic subtype), although a chronic course in some patients has been described (particularly in the depressed subtype). The prognosis is better than that in schizophrenia but is worse than that in mood disorders.

The treatment is with mood stabilisers (such as lithium or valproate), antipsychotics, antidepressants and/or ECT, depending on the predominant symptomatology.

CAPGRAS' SYNDROME (THE DELUSION OF DOUBLES)

Capgras' syndrome is a syndrome that is closely related to delusional disorders and is characterised by a delusional conviction that other persons in the environment are not their real selves but are their own doubles.

It is one of the several delusional misidentification syndromes, of which there are four types described:
1. Typical Capgras' syndrome (*Illusion des sosies*): Here the patient sees a familiar person as a complete stranger who is imposing on him as a familiar person.
2. *Illusion de Fregoli*: The patient falsely identifies stranger(s) as familiar person(s).
3. *Syndrome of subjective doubles*: The patient's own self is perceived as being replaced by a double.
4. *Intermetamorphosis*: Here the patient's misidentification is complete and the patient misidentifies not only the 'external appearance' (as in the previous three types) but also the complete personality.

The syndrome is commonly seen in psychotic conditions with delusional symptomatology, such as paranoid schizophrenia (most frequently), delusional disorders and organic delusional disorder.

The treatment consists of adequately treating the underlying disorder.

REACTIVE PSYCHOSIS

Reactive psychosis is characterised by following features:

1. A sudden onset of symptoms.
2. Presence of a major stress before the onset (the quantum of stress should be severe enough to be stressful to a majority of people).
3. A clear temporal relation between stress and the onset of psychotic symptoms.
4. No organic cause underlying the psychosis.

The usual duration of illness is less than one month and recovery is usually complete.

Currently a majority of cases of reactive psychosis would be classified under acute and transient psychotic disorder with associated stress (in ICD-10) or brief reactive psychosis (in DSM-IV-TR).

Chapter 8

Neurotic, Stress-related and Somatoform Disorders

The terms *neurosis* (Table 8.1) and *psychosis* are currently not widely used. The definitions and descriptions of these terms are far from perfect and there are clearly exceptions to the rules. These terms also have psychodynamic connotations. As current classificatory systems are largely theoretical, any aetiological meaning is not very helpful.

DSM-IV-TR does not use these terms at all and although ICD-10 still mentions the term *neurotic* in the classification, it discourages the use of the terms neurosis and psychosis.

In ICD-10, *'neurotic, stress-related and somatoform disorders* have been classified into the following types:
1. Phobic anxiety disorder,
2. Other anxiety disorders (called simply *anxiety disorder* in this book),
3. Obsessive compulsive disorder.

ANXIETY DISORDER

Anxiety is the commonest psychiatric symptom in clinical practice and anxiety disorders are one of the commonest psychiatric disorders in general population.

Anxiety is a 'normal' phenomenon, which is characterised by a state of apprehension or unease arising out of anticipation of danger. Anxiety is often differentiated from fear, as fear is an apprehension in response to an external danger while in anxiety the danger is largely unknown (or internal).

Table 8.1: Definition of Neurosis

The term *neurosis* has been variously defined as meeting one or more of the following criteria:
1. The presence of a symptom or group of symptoms which cause subjective distress to the patient.
2. The symptom is recognised as undesirable (i.e. insight is present).
3. The personality and behaviour are relatively preserved and not usually grossly disturbed.
4. The contact with reality is preserved.
5. There is an absence of organic causative factors.
6. Reaction to severe stress, and adjustment disorders,
7. Dissociative (conversion) disorders,
8. Somatoform disorders, and
9. Other neurotic disorders.

Normal anxiety becomes pathological when it causes significant subjective distress and/or impairment in functioning of an individual.

Some authors separate anxiety into two types:
1. *Trait anxiety:* This is a habitual tendency to be anxious in general (a trait) and is exemplified by 'I often feel anxious'.
2. *State anxiety:* This is the anxiety felt at the present, cross-sectional moment (state) and is exemplified by 'I feel anxious now'.

Persons with trait anxiety often have episodes of state anxiety. The symptoms of anxiety can be broadly classified in two groups: physical and psychological (psychic) (Table 8.2).

Table 8.2: Symptoms of Anxiety

1. *Physical Symptoms*
   A. *Motoric Symptoms:* Tremors; Restlessness; Muscle twitches; Fearful facial expression
   B. *Autonomic and Visceral Symptoms:* Palpitations; Tachycardia; Sweating; Flushes; Dyspnoea; Hyperventilation; Constriction in the chest; Dry mouth; Frequency and hesitancy of micturition; Dizziness; Diarrhoea; Mydriasis

2. *Psychological Symptoms*
   A. *Cognitive Symptoms:* Poor concentration; Distractibility; Hyperarousal; Vigilance or scanning; Negative automatic thoughts
   B. *Perceptual Symptoms:* Derealisation; Depersonalisation
   C. *Affective Symptoms:* Diffuse, unpleasant, and vague sense of apprehension; Fearfulness; Inability to relax; Irritability; Feeling of impending doom (when severe)
   D. *Other Symptoms:* Insomnia (initial); Increased sensitivity to noise; Exaggerated startle response.

Generalised Anxiety Disorder

This is characterised by an insidious onset in the third decade and a stable, usually chronic course which may or may not be punctuated by repeated panic attacks (episodes of acute anxiety). The symptoms of anxiety should last for at least a period of 6 months for a diagnosis of generalised anxiety disorder to be made.

The one year prevalence of generalised anxiety disorder in the general population is about 2.5-8%. It is the commonest psychiatric disorder in the population. As anxiety is a cardinal feature of almost all psychiatric disorders, it is very important to exclude other diagnoses. The most important differential diagnosis is from depressive disorders and organic anxiety disorder.

Panic Disorder

This is characterised by discrete episodes of acute anxiety. The onset is usually in early third decade with often a chronic course. The panic attacks occur recurrently every few days. There may or may not be an underlying generalised anxiety disorder.

The episode is usually sudden in onset, lasts for a few minutes and is characterised by very severe anxiety. Classically the symptoms begin unexpectedly or 'out-of-the-blue'. Usually there is no apparent precipitating factor, though some patients report exposure to phobic stimuli as a precipitant.

The differential diagnosis is from organic anxiety disorder (Chapter 3) (e.g. secondary to hypoglycaemia, hyperthyroidism, phaeochromocytoma) and cardiac disorders (e.g. MVPS or mitral valve prolapse syndrome).

The life time prevalence of panic disorder is 1.5-2%, with 3-4% reporting subsyndromal panic symptoms (i.e. panic symptoms not severe enough to qualify for panic disorder). Panic disorder is usually seen about 2-3 times more often in females. Panic disorder can present either alone or with agoraphobia.

Aetiology

The cause of anxiety disorders is not clearly known. There are however several theories, of which more than one may be applicable in a particular patient.

1. Psychodynamic Theory

According to this theory, anxiety is a signal that something is disturbing the internal psychological equilibrium. This is called as *signal anxiety*. This signal anxiety arouses the ego to take defensive action which is usually in the form of *repression,* a primary defense mechanism. Ordinarily when repression fails, other secondary defense mechanisms (such as conversion, isolation) are called into action.

In anxiety, repression fails to function adequately but the secondary defense mechanisms are *not* activated. Hence, anxiety comes to the fore-front unopposed. Developmentally, primitive anxiety is manifested as somatic symptomatology while developmentally advanced anxiety is signal anxiety. Panic anxiety, according to this theory, is closely related to the separation anxiety of childhood.

2. Behavioural Theory

According to this theory, anxiety is viewed as an unconditioned inherent response of the organism to painful or dangerous stimuli. In anxiety and phobias, this becomes attached to relatively neutral stimuli by conditioning.

3. Cognitive Behavioural Theory (CBT)

According to cognitive behaviour theory, in anxiety disorders there is evidence of selective information processing (with more attention paid to threat-related information), cognitive distortions, negative automatic thoughts and perception of decreased control over both internal and external stimuli.

4. Biological Theory

i.   Genetic evidence: About 15-20% of first degree relatives of the patients with anxiety disorder exhibit anxiety disorders themselves. The concordance rate in the monozygotic twins of patients with panic disorders is as high as 80% (4 times more than in dizygotic twins).

ii. Chemically induced anxiety states: Infusion of chemicals (such as sodium lactate, isoproterenol and caffeine), ingestion of yohimbine and inhalation of 5% CO_2 can produce panic episodes in predisposed individuals. Administration (oral) of MAOIs before the lactate infusion protects the individual(s) from panic attack, thus providing a probable clue to the biological model of anxiety.

iii. GABA-benzodiazepine receptors: This is one of the most recent advances in the search for the aetiology of anxiety disorders. The benzodiazepine receptors are distributed widely in the central nervous system. Presently, two types of benzodiazepine receptors have been identified. The type I (ω_1) is GABA and chloride independent, while type II (ω_2) is GABA and chloride dependent.

GABA (Gamma amino butyric acid) is the most prevalent inhibitory neurotransmitter in the central nervous system. It has been suggested that an alteration in GABA levels may lead to production of clinical anxiety. The fact that the benzodiazepines (which facilitate GABA transmission, thereby causing a generalised inhibitory effect on the CNS) relieve anxiety and that benzodiazepine-antagonists (e.g. flumazenil) and inverse agonists (e.g. β-carbolines) cause anxiety, lends heavy support to this hypothesis.

iv. Other neurotransmitters: Norepinephrine, 5-HT, dopamine, opioid receptors and neuroendocrine dysfunction have also been implicated in the causation of anxiety disorders.

v.   Neuroanatomical basis: Locus coeruleus, limbic system, and prefrontal cortex are some of the areas implicated in the aetiology of anxiety disorders. Regional cerebral blood flow (rCBF) is increased in anxiety, though vasoconstriction occurs in severe anxiety.

vi. Organic anxiety disorder: This disorder is characterised by the presence of anxiety which is secondary to the various medical disorders (e.g. hyperthyroidism, phaeochromocytoma, coronary artery disease). If anxiety symptoms can occur secondary to medical disorders, it seems possible than that anxiety has a biological basis.

Treatment

The treatment of anxiety disorders is usually multimodal.

1. Psychotherapy

Psychoanalytic psychotherapy is not usually indicated, unless characterological (personality) problems co-exist. Usually supportive psychotherapy is used either alone, when anxiety is mild, or in combination with drug therapy. The establishment of a good therapist-patient relationship is often the first step in psychotherapy.

Recently, there has been an increasing use of CBT in the management of anxiety disorders, particularly panic disorders (with or without agoraphobia). CBT can be used either alone or in conjunction with SSRIs.

2. Relaxation Techniques

In patients with mild to moderate anxiety, relaxation techniques are very useful. These techniques are used by the patient himself as a routine exercise everyday and also whenever anxiety-provoking situation is at hand.

These techniques include Jacobson's progressive relaxation technique, yoga, *pranayama*, self-hypnosis, and meditation (including TM or transcendental meditation).

3. Other Behaviour Therapies

The behaviour therapies include biofeedback and hyperventilation control. These methods are important adjuncts to treatment.

4. Drug Treatment

The differential response of generalised anxiety and panic to drug treatment has lead to what is called as the *pharmacological dissection of anxiety disorders* though this differentiation has become much more diluted recently with antidepressants used in treatment of both conditions.

The drugs of choice for generalised anxiety disorder have traditionally been benzodiazepines, and for panic disorder, antidepressants. Both benzodiazepines and antidepressants are discussed in detail in Chapter 15. It is useful to begin the treatment of panic disorders with small doses of antidepressants, usually SSRIs (e.g. fluoxetine).

Benzodiazepines (such as alprazolam and clonazepam) are useful in short-term treatment of both generalised anxiety and panic disorders. However, tolerance and dependence potential limit the use of these drugs. Several antidepressants (such as sertraline) are now licensed for treatment of anxiety and panic disorders.

β-blockers such as propranolol and atenolol are particularly useful in the management of anticipatory anxiety (e.g. anxiety occurring before going on stage or before examinations). However, due care must be exercised in the use of propranolol in the patients with history of asthma, bradycardia or heart block. Atenolol does not cross the blood brain barrier and takes care of only the peripheral symptoms of anxiety. It also has less likelihood of causing bronchial constriction than propranolol.

Buspirone is an anti-anxiety drug (discussed in Chapter 15) which does not have any dependence potential, unlike benzodiazepines. It takes about 2-3 weeks before its action is apparent. It may be prefer-able to benzodiazepines for the long-term management of anxiety disorder. It, however, has not much role in the management of panic disorder.

PHOBIC DISORDER

Phobia is defined as an irrational fear of a specific object, situation or activity, often leading to persistent avoidance of the feared object, situation or activity.

The characteristic features of phobia are described in Table 8.3. The common types of phobias are:

1. Agoraphobia,
2. Social phobia, and
3. Specific (Simple) phobia.

Agoraphobia

Agoraphobia is an example of irrational fear of situations. It is the commonest type of phobia encountered in clinical practice. Women far out-number men in suffering from agoraphobia in the Western countries.

It is characterised by an irrational fear of being in places away from the familiar setting of home. Although it was earlier thought to be a fear of open spaces only, now it includes fear of open spaces, public places, crowded places, and any other place from *where there is no easy escape to a safe place.*

Table 8.3: Phobia: Some Characteristic Features

1. Presence of the fear of an object, situation or activity.
2. The fear is out of proportion to the dangerousness perceived.
3. Patient recognises the fear as irrational and unjustified (Insight is present).
4. Patient is unable to control the fear and is very distressed by it.
5. This leads to persistent avoidance of the particular object, situation or activity.
6. Gradually, the phobia and the phobic object become a preoccupation with the patient, resulting in marked distress and restriction of the freedom of mobility (afraid to encounter the phobic object; *phobic avoidance*).

In fact, the patient is afraid of all the places or situations from where escape may be perceived to be difficult or help may not be available, if he suddenly develops embarrassing or incapacitating symptoms. These embarrassing or incapacitating symptoms are the classical symptoms of panic.

A full-blown panic attack may occur (*agoraphobia with panic disorder*) or only a few symptoms (such as dizziness or tachycardia) may occur (*agoraphobia without panic disorder*).

As the agoraphobia increases in severity, there is a gradual restriction in the normal day-to-day activities. The activities may become so severely restricted that the person becomes self-imprisoned at his home. One or two persons (usually close relations or friends) may be relied upon, with whom the patient can leave home. Hence, the patient becomes severely dependent on these *phobic companion(s)*.

Social Phobia

This is an example of irrational fear of activities or social interaction, characterised by an irrational fear of performing activities in the presence of other people or interacting with others. The patient is afraid of his own actions being viewed by others critically, resulting in embarrassment or humiliation.

There is marked distress and disturbance in routine daily functioning. Some of the examples include fear of blushing (*erythrophobia*), eating in company of others, public speaking, public performance (e.g. on stage), participating in groups, writing in public (e.g. signing a check), speaking to strangers (e.g. for asking for directions), dating, speaking to authority figures, and urinating in a public lavatory (*shy bladder*). Sometimes, alcohol (and sometimes, other drugs) is used to overcome the anxiety occurring in social situations.

Specific (Simple) Phobia

In contrast to agoraphobia and social phobia where the stimuli are generalised, in specific phobia the stimulus is usually well circumscribed. This is an example of irrational fear of objects or situations.

Specific phobia is characterised by an irrational fear of a specified object or situation. Anticipatory anxiety leads to persistent avoidant behaviour, while confrontation with the avoided object or situation leads to panic attacks. Gradually, the phobia usually spreads to other objects and situations.

The disorder is diagnosed only if there is marked distress and/or disturbance in daily functioning, in addition to fear and avoidance of the specified object or situation. Some of the examples of simple phobia include *acrophobia* (fear of high places), *zoophobia* (fear of animals), *xenophobia* (fear of strangers), *algophobia* (fear of pain), and *claustrophobia* (fear of closed places).

The list of specific phobias is virtually endless.

Course

Phobias are generally more common in women with an onset in late second decade or early third decade. Typically, the onset is sudden without any apparent cause. The course is usually chronic with gradually increasing restriction of daily activities. Sometimes, phobias are spontaneously remitting.

Aetiology

Psychodynamic Theory

As discussed in the aetiology of anxiety disorders, anxiety is usually dealt with the defense mechanism of *repression*. When repression fails to function adequately, other secondary defense mechanisms of ego come into action.

In phobia, this secondary defense mechanism is *displacement*. By using displacement, anxiety is transferred from a really dangerous or frightening object to a neutral object. These two objects are often connected by symbolic associations.

The neutral object chosen unconsciously is the one which can be easily *avoided* in day-to-day life, in contrast to the frightening object (frightening to the patient only, due to oedipal genital drives).

In agoraphobia, loss of parents in childhood and separation anxiety have been theorised to contribute to causation.

From a psychobiological perspective, the traumatic experiences of childhood may affect the child's developing brain in such a manner that the child becomes susceptible to anxiety and fear in childhood and later life.

Behavioural Theories

The behavioural theories explain phobia as a conditioned reflex. Initially, the anxiety provoked by a naturally frightening or dangerous object occurs in contiguity with a second neutral object. If this happens often enough, the neutral object becomes a conditioned stimulus for causing anxiety.

In 1920, John Watson experimentally produced phobia in an 11 month old boy who came to be know as 'Little Albert'. Using classical conditioning, he paired white objects to a loud noise. 'Little Albert' gradually developed a fear of all white objects. Of course, it would be completely unethical to replicate this experiment in the present day.

Although the behavioural theory does not explain all the features of phobic disorders adequately, it is very helpful in planning systematic treatment.

Biological Theories

All phobias, especially agoraphobia, are closely linked to panic disorders. It has been suggested that probably the biological models of panic apply to phobias too.

However, the evidence for this view is not strong at present, except for the importance of genetic factors in specific phobias of blood injury type. There is also some evidence for the presence of familial factors in social phobias.

Differential Diagnosis

The differential diagnoses include anxiety disorder, panic disorder, major depression, avoidant personality disorder, obsessive compulsive disorder, delusional disorder, hypochondriasis, and schizophrenia.

Treatment

Most patients with phobic disorder rely on avoidance to manage their fears and anxieties. As long as they find ways to limit their lives within the limitations imposed by phobias, they experience little, if any, anxiety. When they are forced to face the phobic situation, anxiety mounts and they then seek treatment. The patients with more than one phobia and presence of panic symptoms often seek treatment earlier.

The treatment approach is usually multi-modal.

Psychotherapy

Psychodynamically oriented psychotherapy is not usually helpful in treatment of phobias. This approach is however indicated when there are characterological or personality difficulties as well. *Supportive psychotherapy* is a helpful adjunct to behaviour therapy and drug treatment.

As stated earlier, *cognitive behaviour therapy* (CBT) can be used to break the anxiety patterns in phobic disorder. It is usual to combine CBT with behavioural techniques.

Behaviour Therapy

If properly planned, this mode of treatment is usually successful. The behavioural therapies are discussed in Chapter 18 and only the names of important techniques are mentioned here.

1. Flooding.
2. Systematic desensitisation.
3. Exposure and response prevention.
4. Relaxation techniques.

Drug Treatment

The drugs used in the treatment of phobia are:

1. Benzodiazepines (Chapter 15) are useful in reducing the anticipatory anxiety. *Alprazolam* is stated to have anti-phobic, anti-panic and anti-anxiety properties. So, it is the drug of choice, when benzodiazepines are used. However, long-term, double-blind randomised controlled trials are needed. The other drugs used include clonazepam and diazepam.

   However, long-term use of benzodiazepines is fraught with the dangers of tolerance and dependence.

2. Among the antidepressants (discussed in Chapter 15), SSRIs are currently drugs of choice, with paroxetine being the most widely used drug. Other SSRIs, such as fluoxetine and sertraline are also equally effective. Fluoxetine has the advantage of a longer half-life. Other antidepressants such as imipramine (TCA) and phenelzine (MAOI), are also helpful in treating the panic attacks associated with phobias, thereby decreasing the distress.

As mentioned earlier, multiple approaches are usually combined together in treatment of a particular patient.

OBSESSIVE-COMPULSIVE DISORDER

An *obsession* is defined as:
1. An idea, impulse or image which intrudes into the conscious awareness repeatedly.
2. It is recognised as one's own idea, impulse or image but is perceived as *ego-alien* (foreign to one's personality).
3. It is recognised as irrational and absurd (insight is present).
4. Patient tries to resist against it but is unable to.
5. Failure to resist, leads to marked distress.

Differentiation has to be made clinically from delusion and thought insertion. A *delusion* is recognised as one's own idea but is not recognised as ego-alien. In fact, it is strongly believed; hence it is not thought to be irrational and is never resisted. *Thought insertion* is not thought of as one's own idea, but instead somebody else's thought being forcibly inserted into one's mind.

An obsession is usually associated with compulsion(s). A *compulsion* is defined as:
1. A form of behaviour which usually follows obsessions.
2. It is aimed at either preventing or neutralising the distress or fear arising out of obsession.
3. The behaviour is not realistic and is either irrational or excessive.
4. Insight is present, so the patient realises the irrationality of compulsion.

5. The behaviour is performed with a sense of subjective compulsion (urge or impulse to act).

Compulsions may diminish the anxiety associated with obsessions.

Epidemiology, Course and Outcome

In India, obsessive compulsive disorder (OCD) is more common in unmarried males, while in other countries, no gender differences are reported. This disorder is commoner in persons from upper social strata and with high intelligence. The average age of onset is late third decade (i.e. late 20s) in India, while in the Western countries the onset is usually earlier in life.

Recent studies show the life-time prevalence of OCD to be as high as 2-3%, though the Indian data shows a lower prevalence rate. Although classically thought to have a steady *chronic* course, the longitudinal profile of this disorder can also be *episodic*.

A summary of long-term follow-up studies shows that about 25% remained unimproved over time, 50% had moderate to marked improvement while 25% had recovered completely.

Clinical Syndromes

ICD-10 classifies OCD into three clinical subtypes:
1. Predominantly obsessive thoughts or ruminations,
2. Predominantly compulsive acts (compulsive rituals), and
3. Mixed obsessional thoughts and acts.

Depression is very commonly associated with obsessive compulsive disorder. It is estimated that at least half the patients of OCD have major depressive episodes while many other have mild depression. *Premorbidly* obsessional or anankastic personality disorder or 'traits' may be commoner than in rest of the population.

Four clinical syndromes have been described in literature, although admixtures are commoner than pure syndromes.

Washers

This is the commonest type. Here the *obsession* is of *contamination* with dirt, germs, body excretions and the like. The *compulsion* is *washing* of hands or the whole body, repeatedly many times a day. It usually spreads on to washing of clothes, washing of bathroom, bedroom, door knobs and personal articles, gradually.

The person tries to avoid contamination but is unable to, so washing becomes a ritual.

Checkers

In this type, the person has multiple *doubts,* e.g. the door has not been locked, kitchen gas has been left open, counting of money was not exact, etc. The *compulsion,* of course, is *checking* repeatedly to 'remove' the doubt.

Any attempt to stop the checking leads to mounting anxiety. Before one doubt has been cleared, other doubts may creep in.

Pure Obsessions

This syndrome is characterised by repetitive intrusive thoughts, impulses or images which are *not* associated with compulsive acts. The content is usually sexual or aggressive in nature. The distress associated with these obsessions is dealt usually by *counter-thoughts* (such as counting) and not by behavioural rituals.

A variant is *obsessive rumination*, which is a preoccupation with thoughts. Here, the person repetitively ruminates in his mind about the pros and cons of the thought concerned.

Primary Obsessive Slowness

A relatively rare syndrome, it is characterised by severe obsessive ideas and/or extensive compulsive rituals, in the relative absence of manifested anxiety. This leads to marked slowness in daily activities.

This subtype is quite difficult to diagnose in the routine clinical practice, unless the possibility of this subtype is kept in mind.

In clinical practice, one of the most useful scales is the Y-BOCS (Yale-Brown Obsessive Compulsive Scale). It can be used to elicit the symptomatology and rate the severity of OCD. The Y-BOCS classifies the symptoms and signs of OCD as follows:

1. Aggressive obsessions
2. Contamination obsessions
3. Sexual obsessions
4. Hoarding/Saving obsessions
5. Religious/Scrupulous obsessions
6. Obsession with need for symmetry or exactness
7. Somatic obsessions
8. Miscellaneous obsessions
9. Cleaning/washing compulsions
10. Checking compulsions
11. Repeating rituals
12. Counting compulsions
13. Ordering/arranging compulsions
14. Hoarding/collecting compulsions
15. Miscellaneous compulsions.

Aetiology

Several causative factors have been explored in the past but no clear aetiology of obsessive compulsive disorder is known yet. Some of the important theories include:

Psychodynamic Theory

Sigmund Freud found obsessions and phobias to be psychogenetically related. This theory can be explained in a flow diagram (Fig. 8.1).

Isolation of Affect: By this defense mechanism, ego removes the affect (*isolates the affect*) from the anxiety-causing idea. The idea is thus weakened, but remains still in the consciousness. The affect however becomes free and attaches itself to other *neutral idea(s)* by symbolic associations. Thus, these neutral ideas become anxiety-provoking and turn into *obsessions*.

This happens only when *isolation of affect* is not fully successful (incomplete isolation of affect). When it is fully successful, both the idea and affect are repressed and there are *no* obsessions.

Undoing: This defense mechanism leads to compulsions, which prevent or *undo* the feared consequences of obsessions.

Reaction formation results in the formation of obsessive compulsive personality traits rather than

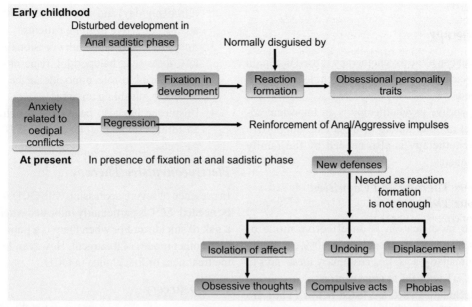

Early childhood
Disturbed development in

Anal sadistic phase

Normally disguised by

Anxiety related to oedipal conflicts

Fixation in development

Reaction formation

Obsessional personality traits

Regression

Reinforcement of Anal/Aggressive impulses

At present In presence of fixation at anal sadistic phase

New defenses

Needed as reaction formation is not enough

Isolation of affect

Undoing

Displacement

Obsessive thoughts

Compulsive acts

Phobias

Fig. 8.1: Psychodynamic Theory of Obsessive Compulsive Disorder: A Brief Summary

contributing to obsessive compulsive symptoms, while *displacement* leads to formation of phobic symptoms. These defense mechanisms are discussed in Table 17.1.

This mechanism has been explained in slight detail as this theory attempts to describe the probable causation of OCD in a remarkably systematic manner. However, it must be remembered that this is only a theory and whether it is true or not, is a matter of conjecture.

Thus, the psychodynamic theory explains OCD by a defensive regression to anal-sadistic phase of development with the use of isolation, undoing and displacement to produce obsessive-compulsive symptoms.

Behavioural Theory

The behavioural theory explains *obsessions* as conditioned stimuli to anxiety (similar to *phobias*). *Compulsions* have been described as learned behaviour which decrease the anxiety associated with obsessions. This decrease in anxiety positively reinforces the compulsive acts and they become 'stable', learned behaviours.

Behavioural or learning theory is *not* able to explain the causation of OCD adequately but is very useful in its treatment.

Biological Theories

1. Obsessive compulsive symptoms can occur secondary to many illnesses such as von Economo's encephalitis, basal ganglia lesions, Gilles de la Tourette syndrome, and hypothalamic and third ventricle lesions.
2. Obsessive compulsive disorder is found in 5-7% of first degree relatives of the patients with OCD.
3. Psychosurgery has been successfully used for treatment of OCD.
4. Biochemically, the central 5-HT system seems to be involved in OCD, as SSRIs are useful in the treatment of OCD.

Some authors pointed at cingulum (gyrus) as the probable site of lesion, while others have found EEG abnormalities most marked over the temporal lobes.

However, at the present moment, there is no conclusive evidence for OCD having a clearly proven organic aetiology.

Treatment

Psychotherapy

1. Psychoanalytic psychotherapy is used in certain selected patients, who are psychologically oriented.
2. Supportive psychotherapy is an important adjunct to other modes of treatment. Supportive psychotherapy is also needed by the family members.

Behaviour Therapy and Cognitive Behaviour Therapy

Behaviour modification is an effective mode of therapy, with a success rate as high as 80%, especially for the compulsive acts. It is customary these days to combine CBT with BT at most centres.

The techniques used are listed below (They are described in Chapter 18):

i. Thought-stopping (and its modifications).
ii. Response prevention.
iii. Systematic desensitisation.
iv. Modelling.

Drug Treatment

1. Benzodiazepines (e.g. alprazolam, clonazepam) have a limited role in controlling anxiety as adjuncts and should be used very sparingly.
2. *Antidepressants:* Some patients may improve dramatically with specific serotonin reuptake inhibitors (SSRIs).

   Clomipramine (75-300 mg/day), a nonspecific serotonin reuptake inhibitor (SRI), was the first drug used effectively in the treatment of OCD. The response is better in the presence of depressive symptoms, but many patients with pure OCD also improve substantially.

   Fluoxetine (20-80 mg/day) is a good alternative to clomipramine and often preferred these days for its better side-effect profile. *Fluvoxamine* (50-200 mg/day) is marketed as a specific anti-obsessional SSRI drug, whilst paroxetine (20-40 mg/day) and sertraline (50-200 mg/day) are also effective in some patients.

3. *Antipsychotics:* These are occasionally used in low doses (e.g. haloperidol, risperidone, olanzapine, aripiprazole, pimozide) in the treatment of severe, disabling anxiety.
4. Buspirone has also been used beneficially as an adjunct for augmentation of SSRIs, in some patients.

Electroconvulsive Therapy

In presence of severe depression with OCD, ECT may be needed. ECT is particularly indicated when there is a risk of suicide and/or when there is a poor response to the other modes of treatment. However, ECT is not the treatment of first choice in OCD.

Psychosurgery

Psychosurgery can be used in treatment of OCD that has become intractable, and is not responding to other methods of treatment. It is worth mentioning that psychosurgery is only available as a treatment choice at a very few centres throughout the world.

The best responders are usually those who have significant associated depression, although pure obsessives also do respond. The main benefit is the marked reduction in associated distress and severe anxiety.

The procedures which can be employed are:

i. Stereotactic limbic leucotomy.
ii. Stereotactic subcaudate tractotomy.

Psychosurgery is usually followed by intensive behaviour therapy aimed at rehabilitation. However, with the easy availability of SSRIs, and a good response of OCD symptoms to SSRIs and other pharmacological measures, psychosurgery is very rarely used in the treatment of OCD.

Very often, a comprehensive treatment of OCD requires that multiple treatment modalities (e.g. drug treatment and BT/CBT) be combined in a specific manner, suitable to the particular patient being treated at the time.

DISSOCIATIVE AND CONVERSION DISORDERS

The word *hysteria* has been used in so many contexts by psychiatrists, physicians and non-professionals that it no longer has any one meaning. These various contexts include:

1. Impulsive, uncontrolled behaviour (impulse dyscontrol).
2. Manipulative, exhibitionistic, emotional, dramatic, and/or seductive behaviour (histrionic personality traits).
3. Absence of objective signs of organic illness.
4. Presence of multiple vague somatic symptoms, especially in a female patient (masked depression, somatisation disorder or Briquet's hysteria).
5. Hypochondriasis.
6. Any mental illness.
7. Presence of certain symptoms which are not explainable in the context of present organic illness (functional overlay, conversion symptoms).
8. Difficult patient; poor doctor-patient communication.
9. 'Sick' role or 'abnormal illness behaviour'.
10. Psychosomatic disorders.
11. Malingering.
12. Psychosexual dysfunctions.

This list is not exhaustive. Therefore, it is not surprising that the word *hysteria* has been removed from DSM-IV-TR as well as the ICD-10. The term hysteria has now been replaced in the ICD-10 by 'conversion and dissociative disorders' and in DSM-IV-TR, by conversion and dissociative disorders.

Epidemiology

Hysteria (comprising of conversion, dissociation and somatisation disorder) constitutes about 6-15% of all outpatient diagnoses and 14-20% of all neurotic disorders. Females usually outnumber males, but in children the percentage tends to be similar in boys and girls.

Conversion Disorder

Conversion disorder is characterised by the following clinical features:

1. Presence of symptoms or deficits affecting motor or sensory function, suggesting a medical or neurological disorder.
2. Sudden onset.
3. Development of symptoms usually in the presence of a significant psychosocial stressor(s).
4. A clear temporal relationship between stressor and development or exacerbation of symptoms.
5. Patient does not intentionally produce the symptoms.
6. There is usually a 'secondary gain' (though not required by ICD-10 for diagnosis).
7. Detailed physical examination and investigations do not reveal any abnormality that can explain the symptoms adequately.
8. The symptom may have a 'symbolic' relationship with the stressor/conflict.

There can be *two* different types of disturbances in conversion disorder; motor and sensory. Autonomic nervous system is typically not involved, except when the voluntary musculature is involved, e.g. vomiting, globus hystericus.

In ICD-10, conversion disorder is subsumed under 'dissociative disorders of movement and sensation', a subtype under 'dissociative (conversion) disorders'. It is further classified in to dissociative motor disorders, dissociative anaesthesia and sensory loss, and dissociative convulsions.

Dissociative Motor Disorders

The *motor disturbance* usually involves either paralysis or abnormal movements. The *'paralysis'* may be a monoplegia, paraplegia or quadriplegia.

Classically, the symptom distribution is according to the patient's knowledge of nervous system. The examination shows normal or voluntarily increased tone and normal reflexes. However, a prolonged 'paralysis' may lead to the development of contractures.

The *abnormal movements* can range from tremors, choreiform movements and gait disturbances, to convulsive movements. These movements either occur or increase when attention is directed towards them, and may disappear when patient is watched unobserved.

These movements do not fit the 'typical' clinical picture of the abnormal involuntary movement disorders. The gait disturbance (*astasia abasia*) is usually characterised by a wide-based, jerky, staggering, dramatic and irregular gait with exaggerated body movements.

Dissociative Anaesthesia and Sensory Loss (Sensory Disorders)

The *sensory disturbance* is exemplified by a 'glove and stocking' anaesthesia (absence of all sensations with an abrupt boundary, not conforming to the distribution of dermatomes, and usually limiting at wrists and ankles), hemi-anaesthesias, blindness or contracted visual fields (tubular vision), and deafness. The detailed examination usually shows absence of objective signs of the particular illness and the disturbance is usually based on patient's knowledge of that illness.

Sensory disturbances are inconsistent with the anatomic patterns expected. Often all sensory modalities (such as touch, pain, temperature and position sense) are affected at the same level. In conversion disorder, the loss of vibration sense maintains a strict midline separation, in spite of the fact that vibrations can be perceived on the other side of body through bone conduction. However, this is not a fool-proof test.

A patient with bilateral conversion blindness is able to go about his way reasonably well and doesn't injure himself by walking into obstacles. In unilateral conversion blindness, the pupillary reflex of the affected eye is normal.

Mixed presentations, with both sensory and motor symptoms, are quite common.

Dissociative Convulsions (Hysterical Fits)

Earlier known as 'hysterical fits' or pseudoseizures, dissociative convulsions are characterised by presence of convulsive movements and partial loss of consciousness. This is a very common disorder in India and other developing countries, though some patients may present with only a partial, brief unresponsiveness, in the absence of convulsive movements (called as *brief dissociative stupor* or *simple dissociative disorder*).

Clearly, differential diagnosis with true seizures is important. The main differentiating points between epileptic seizures and dissociative convulsions are listed in Table 8.4.

Dissociative Disorder

These disorders are characterised by the following clinical features:

1. Disturbance in the normally integrated functions of consciousness, identity and/or memory.
2. Onset is usually sudden and the disturbance is usually temporary. Recovery is often abrupt.
3. Often, there is a precipitating stress before the onset. There is a clear temporal relationship between the stressor and the onset of the illness. A frequent stressful situation is an ongoing war.
4. A 'secondary gain' resulting from the development of symptoms may be found.
5. Detailed physical examination and investigations do not reveal any abnormality that can explain the symptoms adequately.

The common clinical types are described below:

Dissociative Amnesia

This is the commonest clinical type of dissociative disorder. Occurring mostly in adolescent and young adults (females more than males, except in war), it is characterised by a sudden inability to recall important personal information (amnesia), particularly concerning stressful or traumatic life events. The amnesia can not be explained by everyday forgetfulness and there is no evidence of an underlying medical illness.

Most often, dissociative amnesia follows a traumatic or stressful life situation. Sometimes, imagined stressors or expression of 'forbidden' impulses may also precipitate the onset of amnesia.

Table 8.4: Dissociative Convulsions and Epileptic Seizures

	Clinical Features	Epileptic Seizures	Dissociative Convulsions (Hysterical Fits)
1.	Attack pattern	Stereotyped, known clinical patterns	Absence of any established clinical pattern. Purposive body movements occur
2.	Place of occurrence	Anywhere	Usually indoors or at safe places
3.	Warning	Both prodrome and aura are stereotyped	Variable
4.	Time of day	Anytime. Can occur during sleep	Never occur during sleep
5.	Tongue bite	Usually present	Usually absent. Cheek and lip bite may be present
6.	Incontinence of urine and faeces	Can occur	Very rare
7.	Injury	Can occur	Very rare. If occurs, it is minor or may be accidental
8.	Speech	No verbalisation during the seizure	Verbalisation may occur during the fit
9.	Duration	Usually about 30-70 sec. (Short)	20-800 sec. (Prolonged)
10.	Head turning	Unilateral	Side to side turning
11.	Eye gaze	Staring, if eyes are open	Avoidant gaze
12.	Amnesia	Complete	Partial
13.	Neurological signs	Present, e.g. up-going plantars	Absent
14.	Post-ictal confusion	Present	Absent
15.	Stress	Present in 25%	Present much more often
16.	EEG - Inter-ictal	Usually abnormal;	Usually normal
	- Ictal	Abnormal	Normal
17.	Serum prolactin	Increased in post-ictal period (15-20 minutes after seizure; returns back to normal in 1 hour)	Usually normal

This amnesia is of four types (Table 8.5). During the amnesic period, there may be slight clouding of consciousness. In the post-amnesic period, the awareness of disturbance of memory is present.

Dissociative Fugue

Dissociative fugue is characterised by episodes of wandering away (usually away from home). During the episode, the person usually adopts a new identity with complete amnesia for the earlier life. The onset is usually sudden, often in the presence of severe stress. The termination too is abrupt and is followed by amnesia for the episode, but with recovery of memories of earlier life. The characteristic feature is the assumption of a purposeful new identity, with absence of awareness of amnesia.

Table 8.5: Types of Dissociative Amnesia

1. *Circumscribed amnesia* (commonest type): There is an inability to recall all the personal events during a circumscribed period of time, usually corresponding with the presence of the stressor.

2. *Selective amnesia* (less common): This is similar to circumscribed amnesia but there is an inability to recall only some selective personal events during that period while some other events during the same period may be recalled.

3. *Continuous amnesia* (rare): In this type, there is an inability to recall all personal events following the stressful event, till the present time.

4. *Generalised amnesia* (very rare): In this type, there is an inability to recall the personal events of the whole life, in the face of a stressful life event.

An important differential diagnosis is from fugue states seen in complex partial seizures or temporal lobe epilepsy. In complex partial seizures, there is no assumption of a new identity, confusion or disorientation is present during the episode and the episodes are not only linked to any precipitating stress.

Multiple Personality (Dissociative Identity) Disorder

In this dissociative disorder, the person is dominated by two or more personalities, of which only one is being manifest at a time. These personalities are usually different, at times even opposing. Each personality has a full range of higher mental functions, and performs complex behaviour patterns.

Usually one personality is not aware of the existence of the other(s), i.e. there are amnesic barriers between the personalities. Both the onset and termination of control of the each personality is sudden.

Classical examples in the published literature include 'Three faces of Eve' and 'Sybil'.

Trance and Possession Disorders

Trance and possession disorders (*possession hysteria*) are characterised by the control of person's personality by a 'spirit', during the episodes. Usually the person is aware of the existence of the other (i.e. 'possessor'), unlike in multiple personality. This disorder is very commonly seen in India and certain African countries.

Other Dissociative Disorders

Ganser's syndrome (*hysterical pseudodementia*) is commonly found in prison inmates. The characteristic feature is *vorbeireden,* which is also called as 'approximate answers'. The answers are wrong but show that the person understands the nature of question asked. For example; when asked the colour of a red pen, the patient calls it blue.

Aetiology

The aetiological theories of dissociative (and conversion) disorders are predominantly of three types:

Psychodynamic Theory

The explanation given by this theory can be summarised in a flow diagram (Fig. 8.2). For further details regarding the defense mechanisms and Freudian theory, see Tables 17.1 and 17.2.

Behavioural Theory

According to this theory, dissociative (and conversion) symptoms are learned responses in the face of stress. For the first time, the symptom may be learned from the surrounding environment (e.g. seeing a paralysed patient).

The development of the symptom brings about psychological relief by avoidance of stress and is thus secondarily reinforced.

Biological Theory

The biological basis of dissociative (conversion) disorders is far from proven. Some long-term studies (e.g. Slater) have found that up to 80% of patients, diagnosed as 'hysteria', were later found to have physical illnesses. However, replications of such studies have not found such high figures.

Conversion symptoms are frequently seen in the patients with epilepsy and it may at times be difficult to differentiate between true seizures and pseudo-seizures.

Similarly, 'conversion-release' symptoms are seen in some cerebral cortex lesions. However, these are only conversion *symptoms* and are not dissociative (and conversion) *disorders* [i.e. other features for diagnosis of dissociative (conversion) disorders are not present]. Hence, these are of doubtful help in elucidating the aetiology of dissociative (and conversion) disorders.

Diagnosis

Diagnosis is based *not* merely on the absence of objective signs of physical illness, although it is very important to exclude an underlying or associated physical illness. The presence of positive points in history and examination should be present, before a diagnosis of

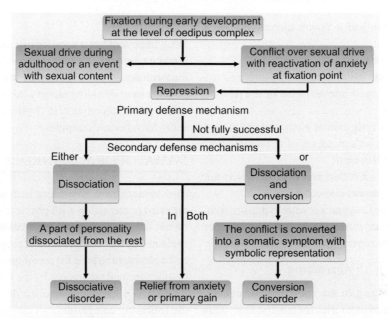

Fig. 8.2: Psychodynamic Theory of Dissociative (Conversion) Disorder

dissociative (and conversion) disorders can be made. These positive points are the characteristic clinical features listed previously.

As dissociative (and conversion) disorders and physical illness can be co-existent, a detailed examination is a must. Dissociative (conversion) symptoms appearing for the first time in an elderly male, especially in a male more than 50 years old, a strong suspicion of underlying physical or major psychiatric illness should be kept in mind.

Other clinical features of dissociative (conversion) disorders include *la-belle-indifférence*, which is a lack of concern towards the symptoms, despite the apparent severity of the disability produced. Although earlier thought to be a hallmark of dissociative (conversion) disorders, it is now known to be present even in physical illnesses. In addition, it is not always present in dissociative (conversion) disorders.

Premorbid histrionic personality traits are often present, although a personality disorder is less commonly present.

Treatment

Behaviour Therapy

Since the patients with dissociative disorders can be *attention seeking* and their symptoms increase with focus of attention, the symptoms should not be unduly focussed on. These patients should be treated as normal, and *not* encouraged to stay in a *sick-role*. Any improvement in symptomatology should be actively encouraged.

Since these patients can also very *suggestible*, they respond quickly to the above-stated methods, with a consistently firm but empathic attitude.

When there is a *sudden, acute symptom*, its prompt removal may prevent habituation and future disability. This may be achieved by one of the following methods:

i. Strong suggestion for a return to normalcy.
ii. *Aversion therapy* (liquor ammonia; aversive electric stimulus; pressure just above eyeballs or tragus of ear; closing the nose and mouth) are occasionally employed carefully in resistant cases.

However, the use of aversion therapy has been decried as it:

a. tends to get over-used;
b. may harm the patient;
c. violates the basic human rights of the patient; and
d. can lend a wrong mental picture of the patient in the physician's mind, i.e. of a 'manipulator' needing punishment!

The current status is that aversion therapy is not a preferred treatment choice.

iii. Amplification of suggestion with hypnosis, free-association, intravenous amytal or thiopentone, or intravenous diazepam.

Psychotherapy with Abreaction

Abreaction is bringing to the conscious awareness, thoughts, affects and memories for the first time. This may be achieved by:

i. Hypnosis.
ii. Free association.
iii. Intravenous thiopentone or diazepam: The aim of abreaction with IV thiopentone is, both, to make the conflicts conscious and to make the patient more suggestible to therapist's advice. Once the conflicts have become conscious and their affects (emotions) have been released, the conversion or dissociative symptom disappears.

Supportive Psychotherapy

Supportive psychotherapy is needed especially when the conflicts (and the current problems) have become conscious and have to be faced in routine life. It is an important adjunct to treatment.

Psychoanalysis

This mode of treatment is chosen not on the basis of conversion/dissociative symptoms but on the total personality structure of the patient. Several patients respond remarkably well. The total length of therapy in classical psychoanalysis is usually five years or more.

Drug Therapy

Drug treatment has a very limited role in dissociative (and conversion) disorders (apart from the use of IV thiopentone, amytal or diazepam in abreaction). A few patients have disabling anxiety (although anxiety as a rule is rather uncommon in 'hysteria') and may need short-term benzodiazepines.

SOMATOFORM DISORDER

The somatoform disorders are characterised by repeated presentation with physical symptoms which do not have any adequate physical basis (and are not explained by the presence of other psychiatric disorders), and a persistent request for investigations and treatment despite repeated assurances by the treating doctors.

In ICD-10, somatoform disorders are divided into the following categories.

Somatisation Disorder

Somatisation disorder is characterised by the following clinical features:

1. Multiple somatic symptoms in the absence of any physical disorder.
2. The symptoms are recurrent and chronic (of many years duration, usually); at least 2 year duration is needed for diagnosis.
3. The symptoms are vague, presented in a dramatic manner, and involve multiple organ systems. The common symptoms include *gastrointestinal* (abdominal pain, beltching, nausea, vomiting, regurgitation), *abnormal skin sensations* (numbness, soreness, itching, tingling, burning), and *sexual and menstrual complaints* (menorrhagia, dysmenorrhoea, dyspareunia).
4. There is frequent change of treating physicians.
5. Persistent refusal to accept the advice or reassurance of several doctors that there is no physical explanation for the symptoms.
6. Some degree of impairment of social and family functioning attributable to the nature of the symptoms and resulting behaviour.
7. Presence of conversion symptoms is common.

This disorder usually begins in second or third decade of life and is much more common in females. In the first degree relatives of patients with somatisation disorder, disorders such as somatisation disorder (in females), and alcoholism and psychopathy (in males) are common. Histrionic personality traits or disorder may also be present.

Differential Diagnosis

It is important to rule out physical disorders before making a diagnosis of somatisation disorder. Particularly those physical disorders, which often present with apparently vague and multiple somatic symptoms, must be kept in mind. This is especially so if the onset of symptoms is in the later part of life (> 35 years of age; more so if > 45 years of age) and in male patients. These physical disorders include:
1. Multiple sclerosis.
2. Hypothyroidism.
3. Acute intermittent porphyria.
4. Systemic lupus erythematosus (SLE).
5. Hyperparathyroidism.
6. Carcinoma pancreas.

Somatisation sometimes presents as an 'idiom of distress' in the absence of a diagnosable psychiatric disorder. However, certain psychiatric disorders must be ruled out.
1. *Schizophrenia:* In the initial (prodromal) stages, multiple somatic symptoms may be present but later typical features of schizophrenia are manifested.
2. *Major depression:* Particularly in developing countries such as India, multiple somatic symptoms are common in major depression. The presence of depressed mood, depressive ideation and disturbances of biological functions in major depression helps in differentiation. Occasionally, differential diagnosis with *masked depression* may be difficult.
3. *Hypochondriasis:* In *somatisation disorder*, there are multiple, vague somatic symptoms, while in *hypochondriasis*, normal body functions or minor

somatic symptoms are interpreted as the presence of a serious body disease.
4. *Conversion disorder:* Although conversion symptoms are common in somatisation disorder, they are classified separately. The number of symptoms in conversion disorder is far less (one or two) than in somatisation disorder (usually more than ten).
5. *Delusional disorders:* Somatic delusions may be present in delusional disorders (e.g. monosymptomatic hypochondriacal psychosis). In delusional disorders, there is a delusional conviction of somatic symptoms, with far fewer symptoms.

Treatment

The treatment is often difficult. It mainly consists of:
1. Supportive psychotherapy: The treatment of choice is usually supportive psychotherapy. The first step is to enlist the patient in the therapeutic alliance by establishing a rapport. It is useful to demonstrate the link between psychosocial conflict(s) and somatic symptoms, if it is apparent. In chronic cases, 'symptom reduction' rather than 'complete cure' might be a reasonable goal.
2. Behaviour modification: After rapport is established, attempts at modifying behaviour are made, for example, not focusing on the symptoms *per se*, and positively reinforcing normal functioning.
3. Relaxation therapy, with graded physical exercises.
4. Drug therapy: Antidepressants and/or benzodiazepines can be given on a short-term basis for associated depression and/or anxiety. Benzodiazepines should be used with great caution, as the risk of dependence and misuse is high in these patients.

Hypochondriasis (Hypochondriacal Disorder)

Hypochondriasis is defined as a persistent preoccupation with a fear (or belief) of having one (or more) serious disease(s), based on person's own interpretation of normal body function or a minor physical abnormality.

The other important features of hypochondriasis are:

1. Complete physical examination and investigations do not show presence of any significant abnormality.
2. The fear or belief persists despite assurance to the contrary by showing normal reports to the patient.
3. The fear or belief is *not* a delusion but is instead an example of an overvalued idea. The patient may agree regarding the possibility of his exaggerating the graveness of situation, at that time.
4. A preoccupation with medical terms and syndromes is quite common. The patient tends to change the physician frequently, in order to get investigated again.

The usual age of onset is in the late third decade. The course is usually chronic with remissions and relapses. Obsessive personality traits and narcissistic personality features are frequently seen, in addition to associated anxiety and depression.

Aetiology

The cause of hypochondriasis is not known. The important theories are mentioned below:

1. Psychodynamic Theory
Hypochondriasis is believed to be based on a narcissistic personality, caused by a narcissistic libido. Here other parts of body become erotogenic zones, which act as substitutes for genitals. Hypochondriacally focused organs symbolise the genitals. It must be remembered that this is only a theoretical psychodynamic construct.

2. As a Symptom of Depression
Hypochondriacal symptoms are commonly present in major depression. In fact, according to some, hypochondriasis is almost always a part of another psychiatric syndrome, most commonly a mood disorder. Thus, hypochondriasis has been visualised as a *masked depression* or *depressive equivalent*, though not everyone agrees with this view.

Treatment

The treatment of hypochondriasis is often difficult. It basically consists of:

1. Supportive psychotherapy.
2. Treatment of associated or underlying depression and/or anxiety, if present.

Somatoform Autonomic Dysfunction

According to ICD-10, in this disorder, symptoms are presented by the patient as if they were due to a physical disorder of an organ system that is predominantly under autonomic control, e.g. heart and cardiovascular system (such as palpitations), upper gastrointestinal tract (such as aerophagy, hiccough), lower gastrointestinal tract (such as flatulence, irritable bowel), respiratory system (such as hyperventilation), genitourinary system (such as dysuria), or other organ systems.

There is preoccupation with, and distress regarding, the possibility of a serious (but often unspecified) disorder of the particular organ system. Physical examination and investigations do not however show presence of any significant abnormality. The preoccupation persists despite repeated assurances and explanations.

Treatment

The treatment consists of:

1. Supportive psychotherapy.
2. Drug treatment: The symptoms of anxiety and/or depression usually respond to short-term use of benzodiazepines and antidepressants.

Some other common disorders are described in some detail below:

Hyperventilation Syndrome (HVS)

This is a very common clinical syndrome which is often missed, particularly when it does not present in its full blown form. The syndrome is characterised by a 'habit' of hyperventilation which becomes particularly marked in the presence of psychosocial stress, or any emotional upheaval.

In its *mild form*, it is characterised by excessive fatigue, chest pain, headache, palpitations, sweating and a feeling of 'lightheadedness'. In *severe* hyperventilation syndrome, carpopaedal spasm (tetany), paraesthesias and loss of consciousness may occur.

These symptoms are produced by hypocapnia (or a decrease in arterial pCO_2). The sequence of events in hyperventilation syndrome is explained in Figure 8.3.

The diagnosis is usually easy, if the possibility of hyperventilation is remembered. Apart from the clinical history and presence of frequent 'sighing' during the interview, a simple test would demonstrate the symptomatology. The patient is asked to breathe rapidly and deeply for 2-3 minutes. This produces the classical physical symptoms. If carried on longer, tetany and unconsciousness would result; therefore, due care should be undertaken in performing this test.

Treatment

1. Relaxation techniques: Jacobson's progressive muscular relaxation, autohypnosis or hypnosis, *yoga,* transcendental meditation (TM), and/or biofeedback.
2. Teaching relaxed breathing techniques, which include:
   i. Breathing more from the abdomen, thus avoiding the use of accessory muscles of expiration.
   ii. Slow respiration with passive expiration, without muscular effort.
   iii. A short rest cycle to be voluntarily introduced after each respiratory cycle.
3. Treatment of underlying anxiety or depression, if present, with antidepressants and/or short-term benzodiazepines.
4. *Breathing-in-bag technique:* The aim of this technique is to have the patient re-breathe the expired air. This prevents the decrease in pCO_2 which causes physical symptoms, or causes an increase in pCO_2 where physical symptoms have already developed. Re-breathing in a paper bag, which is carried by the patient, quickly reverts the symptoms. It is really important to emphasise a safe use of the bag, to prevent the possibility of suffocation. There is some recent evidence doubting the efficacy of this approach.

Irritable Bowel Syndrome (IBS)

This is a common syndrome, often known by a large variety of names, such as spastic colitis, irritable

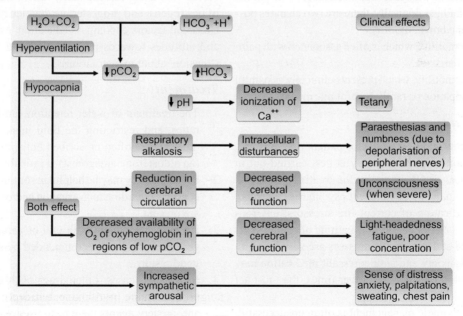

Fig. 8.3: Physiology of Hyperventilation Syndrome

colon syndrome, nervous diarrhoea, mucus colitis, and colon neurosis.

The principal abnormality in IBS is a disturbance of bowel mobility, which is modified by psychosocial factors. The patients usually present with one or more of the following symptoms:

1. Abdominal pain, discomfort or cramps.
2. Alteration of bowel habits (diarrhoea or constipation).
3. A sensation of incomplete evacuation.

Quite often, all three features (abdominal pain and diarrhoea alternating with constipation) are present together; also associated is flatulence. The patients often describe their stools in a dramatic manner.

It is a fairly common disorder occurring in nearly 40% of all patients attending a gastroenterology (GE) clinic. Although females more frequently have IBS in America, in India males are more often affected. It is more or less a stable disorder with frequent exacerbations.

The typical mode of onset or exacerbation is with occurrence of a psychosocial stressor or emotional upheaval. Physiologically, there are two changes possible in the bowel motility.

1. Hypomotility, which is often associated with painless diarrhoea.
2. Hypermotility, which presents clinically as painful constipation or rarely painful diarrhoea.

Treatment

1. A stable and trustful doctor-patient relationship.
2. Supportive psychotherapy is best carried out in medical or GE clinic by the treating physician. These patients often resent psychiatric referrals.
3. Identification of current life stressors, environmental manipulation, and learning of coping skills aimed at dealing with stressors are very helpful.
4. Anti-anxiety and antidepressant medication may be helpful at times. At other times, they just act like placebos.
5. Symptomatic management is often unsuccessful. However, prokinetic agents (e.g. cisapride) may

sometimes be useful. A trial of fibre (wheat bran, psyllium, methylcellulose) is reasonable in some patients with irritable bowel syndrome.

Premenstrual Syndrome

Premenstrual syndrome or *premenstrual tension* (PMT—as it has been commonly called) is characterised by a variety of physical, psychological and behavioural symptoms occurring in the second half of menstrual cycle. Typically, the symptoms start after a few days of ovulation, reach a peak about 4-5 days before menstruation and disappear usually around menstruation. The period between menstruation and next ovulation is normal.

The syndrome is characterised by feelings of irritability, depression, crying spells, restlessness and anxiety. These are associated with changes in appetite, signs and symptoms of water retention (such as pedal oedema, weight gain, swelling of breasts, a sense of bloating of abdomen), gastroenterological changes, headache and fatigue.

The aetiology is probably multifactorial. The biological factors include faulty luteinisation, excess of oestrogens, and progesterone deficiency. The psychosocial factors encompass education, expectations and attitudes towards menstruation and femininity ('tension' about menstruation).

Treatment

1. The treatment of water retention can be by diuretics, and restricting the fluid intake. Thiazide diuretics are often prescribed but spironolactone (an aldosterone antagonist) is probably superior.
2. Psychotherapy may be helpful in some cases where conflicts regarding menstruation and/or femininity are present.
3. Hormonal treatment with oral or parenteral progesterone has been recommended by some, with good results.
4. In resistant cases, other drugs such as lithium, bromocriptine, pyridoxine, antidepressants and anti-anxiety agents have been used with varying success.

Persistent Somatoform Pain Disorder

It was previously called as *psychogenic pain disorder*. In this disorder, persistent, severe and distressing pain is the main feature which is, either grossly in excess of what is expected from the physical findings, or inconsistent with the anatomical distribution of nervous system. Preoccupation with pain is common.

There is often a precipitating stressful event and secondary gain may be present. Repeated change of physicians *(doctor-shopping)* is common. The affected person often assumes a 'sick-role' or an 'invalid-role'. Abuse and dependence of analgesics and minor tranquilisers is common, particularly when the course is chronic.

This disorder is more common in females, with an onset in the third or fourth decade of life.

Treatment

1. The patients usually refuse psychiatric intervention; therefore treatment is often managed by the treating physician.
2. Drug therapy should be avoided if possible as the risk of iatrogenic drug abuse is quite high.
3. In the absence of other modes of successful treatment, a supportive relationship with a physician will prevent doctor-shopping and provide relief.

Other Somatoform Disorders

In ICD-10, this category includes other somatoform disorders not classified in the previous four categories, e.g. 'globus hystericus', psychogenic torticollis, psychogenic pruritus, psychogenic dysmenorrhoea, teeth-grinding.

OTHER NEUROTIC DISORDERS

In ICD-10, the other neurotic disorders are divided into the following categories:

Neurasthenia

According to ICD-10, this disorder is characterised by:

Persisting/distressing complaints of increased fatigue after mental effort, or of weakness/exhaustion after minimal effort; with two or more of the following: feelings of muscular aches/pains, dizziness, tension headaches, sleep disturbances, inability to relax, irritability and dyspepsia. It is important to rule out other mental disorders which may fully explain the symptoms.

This is clearly a poorly defined syndrome and its independence as a diagnosis is doubtful. A differential diagnosis with *CFS (chronic fatigue syndrome),* and other medical and psychiatric disorders presenting with fatigue, is important before diagnosing neurasthenia.

CFS is characterised by profound fatigue (present at rest, and made worse by physical and mental effort), muscle pains, headache, sore throat, functional impairment and nonspecific 'soft' physical signs, e.g. mild fever, mild lymphadenopathy. CFS is diagnosed in the absence of medical or other psychiatric disorder(s), though neuropsychiatric symptoms may be present.

Depersonalisation Disorder (or Depersonalisation-Derealisation Syndrome)

Depersonalisation is characterised by an alteration in the perception or experience of self, so that the feeling of one's own reality is temporarily changed or lost.

It is an *'as if'* phenomenon. The person affected is not delusionally convinced about the change, and instead describes it to have occurred, as-if. This is often accompanied by *derealisation*, which is an alteration in the perception or experience of the external world, so that the feeling of reality of external world is temporarily changed or lost. This too is an *'as if'* phenomenon. Derealisation is a larger concept which also encompasses depersonalisation. As they both often occur together the syndrome is also called as depersonalisation-derealisation syndrome.

As both depersonalisation and derealisation occur in many other disorders (Table 8.6), the term depersonalisation disorder should be used only when other disorders have been ruled out.

The other associated clinical features may include:

1. The episodes of depersonalisation and/or derealisation causing significant social, interpersonal or occupational impairment. The episodes recur frequently.
2. The onset and termination of episodes is usually sudden.
3. Marked distress and anxiety results, as the experience is highly unpleasant.
4. Insight into the illness is usually present.
5. A feeling of loss of control on one's action and speech may occur.
6. The episodes occur in the presence of a clear sensorium.

The age of onset is usually late second or early third decade. The course is usually chronic.

Treatment

The treatment is usually not very successful though co-morbid symptoms of anxiety and depression can often be treated. The various methods which can be tried include:

1. Supportive psychotherapy.
2. Drug therapy with antidepressants; rarely antipsychotics may also be tried.

Other Specified Neurotic Disorders (Culture Bound Syndromes)

In ICD-10, this category includes miscellaneous disorders which are of uncertain aetiology and nosological status, and which occur in certain cultures, e.g. *dhat syndrome, koro, latah, wihtigo, piblokto* and *amok*. These are called as *culture-bound syndromes*, as they are localised to certain geographical areas only, and are not usually seen in the Western, developed countries.

Dhat Syndrome

Dhat syndrome is a culture-bound syndrome, which is prevalent in the Indian subcontinent. This is characterised by:

1. Complaint of passage of *dhat* in urine.
2. Multiple somatic symptoms.
3. Asthenia (physical or mental exhaustion).

Table 8.6: Depersonalisation: Causes

1. Psychiatric Disorders
   i. Depersonalisation disorder
   ii. Phobic-anxiety-depersonalisation (PAD) syndrome
   iii. Anxiety disorder
   iv. Panic disorder
   v. Agoraphobia
   vi. Schizophrenia
   vii. Depression
2. Neurological Disorders
   i. Complex partial seizures
   ii. Migraine
   iii. Cerebral tumours (especially affecting non-dominant parietal lobe)
   iv. Encephalitis
3. Other Causes
   i. Hyperventilation
   ii. Alcohol and drug dependence
   iii. Hypoglycaemia
   iv. Fatigue
   v. Grief
   vi. Sensory deprivation

4. Anxiety or depression may be present.
5. Sexual dysfunction may occur.

Dhat is a whitish discharge passed in urine and believed to be semen by the patient. According to an ancient sociocultural belief prevalent in the Indian society, semen is an 'extremely precious' body element which is produced from several drops of blood. Hence, it follows from this view that loss of semen will be perceived to lead to weakness and sexual dysfunction. Often, masturbatory anxiety and overconcern with nocturnal emissions are also associated with other clinical symptoms.

Treatment

1. *Counselling and Psychotherapy:* This is the most important method of treatment directed towards removing misconceptions regarding apprehension of semen loss. This counselling is combined with general sex education. Specifically, fears regarding masturbation and nocturnal emissions are allayed.

Cognitive behavioural techniques can easily be incorporated in the psychotherapy model applied.

2. *Symptomatic treatment:* The treatment of underlying anxiety, depression, hypochondriasis and/or sexual dysfunction by the usual means may also be necessary. Several patients present with underlying (or co-morbid) depression and anxiety, and may need psychopharmacological management of these symptoms.

Amok

Amok is characterised by a sudden, unprovoked episode of rage, in which the affected person runs about (runs '*amok*') and indiscriminately injures or kills any person who is encountered on the way. This condition is usually seen in south-east Asia (e.g. Malaysia).

Koro

Koro is a culture-bound syndrome seen in Asia (including India). The affected male person has the belief that his penis is shrinking and may disappear in to his abdominal wall and he may then die.

Females are also affected infrequently, with a corresponding belief that their breasts (and/or vulva) are shrinking.

Koro often spreads rapidly to the other members of community in an epidemic form. It is usually based on the culturally elaborated fears regarding nocturnal emission and masturbation (particularly in men).

Wihtigo (Windigo)

This syndrome is seen in native American-Indians. The affected person has the belief that he has been transformed in to a *wihtigo,* a cannibal monster. The episodes are known to have occurred especially during times of starvation.

Piblokto (Arctic Hysteria)

This culture-bound syndrome occurs in Eskimos. The affected person is often a female, who screams and tears-off her clothes, and throws herself on ice in extremely cold conditions. She may imitate the cry of a bird or an animal.

The episode usually lasts for 1-2 hours, followed by amnesia for the events. It is most probably a type of dissociative disorder.

Latah (Startle Reaction)

This syndrome is reported from south-east Asia and Japan. Occurring more often in women, *latah* is typically characterised by the presence of automatic obedience, echolalia, and echopraxia. It is often precipitated by a sudden stimulus, such as loud sound.

Some Indian Culture-bound Syndromes

In addition to dhat syndrome, amok and koro (described above), the other culture-bound syndromes seen in India include *Suchi-bai* (*purity mania*), *ascetic syndrome*, *nupital psychosis*, and *Jhinjhinia*.

REACTION TO STRESS AND ADJUSTMENT DISORDERS

This category in ICD-10 consists of disorders which are temporally related to an exceptionally stressful life event (acute stress reaction and post-traumatic stress disorder) or a significant life change (adjustment disorders) immediately before the onset of illness.

Acute Stress Reaction

According to ICD-10, in this disorder there is an immediate and clear temporal relationship between an exceptional stressor (such as death of a loved one, natural catastrophe, accident, rape) and the onset of symptoms. The symptoms show a mixed and changing picture. This disorder is more likely to develop in presence of physical exhaustion and in extremes of age. It is also more commonly seen in female gender and people with poor coping skills.

The symptoms range from a 'dazed' condition, anxiety, depression, anger, despair, overactivity or withdrawal, and constriction of the field of consciousness. The symptoms resolve rapidly (within few hours usually), if removal from the stressful environment is possible. If the stress continues or cannot be reversed, the resolution of symptoms begins after 1-2 days and is usually minimal after about three days.

Treatment

The treatment consists of removal of the patient from the stressful environment and helping the patient to 'pass through' the stressful experience. IV or oral benzodiazepines (such as diazepam) may be needed in cases with marked agitation.

Post-traumatic Stress Disorder (PTSD)

According to ICD-10, this disorder arises as a delayed and/or protracted response to an exceptionally stressful or catastrophic life event or situation, which is likely to cause pervasive distress in 'almost any person' (e.g. disasters, war, rape or torture, serious accident). The symptoms of PTSD may develop, after a period of latency, within six months after the stress or may be delayed beyond this period.

PTSD is characterised by recurrent and intrusive recollections of the stressful event, either in *flashbacks* (images, thoughts, or perceptions) and/or in dreams. There is an associated sense of re-experiencing of the stressful event. There is marked *avoidance* of the events or situations that arouse recollections of the stressful event, along with marked symptoms of anxiety and increased arousal.

The other important clinical features of PTSD include partial amnesia for some aspects of the stressful event, feeling of numbness, and anhedonia (inability to experience pleasure).

Treatment

The treatment consists of the following measures:

1. *Prevention:* Anticipation of disasters in the high risk areas, with the training of personnel in disaster management.
2. *Disaster management:* Here the speed of providing practical help is of paramount importance. This is also a preventive measure.
3. *Supportive psychotherapy.*

4. *Cognitive behaviour therapy (CBT).*
5. *Drug treatment:* Antidepressants and benzodiazepines (in low doses for short periods) are useful in treatment, if anxiety and/or depression are important components of the clinical picture.

Adjustment Disorders

Adjustment disorders are one of the commoner psychiatric disorders seen in the clinical practice. They are most frequently seen in adolescents and women. Although adjustment disorder is often precipitated by one or more stressors, it usually represents a maladaptive response to the stressful life event(s).

In ICD-10, this disorder is characterised by those disorders which occur within 1 month of a significant life change (stressor). This disorder usually occurs in those individuals who are vulnerable due to poor coping skills or personality factors. It is assumed that the disorder would not have arisen in the absence of the stressor(s). The duration of the disorder is usually less than 6 months, except in the case of prolonged depressive reaction.

The various subtypes include brief or prolonged depressive reaction, mixed anxiety and depressive reaction, and adjustment disorder with predominant disturbance of other emotions and/or predominant disturbance of conduct.

Most patients recover within a period of three months.

Treatment

1. *Supportive psychotherapy* remains the treatment of choice.
2. *Crisis intervention* is useful in some patients, by helping to quickly resolve the stressful life situation which has led to the onset of adjustment disorder.
3. Stress management training and Coping skills training.
4. *Drug treatment* may be needed in some patients for the management of anxiety (benzodiazepines) and/or depressive symptoms (antidepressants).

Chapter 9

Disorders of Adult Personality and Behaviour

SPECIFIC PERSONALITY DISORDERS

Personality is defined as a deeply ingrained pattern of behaviour that includes modes of perception, relating to and thinking about oneself and the surrounding environment. *Personality traits* are normal, prominent aspects of personality. *Personality disorders* result when these personality traits become abnormal, i.e. become inflexible and maladaptive, and cause significant social or occupational impairment, or significant subjective distress.

Although personal distress may occur in some personality disorders, classically the abnormal personality traits are 'ego-syntonic'. This is in sharp contrast to the symptoms in neurotic disorders, which are ego-dystonic and hence cause significant distress to the patient. So, unlike the patients with neurotic disorders, several personality disorder patients do not usually seek psychiatric help unless other psychiatric symptoms co-exist.

Although personality disorders are usually recognisable by early adolescence, they are not typically diagnosed before early adult life. The symptoms continue unchanged through the adult life and usually become less obvious in the later years of life (after 40 years of age).

The life-time prevalence of personality disorders in the general population is about 5-10%. Often symptoms of more than one personality disorder are present in one person. In fact, it is now believed that the occurrence of mixed personality disorders (i.e.

co-morbidity) is commoner than single (pure) personality disorders.

In DSM-IV-TR, the personality disorders (and traits) are coded on Axis II (on the multi-axial system) (see Chapter 1) and have been divided into three clusters.

Cluster A contains disorders which are thought to be "odd and eccentric" and on a "schizophrenic-continuum". These include Paranoid, Schizoid and Schizotypal personality disorders.

Cluster B consists of disorders considered "dramatic, emotional and erratic" and on a "psychopathic continuum". These include Antisocial (or Dissocial), Histrionic, Narcissistic and Borderline (or Emotionally Unstable) personality disorders.

Cluster C has disorders considered "anxious and fearful" and characterised by "introversion". These include Anxious (Avoidant), Dependent and Obsessive Compulsive (or Anankastic) personality disorders.

In addition to these three clusters, some other personality disorders such as passive-aggressive personality disorder and depressive personality disorder have been included in the section on 'Criteria provided for further study' in DSM-IV-TR. In ICD-10, the personality disorders are listed under the section on 'Disorders of adult personality and behaviour'.

Diagnosis

According to ICD-10, the diagnostic guidelines for *specific personality disorder* include conditions not directly attributable to gross brain damage or disease, or to another psychiatric disorder, meeting the following criteria.

1. Markedly disharmonious attitudes and behaviour, involving usually several areas of functioning, e.g. affectivity, arousal, impulse control, ways of perceiving and thinking, and style of relating to others;

2. The abnormal behaviour pattern is enduring, of long standing, and not limited to episodes of mental illness;

3. The abnormal behaviour pattern is pervasive and clearly maladaptive to a broad range of personal and social situations;

4. The above manifestations always appear during childhood or adolescence and continue into adulthood;

5. The disorder leads to considerable personal distress but this may only become apparent late in its course;

6. The disorder is usually, but not invariably, associated with significant problems in occupational and social performance.

Clinical Subtypes

Paranoid Personality Disorder

According to ICD-10, the diagnostic guidelines for paranoid personality disorder include the following features (in addition to features of personality disorders in general, described above).

Clear evidence is usually required of the presence of at least three out of seven traits or behaviours given in the clinical description in ICD-10. These traits include excessive sensitiveness, tendency to persistently bear grudges, significant suspiciousness, a combative and tenacious sense of personal 'right', recurrent suspicions about fidelity of partner without justification, tendency to experience excessive self-importance, and preoccupation with unsubstantiated 'conspiratorial' explanations of events.

The patients may become involved in litigation on small issues. The disorder is commoner in men, and it is more common in minority groups and immigrants.

Psychodynamically, the underlying defense mechanism is *projection*.

Paranoid personality disorder is common in the premorbid personality of some patients of paranoid schizophrenia. However whether its presence predisposes to the development of paranoid schizophrenia is not known. The differential diagnosis is from delusional (paranoid) disorders and paranoid schizophrenia.

Treatment

1. Individual psychotherapy.
2. Supportive psychotherapy.

The response to treatment is usually poor. The patients often do not seek treatment on their own and may resent treatment. Drug treatment has a very limited role.

Schizoid Personality Disorder

According to ICD-10, the diagnostic guidelines for schizoid personality disorder include the following features (in addition to the general features of personality disorders). Clear evidence is usually required of the presence of at least three out of nine traits or behaviours given in the clinical description. These traits include emotional coldness, lack of pleasure from activities, limited capacity to express feelings towards others, apparent indifference to praise or criticism, little interest in sexual experiences, preference for solitary activities, excessive preoccupation with fantasy and introspection, lack of close friends, and marked insensitivity to prevailing social norms and conventions.

The features of this disorder may overlap with paranoid and schizotypal personality disorders, which too belong to the Cluster-A. Psychotic features are typically absent. The disorder is usually more common in men.

Psychodynamically, the disorder is supposed to result from 'cold and aloof' parenting in a child with introverted temperament. However, this hypothesis is far from proven in the research conducted so far.

Like all personality disorders, schizoid personality disorder has an onset in early childhood with stable course over the years. Earlier, it was believed to pre-dispose to the development of schizophrenia, but later studies have failed to replicate the findings.

Treatment
1. Individual psychotherapy.
2. Psychoanalysis or psychoanalytical psycho-therapy.
3. Gradual involvement in group psychotherapy.

The patients often do not seek treatment on their own. The response to treatment is usually not good. Drug treatment clearly has a very limited role.

Schizotypal (Personality) Disorder

According to ICD-10, this disorder is not classified under specific personality disorders but instead along with schizophrenia. However, in DSM-IV-TR, it is considered to be a personality disorder.

The diagnostic guidelines for schizotypal (per-sonality) disorder include the following features. A disorder characterised by eccentric behaviour, and anomalies of thinking and affect, which resemble those seen in schizophrenia, though no definite and characteristic schizophrenic anomalies have occurred at any stage. At least three or four out of nine should be present continuously or episodically for a period of at least 2 years. These include inappropriate or con-stricted affect, odd, eccentric, or peculiar behaviour, poor rapport with others and social withdrawal, odd beliefs or magical thinking, suspiciousness or paranoid ideas, obsessive ruminations without inner resistance, unusual perceptual experiences, vague, circumstantial, metaphorical, or stereotyped thinking, and occasional transient quasi-psychotic episodes (with intense illu-sions, hallucinations, and delusion-like ideas).

This disorder lies between schizoid personality disorder and schizophrenia on a schizophrenic con-tinuum. Differentiation from simple schizophrenia, schizoid personality disorder, and paranoid person-ality disorder is not clearly demarcated. It is more commonly seen in individuals related to patients with schizophrenia and is believed to be a part of the genetic 'spectrum' of schizophrenia. However, its onset, evolution and course are usually those of a personality disorder. It usually runs a chronic course.

Treatment
The response to treatment is usually poor, except for brief psychotic episodes.
1. Psychoanalysis or psychoanalytical psycho-therapy.
2. Individual psychotherapy.
3. Drug therapy: Antipsychotics have been used with-out much benefit. The role of antipsychotics in the treatment is limited to brief psychotic episodes.

Antisocial or Dissocial Personality Disorder

According to ICD-10, the diagnostic guidelines for dissocial (antisocial) personality disorder include the following clinical features. Clear evidence is usually required of the presence of at least three of six traits or behaviours given in the clinical description. This disorder is synonymous with previously used terms such as psychopathy and sociopathy, but does not always mean criminal behaviour. These traits include callous unconcern for the feelings of others, gross and persistent attitude of irresponsibility and disregard for social norms, rules and obligations, incapacity to maintain enduring relationships, very low tolerance to frustration and a low threshold for discharge of aggression, incapacity to experience guilt and to profit from experience, particularly punishment, and marked proneness to blame others.

There may also be persistent irritability as an associated feature. History of conduct disorder in childhood and adolescence, though not invariably present, may further support the diagnosis. There are no psychotic features in this disorder.

Earlier antisocial personality disorder or psycho-pathy was divided into four clinical types, namely:
1. Aggressive psychopath,
2. Inadequate psychopath,
3. Creative psychopath, and
4. Sexual psychopath.

As these are not discrete groups and their charac-teristic symptoms merge with one another, they are no longer classified in this manner. Although no clear aetiology is known, several genetic, environmental and biological factors are associated with this disorder. These factors include more than a 'normal' prevalence of antisocial personality disorder in father; presence of impulsive and inconsistent parents; presence of soft neurological signs, nonspecific EEG abnormalities; and presence of conduct and/or attention deficit disorder in childhood.

This disorder is diagnosed more commonly in males. The course is usually chronic; however, there is some decrease in the symptoms after the fifth decade of life in some patients.

Treatment

Patients often do not seek psychiatric help and if they do, it is usually under pressure from the legal authorities. The therapeutic alliance is often not sustained. The treatment methods include:

1. Individual psychotherapy.
2. Psychoanalysis or psychoanalytical psychotherapy.
3. Group psychotherapy and self-help groups.
4. Drug therapy: Pharmacotherapy is of little help. Earlier claims of beneficial effect of *pericyazine* (an antipsychotic drug) in certain behaviour patterns of antisocial personality disorder have not been substantiated.

Histrionic Personality Disorder

According to ICD-10, the diagnostic guidelines for histrionic personality disorder include the following clinical features. Clear evidence is usually required of the presence of at least three of six traits or behaviours given in the clinical description. These include self-dramatisation and exaggerated expression of emotions, suggestibility (easily influenced by others), shallow and labile affectivity, continual attention-seeking attitude, inappropriate seductiveness, and over-concern with physical attractiveness. Associated features may include egocentricity, self-indulgence, continuous longing for appreciation, feelings that are easily hurt, and persistent manipulative behaviour to achieve own needs.

Tantrums or anger outbursts are common. The actions are not planned for any long-term goals; instead they seek instant satisfaction and approval. Exhibitionistic traits such as dressing flamboyantly, mannerisms

of speech and motor behaviour are present. There is an attempt to look charming, beautiful and seductive. Suicidal gestures may be made at times. Interpersonal relationships are often stormy and ungratifying.

This disorder is more common in female gender. Hysteria (conversion and dissociation disorder) was previously thought to be more common in the presence of histrionic personality disorder, but recent studies have failed to prove this relationship. Psychodynamically, there are usually intense dependency needs. The defense mechanisms used most often are *acting out* and *dissociation*.

Treatment

Psychoanalysis and psychoanalytic psychotherapy are the modes of treatment which are most successful.

Narcissistic Personality Disorder

A relatively new concept in classification, this disorder is characterised by:

1. Ideas of grandiosity and inflated sense of self-importance.
2. Preoccupation with fantasies of unlimited success.
3. Attention seeking, dramatic behaviour, needs constant praise, and unable to face criticism.
4. Lack of empathy with others, with exploitative behaviour.
5. Shaky self-esteem, underlying sense of inferiority, easily depressed by minor events.

Treatment

Psychodynamic/psychoanalytical psychotherapy is the treatment of choice in a psychologically-minded patient.

Emotionally Unstable Personality Disorder

According to ICD-10, emotionally unstable personality disorder is described as a disorder in which there is a marked tendency to act impulsively without consideration of the consequences, together with affective instability. This disorder is further classified into two types: Impulsive type and borderline type.

The *impulsive type* is characterised by emotional instability and lack of impulse control. Outbursts of violence or threatening behaviour are common, particularly in response to criticism by others.

The *borderline type* is characterised by emotional instability. In addition, patient's own self-image, aims, and internal preferences (including sexual) are often unclear or disturbed. There are usually chronic feelings of emptiness. A liability to become involved in intense and unstable relationships may cause repeated emotional crises and may be associated with excessive efforts to avoid abandonment and a series of suicidal threats or acts of self-harm, (although these may occur without obvious precipitants).

The borderline type is also known as *borderline personality disorder* (DSM-IV-TR), the characteristic features of which include the following:

1. Significant and persistent disturbance of identity of self, e.g. 'who am I'. There is marked uncertainty about major issues in life.
2. Unstable and intense interpersonal relationship patterns.
3. Impulsivity.
4. Unstable emotional responses, with rapid shifts. Anger outbursts may occur.
5. Chronic feelings of boredom or emptiness with inability to stay alone.
6. Deliberate self-harm is common in the form of self-mutilation, suicidal gestures, or accident-proneness.

The term *borderline personality disorder* currently includes *ambulatory schizophrenia* and *pseudoneurotic schizophrenia*, which were earlier thought to be subtypes of schizophrenia. Psychodynamically, *splitting* is the primary defense mechanism employed in borderline personality disorder.

There is a considerable overlap between borderline, narcissistic and antisocial (dissocial) personality disorders (they belong to the same Cluster of personality disorders, i.e. Cluster B). Major depressive episodes occur commonly in this disorder.

Treatment

1. Psychoanalysis or psychoanalytical psychotherapy.
2. Supportive psychotherapy.

3. Cognitive behaviour therapy (CBT) or dialectical behaviour therapy (DBT) approaches or principles have been used with some success in treatment.
4. *Drug therapy:* Antidepressants have been used with success in certain patients with depression. Major depressive episode, if occurs, necessitates antidepressant therapy. Occasionally antipsychotics, lithium, valproate or carbamazepine have been used when aggression or impulsivity are prominent.

Drug therapy is not the treatment of first choice in borderline personality disorder.

Anxious (Avoidant) Personality Disorder

According to ICD-10, the diagnostic guidelines for anxious (avoidant) personality disorder include the following features. Clear evidence is usually required of the presence of at least three of six traits or behaviours given in the clinical description. These include persistent and pervasive feelings of tension and apprehension, belief that one is socially inept, personally unappealing, or inferior to others, excessive preoccupation with being criticised or rejected in social situations, unwillingness to become involved with people unless certain of being liked, restrictions in lifestyle because of need to have physical security, and avoidance of social or occupational activities that involve significant inter-personal contact because of fear of criticism, disapproval, or rejection.

Associated features may include hypersensitivity to rejection and criticism. These patients do not enter into interpersonal relationships unless they are very sure of uncritical approval. This disorder is an epitome of what is often called as *inferiority complex*. Understandably, secondary depression is very common.

Treatment

1. Individual psychotherapy.
2. Group psychotherapy.
3. Behaviour therapy: In particular, social skills training and assertiveness training are useful.
4. CBT: The focus is on negative thoughts and negative self-appraisal.

Dependent Personality Disorder

According to ICD-10, the diagnostic guidelines for dependent personality disorder include the following features. Clear evidence is usually required of the presence of at least three of six traits or behaviours given in the clinical description. These include allowing others to make decisions for them, subordination of one's own needs to those of others and undue compliance with their wishes, unwillingness to make even reasonable demands on the people one depends on, feeling uncomfortable or helpless when alone, preoccupation with fears of being abandoned by a person with whom one has a close relationship, and limited capacity to make everyday decisions without an excessive amount of advice and reassurance from others.

Associated features may include perceiving oneself as helpless, incompetent, and lacking stamina. There may be an overlap with avoidant and passive-aggressive personality disorders. Some patients exhibit *masochistic character*. They repetitively establish close interpersonal relationships which result in punishment.

Treatment
1. Individual psychotherapy.
2. Group psychotherapy.
3. Behaviour therapy (such as assertiveness training and social skills training) is often useful.
4. CBT: The focus is on negative thoughts and negative self-appraisal.

Obsessive-Compulsive (Anankastic) Personality Disorder

According to ICD-10, the diagnostic guidelines for anankastic personality disorder include the following clinical features. Clear evidence is usually required of the presence of at least three of eight traits or behaviours given in the clinical description. These include feelings of excessive doubt, preoccupation with details, perfectionism that interferes with task completion, excessive conscientiousness, excessive pedantry and adherence to social conventions, rigidity and stubbornness, unreasonable insistence that

others submit to exactly their way of doing things, and intrusion of insistent and unwelcome thoughts or impulses.

This disorder is more often diagnosed in males, and is common in premorbid personality of patients with obsessive compulsive disorder. Major depressive episodes are frequent. Psychodynamically, this disorder is believed to result from fixation at the anal sadistic phase, with the employment of *reaction formation* as a defense mechanism.

Treatment
These patients usually retain insight, and hence seek psychiatric help on their own.
1. Psychoanalysis or psychoanalytical psychotherapy.
2. Group psychotherapy.

Passive-Aggressive Personality Disorder

This disorder is not listed as a personality disorder in both ICD-10 and DSM-IV-TR, though it is listed in DSM-IV-TR under the section on 'Criteria provided for further study'. It is characterised by the following clinical features:
1. Significant and persistent *passive resistance* to demands for adequate social and occupational performance.
2. Stubbornness, intentional inefficiency, procrastination, unjustified protests, 'forgetfulness' and/or dawdling are used to achieve the purpose.

Passive resistance is viewed as an expression of 'covert anger' or 'retroflexed anger'. This behaviour is often 'chosen' in spite of the fact that a more direct and active way of showing an opinion and/or resisting was possible. An overlap with dependent personality disorder is common. Secondary depression may develop.

Treatment
1. Supportive psychotherapy.
2. Behaviour therapy: Social skills training and assertiveness training are helpful.
3. Group therapy.
4. Drug therapy: Antidepressants may be needed for secondary depression.

ENDURING PERSONALITY CHANGES, NOT ATTRIBUTABLE TO BRAIN DAMAGE AND DISEASE

This new category in ICD-10 includes disorders of adult personality and behaviour which develop following catastrophic or excessive prolonged stress, or following a severe psychiatric illness, in people with no personality disorder. The presence of brain damage or disease which may cause similar clinical features should be ruled out.

HABIT AND IMPULSE DISORDERS

This category includes disorders such as pathological gambling, pyromania, kleptomania, trichotillomania, and intermittent explosive disorder. The disorders in this heterogeneous group are characterised by impulsive behaviour which the patient cannot resist or control. There may be a feeling of release of tension by doing the act and a feeling of guilt after the act is over.

Pathological gambling is characterised by two or more episodes of gambling per year which have no profitable outcome, but are continued despite personal distress and interference with personal functioning in daily living. The person has an intense urge to gamble which is difficult to control and cannot stop gambling by effort of will. Preoccupation with thoughts or mental images of gambling and situations surrounding gambling is often present.

Pyromania (pathological fire-setting) is characterised by two or more acts of fire-setting without an apparent motive. There is an intense urge to set fire to objects, with a feeling of tension before the act and a sense of relief afterwards. There is often a preoccupation with thoughts or mental images of fire-setting and situations surrounding fire-setting.

Kleptomania (pathological stealing) is characterised by two or more thefts, in which there is stealing without apparent motive of personal gain or gain for another person. There is an intense urge to steal, with a feeling of tension before the act and a sense of relief afterwards.

Trichotillomania (compulsive hair-pulling) is characterised by noticeable hair loss caused by person's persistent and recurrent failure to resist impulses to pullout hair. There is an intense urge to pull out hair with mounting tension before the act and a sense of relief afterwards. There is no pre-existent skin lesion or inflammation, and hair pulling is not secondary to any delusion or hallucination.

The management of impulse control disorders consists of behaviour therapy (e.g. aversion therapy), cognitive behaviour therapy (CBT), individual psychotherapy, and occasionally pharmacotherapy (e.g. carbamazepine for intermittent explosive disorder; fluoxetine for trichotillomania).

GENDER IDENTITY DISORDERS

These disorders of adult personality and behaviour are discussed in detail in Chapter 10.

DISORDERS OF SEXUAL PREFERENCE

These disorders of adult personality and behaviour are discussed in detail in Chapter 10.

PSYCHOLOGICAL AND BEHAVIOURAL DISORDERS ASSOCIATED WITH SEXUAL DEVELOPMENT AND ORIENTATION

These disorders of adult personality and behaviour are discussed in detail in Chapter 10.

FACTITIOUS DISORDER (MUNCHAUSEN SYNDROME)

Munchausen syndrome (also known variously as *hospital addiction*, *hospital hoboes*, or *professional patients*) is used for those patients who repeatedly simulate or fake diseases for the sole purpose of obtaining medical attention. There is no other recognisable motive (hence, it is different from *malingering*).

Factitious disorders can present with predominantly physical signs and symptoms, or psychological signs and symptoms, or combined signs and symptoms. The patients distort their clinical histories, laboratory tests' reports, and even facts about other aspects of their lives *(pseudologia fantastica)*. Sometimes, they distort physical signs by self-inflicted injuries and secondary infections. Drug abuse, especially abuse of prescription drugs, is common.

These patients often have a detailed though superficial knowledge of many medical terms and procedures. Evidence of earlier treatment, usually surgical procedures, is often available in the form of multiple scars (e.g. *'grid-iron abdomen'*). These patients are often manipulative and convincingly tell lies, create problems in the inpatient setting and often leave against medical advice, usually after the surgical procedure has been performed.

The cause is not clear. Probably these patients are masochistic, seek dependency from a father-figure (e.g. the physician), attempt to manoeuvre control over the father-figure and see the surgical procedure as partial suicide. The early childhood of these patients is characterised by deprivation and neglect. The prognosis is usually poor and treatment often unsuccessful.

Certain points must be kept in mind by the physician (or surgeon), after the diagnosis has been made. These include:

1. Avoid the feelings of anger, hostility and ridicule which are aroused by the discovery of factitious illness.

2. Patients should not be confronted or labelled as liars. Instead, a psychiatric or psychological consultation should be sought, as these patients may need help.

3. Of course, the unnecessary surgical procedure(s) should not be carried out.

Chapter 10

Sexual Disorders

The sexual disorders can be classified into four main types:
1. Gender identity disorders.
2. Psychological and behavioural disorders associated with sexual development and maturation.
3. Paraphilias (disorders of sexual preference).
4. Sexual dysfunctions.

In ICD-10, gender identity disorders, disorders of sexual preference, and sexual development and orientation disorders are listed under the disorders of adult personality and behaviour, while sexual dysfunctions (not caused by organic disorder or disease) are listed under the behavioural syndromes associated with physiological disturbances and physical factors.

GENDER IDENTITY DISORDERS

These disorders are characterised by disturbance in gender identity, i.e. the sense of one's masculinity or femininity is disturbed. This group includes:
1. Transexualism: Male and female; primary and secondary.
2. Gender identity disorder of childhood.
3. Dual-role transvestism.
4. Intersexuality.

Transexualism

Transexualism, the severest form of gender identity disorders, is characterised by the following clinical features:

1. Normal anatomic sex.
2. Persistent and significant sense of discomfort regarding one's anatomic sex and a feeling that it is inappropriate to one's perceived-gender.
3. Marked preoccupation with the wish to get rid of one's genitals and secondary sex characteristics, and to adopt sex characteristics of the *other sex* (perceived-gender).
4. Diagnosis is made after puberty.

Transexualism is of two main types: Primary and secondary.

Primary Transexualism

This condition has an onset in early childhood and has a stable course over time. This is a relatively homogeneous category. Primary transexuals, more than secondary transexuals, are preoccupied with sex-change or sex-reassignment surgery. There are two main types:
  i. Male (or, male-to-female) primary transexualism.
  ii. Female (or, female-to-male) primary transexualism.

Secondary Transexualism

In contrast to the primary type, secondary transexualism usually has an onset later in life. This is a less severe and more heterogeneous category. The only common feature is a wish to change the anatomic sex.

This category includes effeminate homosexuals, transvestites who secondarily become transexuals and others. A majority of these patients are male (or, male-to-female) transexuals. The prevalence of transexualism is 1:100,000 in males and 1:400,000 in females.

Differential Diagnosis

Differential diagnosis is from the following conditions:

Transvestism (Fetishistic Transvestism)
Transvestism (or fetishistic cross-dressing) is the wearing or using of clothes traditionally of the other gender (cross-dressing), for the purpose of sexual excitement. This is almost exclusively seen in males.

In contrast, transexuals wear clothes of other sex, because they feel a part of the other sex and, not for sexual excitement.

Cross-gender Homosexuality
Effeminate male homosexuals and masculine female homosexuals sometimes cross-dress and occasionally want a sex-change (called *pseudo-transexualism*). But unlike true primary transexualism, these patients do not feel a part of the other sex and always acknowledge themselves as homosexuals (This is in contrast to transexualism. For example, a male transexual who feels like a female, even if he has a homosexual relationship with another male, justifies it as heterosexual because 'he himself feels like a female'), and seek sex-change only rarely, to rationalise or justify their primary homosexual behaviour.

Treatment

The treatment can aim at two opposite ends by either making the person reconcile with the anatomic sex, or arrange sex-change to the desired gender.

Reconciliation with the Anatomic Sex
There are only occasional reports of achieving this purpose in primary transexuals. However, in secondary transexuals, this method may be more effective and should be employed first if possible though this decision is best made by the patient.

The methods include:
  i. Psychotherapy.
  ii. Behaviour therapy.

Sex-change to the Desired Gender
This procedure is known as sex reassignment surgery (SRS). The first procedure was done in 1951 (Denmark) on an American soldier, George Jorgensen who become Christine Jorgensen after SRS. The first female-to-male SRS was performed in 1956.

The procedures include hormonal treatment, phalloplasty, castration, mastectomy, and hysterectomy with salpingo-ophorectomy, which have been used in different combinations. The procedure is performed more often in primary transexuals.

As SRS is an almost irreversible process, the following steps are taken before assigning a patient to surgery:

1. The diagnosis of primary, stable, long-standing transexualism is confirmed.
2. A possibility of stress-induced transexualism is considered and eliminated.
3. The patient has to undergo psychotherapy for at least 3-6 months preoperatively.
4. Experimental trial in the new gender role preoperatively, to assess patient's ability to adjust in the 'new' role.
5. The limitations of SRS should be explained, e.g. infertility, nonfunctional testes, etc.

The success rate in carefully planned SRS can be up to 80-90%. Postoperative psychotherapy is of utmost importance in prevention of psychiatric morbidity.

Dual-role Transvestism

Dual-role transvestism is characterised by wearing of clothes of the opposite sex in order to enjoy the temporary experience of membership of the opposite sex, but without any desire for a more permanent sex change (unlike transexualism). No sexual excitement accompanies the cross-dressing (unlike in fetishistic transvestism).

Gender-identity Disorder of Childhood

This is a disorder similar to transexualism, with a very early age of onset (2-4 years of age). This is characterised by the following clinical features:

1. Persistent and significant desire to be of the other gender, or insistence on being of the other gender.
2. Marked distress regarding the anatomic sex, with strong denial of anatomic sex (in contrast, there is no denial of anatomic sex in transexualism).
3. Involvement in traditional activities, games and clothing pattern of the perceived gender.
4. Onset before puberty.

Although a majority of primary transexuals have gender-identity disorder of childhood in their past history, only a very few of the children with gender-identity disorder, in prospective studies, actually develop transexualism.

Treatment

Treatment of gender identity disorders is similar to transexualism. When the anatomic sex and the gender-identity are opposing, decision on treatment should be based on the gender-identity of the patient.

Inter-sexuality

The patients with this disorder have gross anatomical and/or physiological aspects of the other sex. These aspects can be in:

1. External genitals, e.g. pseudo-hermaphroditism.
2. Gonads, e.g. ovotestes.
3. Internal sex organs, e.g. true hermaphrodite.
4. Hormonal disturbances, e.g. testicular feminisation syndrome, congenital adrenal hypoplasia.
5. Chromosomes, e.g. Turner's syndrome, Klinefelter's syndrome.

PSYCHOLOGICAL AND BEHAVIOURAL DISORDERS ASSOCIATED WITH SEXUAL DEVELOPMENT AND MATURATION

Disorders of sexual development and maturation include disorders where sexual orientation (heterosexual,

homosexual, or bisexual) causes significant distress to the individual or disturbances in the relationships.

It is important to remember that any type of sexual orientation by itself is not a disorder unless it causes distress or disability.

Sexual Maturation Disorder

This disorder usually begins in adolescence and is characterised by uncertainty regarding the gender identity or sexual orientation (heterosexual, homosexual, or bisexual). This uncertainty often leads to anxiety and depression. Sometimes, this disorder arises for the time in an individual after a period of apparently stable sexual orientation.

Egodystonic Sexual Orientation

In this disorder, the sexual orientation is clear. However, the individual wishes to change the orientation because of the associated distress and/or psychological symptoms. This disorder is seen most commonly in homosexuality.

Homosexuality

Homosexuality, in contrast to heterosexuality, is the sexual relationship between persons of the same sex. This is a disorder only when it is the predominant, significant and persistent mode of sexual relationship for that person and it is ego-dystonic (causes significant distress to the individual).

It is obviously of two types: Male homosexuality, and female homosexuality. Female homosexuals are also called as lesbians or sapphic after Sappho, a female homosexual who lived on the Isle of Lesbos in ancient Greece, while male homosexuals are called gay.

The prevalence of homosexuality (in USA) is 4-6% of males and 1-2% of females. Another 5-10% may show bisexual orientation. Homosexual behaviour can be divided into the following types:

1. Obligatory homosexuality
   - Only homosexuality
   - No heterosexuality.

2. Preferred homosexuality
   - Predominant homosexuality
   - Occasional heterosexuality.
3. Bisexuality
   - Almost equal homosexuality and hetero-sexuality.
4. Situational homosexuality
   - Predominant heterosexuality
   - Occasional homosexuality.
5. Latent homosexuality
   - Only heterosexuality
   - Fantasies of homosexuality.

Last few decades have seen a raging controversy on whether homosexuality is a normal phenomenon or a psychiatric disorder. At first, homosexuality was divided into two types (DSM-III, 1980):

1. Ego-syntonic homosexuality (no distress about homosexual behaviour).
2. Ego-dystonic homosexuality (associated with marked distress), and only ego-dystonic type was called abnormal.

   Later (DSM-III-R, 1987), homosexuality was completely dropped from the psychiatric nomenclature, under social and political pressure. DSM-IV-TR does not list homosexuality as a disorder, while ICD-10 only mentions homosexuality under ego-dystonic sexual orientation.

Treatment

Some people with homosexual orientation, who have significant distress about their homosexual orientation and themselves seek psychiatric help, should be offered treatment.

   At present, the treatment is generally offered under the following conditions only.

1. Self-referral by a person with homosexual orienta-tion, for seeking a change in the sexual orientation towards heterosexuality.
2. Self-referral by a person with homosexual ori-entation, for removal of distress associated with homosexuality but not for a change in sexual orientation.
3. Referred by parents, relatives or significant others. However, treatment can generally be offered only if the individual seeks help.

1. For seeking a Change in Sexual Orientation
The methods employed include:

   i. Psychoanalytic psychotherapy (especially when associated with personality issues).
   ii. Behaviour therapy: Aversion therapy (rarely used), covert sensitisation, systematic desen-sitisation (especially if there is a phobia of heterosexual relationship).
   iii. Supportive psychotherapy.
   iv. Androgen therapy (occasionally).

2. For Seeking Removal of Distress Only
The following methods may be useful:

   i. Psychotherapy: Psychoanalytic and supportive, depending on the personality character.
   ii. Drug therapy: Antidepressants and/or benzodi-azepines can be used for treatment of associated depression and anxiety.

3. Referred by Others
The decision regarding treatment for this group is highly debatable. The opinions range from 'no treat-ment at all' to 'treatment as early as possible'. The final approach depends on the sociocultural background of the patient and the viewpoint of the therapist.

   The current viewpoint is that the individuals should be informed regarding sexuality and sexual orientation in as much detail as they wish and the final decision of choosing the sexual orientation should be left to the individual. Obviously, further treatment would depend on that final choice. The individual's motivation and presence of significant distress are important factors in therapy.

Sexual Relationship Disorder

The gender identity disorder or disorder of sexual preference leads to difficulties in establishing and/or maintaining sexual relationships. In such a case, both diagnoses should be made.

PARAPHILIAS (DISORDERS OF SEXUAL PREFERENCE)

Paraphilias (sexual deviations; perversions) are disorders of sexual preference in which sexual arousal occurs persistently and significantly in response to objects which are not a part of normal sexual arousal (e.g. nonhuman objects; suffering or humiliation of self and/or sexual partner; children or nonconsenting person).

These disorders include: Fetishism; fetishistic transvestism; sexual sadism; sexual masochism; exhibitionism; voyeurism; frotteurism; pedophilia; zoophilia (bestiality); and others.

Fetishism

In fetishism, the sexual arousal occurs either solely or predominantly with a nonliving object, which is usually intimately associated with the human body.

The word fetish means magical, i.e. the nonliving object 'magically' becomes phallic for that person. This disorder is almost exclusively seen in males. The fetish object may include shoes, gloves, bras, underpants, stockings, etc.

Fetishism is not diagnosed if the sexual object is the wearing of clothes of opposite sex (fetishistic transvestism), the use of a human body part (masturbation), or the use of a genital-stimulating object (e.g. vibrator). Fetishism is very often associated with masturbation.

Fetishistic Transvestism

This disorder occurs exclusively in heterosexual males. The person actually or in fantasy wears clothes of the opposite sex (cross-dressing) for sexual arousal. This disorder should be differentiated from dual-role transvestism and transexualism.

This disorder may be associated with fantasies of other males approaching the person who is in a female dress. Masturbation or rarely coitus is associated with cross-dressing to achieve orgasm. To be called a disorder, this should be a persistent and significant mode of sexual arousal in the person.

Sexual Sadism

In this disorder, the person (the 'sadist') is sexually aroused by physical and/or psychological humiliation, suffering or injury of the sexual partner (the 'victim'). Most often the person inflicting the suffering is male,

although this is not essential. The methods used range from restraining by tying, beating, burning, cutting, stabbing, to rape and even killing.

Sexual Masochism

This is just the reverse of sexual sadism. Here the person (the 'masochist') is sexually aroused by physical and/or psychological humiliation, suffering or injury inflicted on self by others (usually 'sadists'). Most often the masochist is a female though any pattern is possible. The methods used are the same as the ones used in sexual sadism. Only there is a role reversal.

To be called a disorder, this should be a persistent and significant mode of sexual arousal in the person. Sexual sadism and sexual masochism are often seen in the same individual and are on a continuum; therefore they are classified together as sadomasochism in ICD-10.

Exhibitionism

Exhibitionism is a persistent (or recurrent) and significant method of sexual arousal by the exposure of one's genitalia to an unsuspecting stranger.

This is often followed by masturbation to achieve orgasm. The disorder is almost exclusively seen in males, and the 'unsuspecting stranger' is usually a female (child or adult).

Voyeurism

This is a persistent or recurrent tendency to observe unsuspecting persons (usually of the other sex) naked, disrobing or engaged in sexual activity.

This is often followed by masturbation to achieve orgasm without the observed person(s) being aware. This is almost always seen in males. Watching pornography is not included here.

Frotteurism

This is a persistent or recurrent involvement in the act of touching and rubbing against an unsuspecting, nonconsenting person (usually of the other sex).

Frottage is often employed in crowded places, e.g. buses, where the victim does not protest because she cannot suspect that frottage can be committed there. This is often seen in adolescent males.

Paedophilia

Paedophilia is a persistent or recurrent involvement of an adult (age >16 years and at least 5 years older than the child) in sexual activity with prepubertal children, either heterosexual or homosexual.

This may be associated with sexual sadism. The paedophilic behaviour may be either limited to incest or may spread to children outside the family. In most civilised societies, paedophilia is a serious offense and the convicted paedophile's name remains on a sex offenders' register in order to protect the society.

Zoophilia (Bestiality)

Zoophilia as a persistent and significant involvement in sexual activity with animals is rare. Occasional or situational zoophilia is much more common.

Other Paraphilias

These include sexual arousal with urine (urophilia); faeces (coprophilia); enemas (klismaphilia); corpses (necrophilia), among many others.

Treatment

1. Psychoanalysis and psychoanalytic psychotherapy: This is of particular help if the patient is psychologically minded and has good ego strength for therapy
2. Behaviour therapy: Aversion therapy is the treatment of choice in severe, distressing paraphilia, with the patient's consent.
3. Drug therapy: Antipsychotics have sometimes been used for severe or dangerous aggression associated with paraphilias. Benperidol was earlier believed to be particularly useful but the claim has not been substantiated, and the drug is not available in the market. Antiandrogens (cyproterone acetate or medroxy-progesterone acetate) can be used in paraphilias with excessive sexual activity.

4. Other treatments: Castration and psychosurgery are extremely rare choices these days.

SEXUAL DYSFUNCTIONS

Sexual dysfunction is a significant disturbance in the sexual response cycle, which is not due to an underlying organic cause.

To understand sexual dysfunction, a brief outline of normal human sexual response cycle is in order (Table 10.1). In the light of normal human sexual response cycle, it is easier to understand sexual dysfunctions.

The common dysfunctions include the following:

Disorders of Appetitive Phase (Sexual Desire Disorders)

Hypoactive sexual desire disorder

This disorder is characterised by an absence of fantasies and desire for sexual activity which is not secondary to other sexual dysfunctions, such as premature ejaculation or dyspareunia. Lack or diminution of sexual desire does not imply an inability to experience sexual pleasure; it makes the initiation of sexual act less likely.

This disorder is many times more common in females (previously called as frigidity) and its prevalence increases with age. The contributing factors may include fear of pregnancy, unsatisfactory past sexual experiences, marital disharmony, or fatigue. If the disorder is secondary to biological factors (such as drugs, chronic medical illnesses), it should be listed under 'sexual disorders due to a general medical condition'.

Sexual aversion disorder and lack of sexual enjoyment disorder

In the sexual aversion disorder, there is an aversion to and avoidance of all sexual activity with a sexual partner. The thought of sexual interaction is associated with negative feelings and causes anxiety. The contributing factors may include history of sexual abuse/molestation (especially in childhood), unsatisfactory past sexual experiences, or culturally induced negative feelings towards sexual matters.

Table 10.1: Normal Human Sexual Response Cycle

A normal human sexual response cycle can be divided into five phases:

1. *Appetitive Phase:* The phase before the actual sexual response cycle. This consists of sexual fantasies and a desire to have sexual activity.

2. *Excitement Phase:* The first true phase of the cycle, which starts with physical stimulation and/or by appetitive phase. The major changes during this phase are:
   Males: Penile erection, due to vasocongestion of corpus cavernosa; elevation of testes with scrotal sac.
   Females: Lubrication of vagina by a transudate; erection of nipples (in most women); erection of clitoris; thickening of labia minora.
   The duration of this phase is highly variable and may last for several minutes (or longer).

3. *Plateau Phase:* The intermediate phase just before actual orgasm, at the height of excitement. It is often difficult to differentiate the plateau phase from the excitement phase. The following important changes occur during this phase:
   Males: Sexual flush (inconsistent); autonomic hyperactivity; erection and engorgement of penis to full size; elevation and enlargement of testes; dew drops on glans penis (2-3 drops of mucoid fluid with spermatozoa).
   Females: Sexual flush (inconsistent); Autonomic hyperactivity; retraction of clitoris behind the prepuce; development of orgasmic platform in the lower 1/3rd of vagina, with lengthening and ballooning of vagina; enlargement of breasts and labia minora; increased vaginal transudate.

The duration of this phase may last from half to several minutes.

4. *Orgasmic Phase:* The phase with peak of sexual excitement followed by release of sexual tension, and rhythmic contractions of pelvic reproductive organs. The important changes are as follows:
   Males: 4-10 contractions of penile urethra, prostate, vas, and seminal vesicles; at about 0.8 sec intervals; autonomic excitement becomes marked in this phase. Doubling of pulse rate and respiratory rate, and 10-40 mm increase in systolic and diastolic BP occur; ejaculatory inevitability precedes orgasm; Ejaculatory spurt (30-60 cm; decreases with age); contractions of external and internal sphincters.
   Females: 3-15 contractions of lower 1/3rd of vagina, cervix and uterus; at about 0.8 sec intervals. No contractions occur in clitoris; autonomic excitement becomes marked in this phase. Doubling of pulse rate and respiratory rate, and 10-40 mm increase in systolic and diastolic BP occur; contractions of external and internal sphincters.
   The duration of this phase may last from 3-15 seconds.

5. *Resolution Phase:* This phase is characterised by the following common features in both sexes: A general sense of relaxation and well-being, after the slight clouding of consciousness during the orgasmic phase; disappearance of sexual flush followed by fine perspiration; gradual decrease in vasocongestion from sexual organs and rest of the body; refractory period for further orgasm in males varies from few minutes to many hours; there is usually no refractory period in females.

In the lack of sexual enjoyment disorder (sexual anhedonia), the sexual response is usually normal (which may include a normal orgasm). However, there is a feeling of lack of subjective sexual pleasure. This disorder is more common in females.

Excessive sexual drive

Rarely, both men (satyriasis) and women (nymphomania) may complain of excessive sexual drive as a problem.

Disorders of Excitement and Plateau Phase (Sexual Arousal Disorders or Failure of Genital Response)

Male erectile disorder (Impotence; Erectile dysfunction)

This disorder is characterised by an inability to have or sustain penile erection till the completion of satisfactory sexual activity. It is a relatively common disorder.

Although a large number of physical disorders have been aetiologically incriminated in the causation of male erectile disorder, some important ones are mentioned below. If the disorder is secondary to biological factors (such as drugs, chronic medical illnesses), it should be listed under 'sexual disorders due to a general medical condition' (Table 10.2).

Since many drugs impair the normal sexual functioning and often cause more than one sexual dysfunction, these are listed separately in Table 10.3. The secondary sexual dysfunction is usually more profound in males. In cases of male erectile dysfunction where biological causes have been ruled out, psychological factors should be considered in causation.

Psychological impotence usually occurs acutely. The early morning erections and erections during REM sleep (nocturnal penile tumescence; NPT) are usually preserved. These psychological factors may include one of the following conditions.

1. Ignorance regarding the sexual act.
2. Fear of failure and performance anxiety (e.g. during 'honeymoon').
3. Interpersonal difficulties between the sexual partners (e.g. marital conflict).
4. Anxiety disorder.
5. Mood disorder.
6. Masturbatory anxiety (and 'dhat syndrome' in India).
7. Fatigue (e.g. after the day's hard work).
8. Fear of pregnancy, or sexually transmitted disease.
9. Fear of 'damaging' the sexual partner or one-self.
10. Certain environmental factors (e.g. lack of privacy).
11. Lack of a consistent sexual partner.
12. Fear of commitment (in premarital and extramarital sexual relationships).
13. Poor self-image or 'inferiority complex'.
14. Sexual abuse in childhood.

In many cases of erectile dysfunction, aetiology can be mixed (i.e. both organic as well as psychogenic factors can be present).

Table 10.2: Physical Causes of Male Erectile Disorder/Impotence

I. Local Genital Pathology
  1. Priapism
  2. Congenital malformations
  3. Surgical procedures on pelvic region, e.g. perineal prostatectomy
  4. Mumps
  5. Elephantiasis
  6. Hydrocele or varicocele.

II. Endocrine Disorders
  1. Diabetes mellitus
  2. Dysfunction of pituitary-adrenal-testis axis
  3. Testicular atrophy, e.g. secondary to cirrhosis, dystrophia myotonica, haemochromatosis
  4. Thyroid dysfunction.

III. Neurological Disorders
  1. Autonomic neuropathy, e.g. in diabetes mellitus
  2. Spinal cord lesions, e.g. transverse myelitis
  3. 3rd ventricle tumours
  4. Brain damage, especially in temporal lobe
  5. Multiple sclerosis.

IV. Cardiovascular Disorders
  1. Leriche syndrome.

V. Any Severe or Debilitating Systemic Illness

VI. Alcohol and Drugs.

Female sexual arousal disorder
This disorder is characterised by subjective as well as objective lack of sexual arousal in the form of lack of lubrication or vaginal dryness.

The causes can be biological (e.g. postmenopausal) or psychological (uncommon).

Disorders of Orgasmic Phase (Orgasmic Disorders/Dysfunctions)

Male orgasmic disorder (Male anorgasmia)
Failure or marked difficulty to have orgasm, despite normal sexual excitement, during coitus. An uncommon disorder, it often presents as retarded ejaculation. The causes can be biological (e.g. post-prostate surgery, drug-induced) or psychological (e.g. marital conflicts).

Table 10.3: Sexual Dysfunctions Caused by Drugs

Drugs	Effect on Sexual Desire	Effect on Erectile Function	Effect on Ejaculation
I. Antihypertensives			
1. Methyldopa	Inhibited	Impaired	Impaired
2. Clonidine	—	Impaired	Impaired
3. Propranolol	Inhibited	Impaired	—
4. Thiazide diuretics	—	Impaired	—
5. Spironolactone	Inhibited	Impaired	Impaired
6. Guanethidine	—	Impaired	Impaired; Retrograde ejaculation
7. Hexamethonium	—	Impaired	Impaired; Retrograde ejaculation
II. Hormonal Preparations			
1. Corticosteroids	Inhibited	Impaired	Impaired
2. Oestrogens	Inhibited (in males)	Impaired	Impaired
3. Androgens	Increased (in both sexes)		
III. Psychotropic Medications			
1. Tricyclic antidepressants and MAO inhibitors	+/−	Impaired	Impaired
2. SSRI antidepressants (e.g. paroxetine, fluoxetine)	+/−	Impaired	Delayed ejaculation
3. Thioridazine	Inhibited	Impaired	Retrograde and Delayed ejaculation
4. Chlorpromazine	Inhibited	Impaired	—
5. Haloperidol	—	Impaired	—
6. Trazodone	—	Priapism	—
7. Barbiturates and benzodiazepines	Increased (with low dose, due to decrease in anxiety) Decreased (with high dose)	Impaired (with high dose)	Impaired (with high dose)
8. Lithium	—	Impaired	—
9. Disulfiram	—	—	Delayed ejaculation
IV. Psychoactive Substance Use			
1. Alcohol	Increased (with low dose)	Impaired	Impaired
2. Opiates and cocaine	Inhibited	Impaired (with high dose)	Impaired
V. Others			
1. Anti-inflammatory drugs (e.g. indomethacin)	Inhibited	Impaired	—
2. L-dopa	Inhibited	—	—
3. Anticholinergic drugs (e.g. trihexiphenidyl)	—	Impaired	Impaired

Female orgasmic disorder (Female anorgasmia)

Failure or marked difficulty to have orgasm, despite normal sexual excitement, during coitus. This is a very common disorder.

Anorgasmia can be either primary or secondary. Although the disorder causes marked distress, it is rarely complained of in the clinical setting, particularly in India. This is probably due to cultural factors.

The causes can be biological (e.g. endocrinal disorders such as hypothyroidism, drug-induced) or psychological (e.g. marital conflicts).

Premature ejaculation

This disorder is defined as ejaculation before the completion of satisfactory sexual activity for both partners. In severe cases, it is characterised by ejaculation either before penile entry into vagina or soon after penetration. It is a very common disorder in the clinical setting.

The causes can be biological (relatively uncommon) or psychological (e.g. performance anxiety).

Sexual Pain Disorders

Nonorganic vaginismus

This disorder is characterised by an involuntary spasm of the lower 1/3rd of vagina, interfering with coitus. Penile entry is either painful or impossible.

Before a presumption of nonorganic vaginismus, it is important to rule out organic factors (e.g. local pathology causing pain).

Nonorganic dyspareunia

This disorder is characterised by pain in the genital area of either male or female, during coitus. Before a presumption of nonorganic dyspareunia, it is particularly important to rule out organic factors (e.g. local pathology causing pain) in both males and females.

Sexual Disorders Due to a General Medical Condition

The disorders listed above may occur secondary to a general medical condition; they should then be coded here. These dysfunctions are called disorders only when they occur recurrently and persistently. Also if the sexual dysfunction is due to sexual stimulation being inadequate either in focus, intensity or duration, a diagnosis of excitement and orgasmic phase disorders is not made.

Diagnosis and Differential Diagnosis

Before making a diagnosis of sexual dysfunction, it is of paramount importance to rule out an underlying physical cause, which would need treatment.

Although the diagnosis is clinical, a detailed physical examination and laboratory investigations (e.g. blood counts, blood sugar, liver function tests, thyroid function tests, hormonal profile, and rarely, routine examination and culture of prostatic fluid) coupled with a good history is a must in every patient to rule out an underlying physical cause.

Certain laboratory techniques (e.g. penile plethysmograph, penile tumescence monitoring during sleep) may help in differentiating organic and nonorganic sexual dysfunctions. If NPT (nocturnal penile tumescence) is abnormal, then ancillary investigations such as penile vascular investigations (e.g. penile pulse pressure, penile Doppler, duplex ultrasonography, diagnostic intracavernosal vasoactive substance-papaverine injection test, arteriography, DICC-dynamic infusion cavernosomatogram and cavernosogram, and cavernosography) and penile neurological investigations (e.g. penile sensory threshold test or penile biothesiometry) may be employed.

Though searching for an organic factor responsible for the sexual dysfunction is very important, a large majority of dysfunctions are psychosexual in nature. A detailed sexual and personal history is important in finding out the underlying causes. The common psychological causes of sexual dysfunction have been discussed earlier.

It should be specified whether the sexual dysfunction is psychogenic alone or biogenic factors co-exist; whether the dysfunction is life-long or acquired; and whether the dysfunction is situational or generalised.

Treatment

The treatment usually consists of one or more of the following methods:

1. *Treatment of the underlying physical or psychiatric disorder, if present.*

2. *Psychoanalysis*: This is particularly indicated when the dysfunction is more pervasive and involves personality difficulties. The goal is not symptom removal but is resolution of the underlying unconscious conflicts.

3. *Hypnosis*: Hypnosis can be used either alone or in conjunction with other therapies aiming at symptom removal. However, only suggestible patients can be hypnotised.

4. *Group psychotherapy*: Patients of same sex with different sexual problems or of both sexes with similar sexual problems can be treated in group therapy sessions. The focus is usually on providing education regarding normal sexuality and to remove anxiety or guilt by sharing viewpoints in a group setting. Although occasionally used alone, it is more helpful as an adjunct to other methods of treatment.

5. *Behaviour therapy*: The methods commonly employed include the following:

   i. Relaxation training, e.g. Jacobson's progressive relaxation technique.

   ii. Assertiveness training.

   iii. Systematic desensitisation, aimed at reducing the phobic anxiety related to the sexual act, e.g. in sexual aversion disorder.

   iv. Biofeedback, using a penile plethysmograph.

6. *Masters' and Johnson's technique*: This is one of the most popular and successful methods of treatment for psychosexual dysfunctions. The patient is not treated alone, but both the partners are treated together. This is called as dual-sex therapy, where both the sexual partners are treated by a team of therapists (one male and one female), although later modifications of this technique use only one therapist.

The goal of the treatment is symptom removal, using simple behavioural techniques. The couple is usually seen on a weekly basis; however, the sessions can be more frequent if the couple is encountering particular difficulties during treatment. Some common steps before starting therapy include:

i. Detailed history taking (sexual history) from each partner separately.

ii. Round-table discussions aiming at:

   a. Education about normal sexuality.

   b. Understanding of the couple's current sexual problem(s).

   c. Enhancing communication between the partners regarding sexual matters.

iii. Behaviour modification steps, depending on the type of psychosexual dysfunction.

Brief examples of the techniques used are:

   a. *Sensate focus technique*: This is used particularly for treatment of impotence, although it is also useful in management of other dysfunctions as well. The aim is to 'discover' on body (excluding genital area) 'sensate focuses' (body areas where manipulation leads to sexual arousal). This is usually a general exercise before any sex therapy.

   b. *Squeeze technique (Seman's technique)*: This has been used in treatment of premature ejaculation. The female partner is asked to manually stimulate the penis causing erection. When the male partner experiences 'ejaculatory inevitability', the female partner 'squeezes' the penis on the coronal ridge thus delaying ejaculation.

There are similar simple techniques (such as orgasmic conditioning, desensitisation) for treatment of other psychosexual dysfunctions. The response rate is close to 80%, with maximum success in the treatment of premature ejaculation.

7. *Oral drug therapy*: Till very recently, this was rarely a treatment of first choice in sexual dysfunctions. Current indications of drug treatment include:

   i. Treatment of underlying psychiatric disorder.

   ii. Intense anxiety related to sexual activity may require use of low dose benzodiazepines (such as alprazolam) for a very limited period (to prevent benzodiazepine misuse or dependence).

   iii. Premature ejaculation may sometimes require treatment with fluoxetine, trazodone, or tricyclic antidepressants such as clomipramine (to retard ejaculation).

   iv. Several drugs have been used in the treatment of impotence with varying degrees of efficacy, e.g. alpha-blockers (such as yohimbine, idazoxan), opiate antagonists (such as naltrexone), dopamine agonists (such as bromocriptine, apomorphine), pentoxifylline, and topical drugs (glyceryl trinitrate, minoxidil, papaverine and PgE_1 and E_2).

v. Sildenafil citrate has been used for treatment of erectile dysfunction. Rapidly absorbed after oral administration, the maximum plasma concentration is reached in 30-120 minutes. It is metabolised in liver (mainly by cytochrome P450 3A4) and is converted to an active metabolite. Sildenafil has a terminal half life of about 4 hours. It is highly bound to plasma proteins and is not dialysable. It is a competitive and selective inhibitor of cGMP (cyclic guanosine monophosphate)-specific PDE-5 (phosphodiesterase type 5). It prevents the rate of breakdown of cGMP causing enhanced relaxation of cavernosal smooth muscle, increase in arterial flow in to corpus cavernosa, compression of subtunical veins, and hence penile erection. The typical dose is 50 mg (25-100 mg), 1 hour before sexual activity. The maximum recommended dosing frequency is once a day. The drug acts only in the presence of sexual stimulation. The adverse effects include transient and mild headache, flushing, dyspepsia, and nasal congestion. Caution needs to be exercised in patients with known history of hypersensitivity, with poor cardiovascular status, with anatomical deformation of penis, with conditions that predispose to priapism, and especially those on nitrates.

Other similar drugs include tadalafil and verdenafil.

vi. Hormonal treatment (e.g. androgens) should not be employed unless there is an evidence of hormonal dysfunction.

It should always be remembered that prescription of the non-essential drugs may worsen sexual dysfunction.

8. *Intracavernosal Injection of Vasoactive Drugs (IIVD)*: Papaverine, an alkaloid and a vasoactive substance, has been used as an intracavernosal injection in the differential diagnosis of organic and non-organic impotence and also for treatment of impotence (either alone; or along with phentolamine, phenoxy-benzamine, alprostadil or prostaglandin E_1, and/or atropine).

9. *Physical devices:* Various suction devices (for producing artificial penile tumescence) and penile prosthetic implants are available. Their use, however, should be limited to only those patients who suffer from *organic sexual disorder* or in whom a sufficient and regular trial of psychological management has been completing, with distress persisting.

10. *Vascular surgery:* Rarely, vascular surgery may be needed for some patients with underlying vascular insufficiency (*organic sexual disorder*).

Chapter 11

Sleep Disorders

SLEEP

Nearly one third of human life is spent in sleep, an easily reversible state of relative unresponsiveness and serenity which occurs more or less regularly and repetitively each day. The EEG recordings show typical features of sleep which is broadly divided into two broadly different phases:

1. *D-sleep* (desynchronised or dreaming sleep), also called as REM-sleep (rapid eye movement sleep), active sleep, or paradoxical sleep.
2. *S-sleep* (synchronised sleep), also called as NREM-sleep (non-REM sleep), quiet sleep, or orthodox sleep. S-sleep or NREM-sleep is further divided into four stages, ranging from stages 1 to 4. As the person falls asleep, the person first passes through these stages of NREM-sleep.

The EEG recording during the waking state shows alpha waves of 8-12 cycles/sec. frequency. The onset of sleep is characterised by a disappearance of the alpha-activity.

Stage 1, NREM-sleep is the first and the lightest stage of sleep characterised by an absence of alpha-waves, and low voltage, predominantly theta activity.

Stage 2, NREM-sleep follows the stage 1 within a few minutes and is characterised by two typical EEG changes:

  i. *Sleep spindles:* Regular spindle shaped waves of 13-15 cycles/sec. frequency, lasting 0.5-2.0 seconds, with a characteristic waxing and waning amplitude.

  ii. *K-complexes:* High voltage spikes present intermittently.

Stage 3, NREM-sleep shows appearance of high voltage, 75 μV, δ-waves of 0.5-3.0 cycles/sec.

Stage 4, NREM-sleep shows predominant δ-activity in EEG.

NREM-sleep is followed by REM-sleep, which is a light phase of sleep. The EEG is characterised by a return of α-waves (α-wave sleep); other changes are similar to stage 1 NREM-sleep. One of the most characteristic features of the REM-sleep is presence of REM or rapid (conjugate) eye movements. The other features include generalised muscular atony, penile erection, autonomic hyperactivity (increase in pulse rate, respiratory rate and blood pressure), and movements of small muscle groups, occurring intermittently. Although it is a light stage of sleep, arousal is difficult.

These stages occur regularly throughout the whole duration of sleep. The first REM period occurs typically after 90 minutes of the onset of sleep, although it can start as early as 7 minutes after going-off to sleep, e.g. in narcolepsy, in major depression, and after sleep deprivation.

The important time periods of the various sleep stages are summarised below:

1. In an 8 hour sleep, usually 6-6½ hours are spent in the NREM-sleep while 1½-2 hours are in the REM-sleep.
2. Out of 6-6½ hours NREM-sleep period, only about 70-80 minutes are spent in Stage 4 sleep.

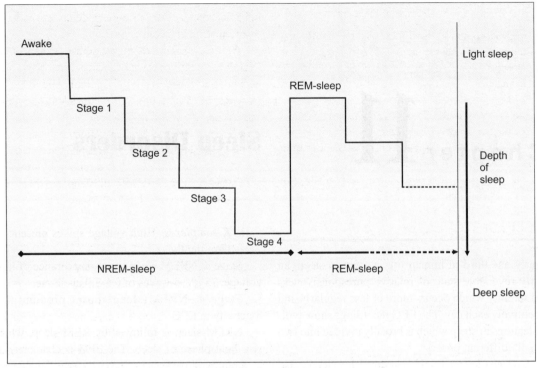

Fig. 11.1: Stages of Sleep

3. The maximum Stage 4 sleep occurs in the first one-third of the night. In the later part, the REM-sleep follows the Stage 3 NREM-sleep directly.

4. The REM-sleep occurs maximally in the last one-third of the night. The REM-sleep occurs regularly after every 90-100 minutes, with progressive lengthening of each REM period. The first REM period typically lasts for less than 10 minutes. Usually, there are 4-5 REM periods in the whole night of sleep.

5. A younger person may typically need more sleep. The usual sleep duration in newborn children is 16-18 hours/day, with nearly 8-10 hours spent in the REM-sleep. As the age advances, the sleep duration tends to reduce.

Certain phenomena are common just before going-off to sleep (hypnagogic phenomena) and just after waking-up (hypnopompic phenomena). These phenomena include a variety of illusions and simple hallucinations (both visual and auditory), jerky muscle movements involving small muscle groups, and deper-sonalisation and derealisation. Some of the methods of sleep study are listed in Table 11.1.

Depending on the duration of total sleep, two extremes of 'normal' sleeping patterns have been described.

1. *Long-sleepers:* These persons regularly and habitually sleep for more than 9 hours/night, and this pattern of sleep does not cause any symptoms or dysfunction.

2. *Short-sleepers:* These persons regularly and habitually sleep for less than 6 hours/night, and this pattern of sleep does not cause any symptoms or dysfunction.

On comparing long-sleepers and short-sleepers, it has been found that the time spent in stage 3 and 4 of NREM-sleep is the same in both. The maximum difference is in the duration of the REM-sleep. The

Table 11.1: Methods of Sleep Study

To study sleep and its associated phenomena, the following techniques can be used.
1. Observation of a sleeping person for externally visible changes.
2. EEG.
3. Polysomnography (This is usually the preferred method in the sleep research centers). It consists of:
   i. Continuous EEG recording, particularly from occipital and parietal leads.
   ii. EOG (electro-oculography) to record the eye movements.
   iii. EMG (electromyography) for muscle potential and activities.
   iv. ECG for changes in cardiac status.
   v. In certain cases, respiratory tracings of various kinds are used, such as oxymetry, expired CO_2, O_2 saturation.
   vi. MSLT (Multiple sleep latency test): It involves repeated measures of the sleep latency (i.e. time to onset of sleep).
   vii. Penile tumescence, body temperature, GSR (galvanic skin response), and body movements are also sometimes studied.
The recordings are made throughout the night sleep.

long-sleeper, on an average, has almost double the duration of REM-sleep as compared to a short-sleeper.

SLEEP DEPRIVATION

Experimental deprivation of sleep is an important method of studying the functions of sleep. After a few days of sleep deprivation, EEG recordings show a gradual diminishing of α activity, with an increase in the lower frequency activity.

After 4-5 days of sleep deprivation, psychological symptoms become prominent. Initially, there is a decrease in attention span, with easy distractibility, drowsiness, decreased initiative to perform and 'micro-sleeps' lasting but a few seconds. In predisposed individuals, psychotic symptoms may appear on the fifth night, characterised by break with reality, illusions and hallucinations, grossly disorganised behaviour, persecutory ideation or delusions, and mild disorientation and confusion.

As time progresses, frank delirium may occur. Whether this type of psychosis can occur in previously normal individuals is doubtful, mainly due to lack of sufficient research data. Clearly, ethical considerations prevent this kind of research.

Recovery after sleep deprivation is characterised by an increase in total sleep duration, usually lasting for 15-16 hours. There is also a rebound increase in the stages 3 and 4 of the NREM-sleep in the first few hours and an increase in the REM-sleep later.

FUNCTIONS OF SLEEP

Despite accumulation of vast amount of research data regarding physiology and biochemistry of sleep, functions of sleep are still far from clear.

It has been observed that persons sleeping for 7-9 hours per day have significantly lower rates of illness. On the other hand, certain disorders carry a higher mortality when present during sleep (especially during early hours of morning), for example, coronary artery disease, nocturnal asthma, sudden nocturnal death (in south-east Asian men), and sleep apnoea.

It has been observed that there is a 5-25% decrease in metabolic rate during night sleep. Conservation of energy therefore appears to be one of the important functions of sleep. It also serves a restorative function for the whole body (particularly during NREM-sleep) and for the brain (cognitive functions; especially during REM-sleep). Further research is likely to clarify exact functions of various components of the sleep cycle.

SLEEP DISORDERS

There are several types of sleep disorders known. The ASDC (Association for Sleep Disorders Centre) has done a lot of work in classifying the various sleep disorders and their classification has been adapted for use both by DSM-IV-TR and ICD-10. The sleep disorders are known as *non-organic sleep disorders* in ICD-10.

The various sleep disorders are divided in 2 sub-types:

I. Dyssomnias
    1. Insomnia
    2. Hypersomnia
    3. Disorders of sleep-wake schedule.
II. Parasomnias
    1. Stage 4 sleep disorders
    2. Other sleep disorders.

Dyssomnias

Dyssomnias are sleep disorders that are characterised by disturbances in the amount, quality or timing of sleep. These are the commonest disorders of sleep.

Insomnia

Insomnia is also known as the Disorder of Initiation and/or Maintenance of Sleep (DIMS). Insomnia means one or more of the following:

1. Difficulty in initiating sleep (going-off to sleep).
2. Difficulty in maintaining sleep (remaining asleep). This can include both:
    a. Frequent awakenings during the night, and
    b. Early morning awakening.
3. Non-restorative sleep where despite an adequate duration of sleep, there is a feeling of not having rested fully (poor quality sleep).

Insomnia is very common, with nearly 15-30% of general population complaining of a period of insomnia per year requiring treatment. It is required for diagnosis that sleep disturbance occurs at least three times a week for at least 1 month, and that it causes either marked distress or interferes with social and occupational functioning.

Aetiology

The common causes of insomnia are listed in Table 11.2.

A person suffering from insomnia should be differentiated from a short-sleeper, who needs less than 6 hours of sleep per night and has no symptoms or dysfunction. A short-sleeper does not need any treatment.

Table 11.2: Common Causes of Insomnia

1. Medical illnesses
    i.   Any painful or uncomfortable condition
    ii. Heart diseases
    iii. Respiratory diseases
    iv. Rheumatic and musculo-skeletal disease
    v.   Old age
    vi. Brain stem or hypothalamic lesions
    vii. Delirium
    viii. PMS (Periodic movements in sleep)
2. Alcohol and drug use
    i.   Drug or alcohol withdrawal syndrome
    ii. Delirium tremens
    iii. Amphetamine or other stimulants, e.g. caffeine
    iv. Chronic alcoholism
3. Current medication, e.g. fluoxetine, steroids, theophylline, propranolol
4. Psychiatric disorders
    i.   Mania (may not complain of decrease in sleep, as there is often a decreased need for sleep)
    ii. Major depression (difficulty in maintenance of sleep is more prominent, although difficulty in initiating sleep is also present)
    iii. Dysthymia (difficulty in initiating sleep is characteristic)
    iv. Anxiety disorder (difficulty in initiating sleep is common)
    v.   Stressful life situation (may cause temporary insomnia).
5. Idiopathic insomnia

One cause of insomnia, PMS (periodic movements in sleep) needs further mention. PMS actually consists of two different syndromes, which often occur together:

1. Periodic Limb Movement Disorder (PLMD), and
2. 'Restless Legs' Syndrome (RLS or *Ekbom syndrome*).

Periodic Limb Movement Disorder (PLMD)

It is characterised by sudden, repeated contraction of one or more of muscle groups (usually of the legs) during sleep. Often occurring bilaterally, it is followed by partial (most commonly) or complete arousal. Since each individual contraction lasts for a few seconds and is repeated at an interval of 20-60sec. during a long sleep-period, partial or complete awakenings occur many times in one night sleep.

The patient is usually not aware of the myoclonus and usually complains of non-restorative sleep or of frequent awakenings. The myoclonus is observed, if at all, by the bed partner. This is commonly seen in middle-aged and elderly people. Due to night-time insomnia, daytime hypersomnia can occur and, at times, may be the only presenting symptom.

'Restless Legs' Syndrome (Ekbom syndrome)

RLS is a condition in which the person experiences, during waking, an extremely uncomfortable feeling in the leg muscles. Sometimes, it may resemble painful creeping sensations deep inside the calf muscles.

Classically, these abnormal sensations occur while sitting or lying down and cause an irresistible urge to move the legs. Moving about or standing provides immediate, temporary relief. This is often associated with periodic limb movement disorder (PLMD) during night sleep. Daily, regular exercises can lead to marked improvement in certain cases.

Treatment

1. A thorough medical and psychiatric assessment.
2. Polysomnography (see Table 11.1) may be needed in some patients to reach a diagnosis.
3. Treatment of the underlying physical and/or psychiatric disorder, if present.
4. Withdrawal of current medications, if any.
5. Relaxation techniques before sleep time and education regarding sleep hygiene (see Table 11.3). Sleep hygiene consists of general guidelines for promoting good sleep. In itself, it is not a treatment for insomnia.
6. Psychotherapy, if indicated.
7. Benzodiazepines may be used, either alone, e.g. in primary insomnia, or may be used with the treatment of underlying physical or psychiatric disorder(s). The use of benzodiazepines should only be for short-term periods, not more than for 4-6 weeks at one time.

Table 11.3: Sleep Hygiene

Some basic components of sleep hygiene are:
1. Regular, daily physical exercises (preferably not in the evening).
2. Minimise daytime napping.
3. Avoid fluid intake and heavy meals just before bed-time.
4. Avoid caffeine intake (e.g. tea, coffee, cola drinks) before sleeping hours.
5. Avoid regular use of alcohol (especially avoid use of alcohol as a hypnotic for promoting sleep).
6. Avoid reading or watching television while in bed.
7. Sleep in a dark, quiet, and comfortable environment.
8. Regular times for going to sleep and waking-up
9. Try relaxation techniques

If the difficulty in initiating sleep is the main symptom, then a benzodiazepine with shorter half-life should be used, such as temazepam, oxazepam or lorazepam.

If the difficulty in maintaining sleep is the predominant symptom, then a longer acting benzodiazepine, such as nitrazepam, flurazepam or even diazepam, should be used (see Chapter 15 for details).

Physicians should be careful to avoid benzodiazepine abuse or dependence in patients presenting with insomnia. Non-benzodiazepine hypnotics (e.g. zopiclone, zolpidem, zalpelon and trazodone) are useful alternatives (see Chapter 15).

8. L-tryptophan, an amino-acid present in many vegetables, is an apparently non-dependence producing hypnotic. The usual dose is 0.5g at night time.

Hypersomnia

Hypersomnia is also known as Disorder of excessive somnolence (DOES). Hypersomnia means one or more of the following:
1. Excessive day time sleepiness.
2. 'Sleep attacks' during day time (falling asleep unintentionally).

3. 'Sleep drunkenness' (person needs much more time to awaken; and during this period is confused or disoriented).

Hypersomnia is seen in about 1-2% of general population at any given time. As insomnia and hypersomnia may be present at the same time, the underlying causes may be common to both. It is required for the diagnosis that the sleep disturbance occurs daily for at least 1 month or for recurrent periods of shorter duration, and that it causes either marked distress or interferes with social and occupational functioning.

Aetiology

The common causes of hypersomnia are listed in Table 11.4.

A person suffering from hypersomnia should be differentiated from a long-sleeper, who needs more than 9 hours of sleep per night and has no symptoms or dysfunction. A long-sleeper does not need any treatment.

A few important causes of hypersomnia are discussed below:

1. Narcolepsy

This is a disorder characterised by excessive daytime sleepiness, often disturbed night-time sleep and disturbances in the REM-sleep. The hallmark of this disorder is decreased REM latency, i.e. decreased latent period before the first REM period occurs. Normal REM latency is 90-100 minutes. In narcolepsy, REM-sleep usually occurs within 10 minutes of the onset of sleep.

The common age of onset is 15-25 years, with usually a stable course throughout life. The prevalence rate of narcolepsy is about 4 per 10,000.

The classical tetrad of symptoms is:

i. *Sleep attacks* (most common)*:* The person is unable to resist a sleep attack or 'nap', from which he or she awakens refreshed. These 'attacks' can occur during any time of the day, even whilst driving. Usually, there is a gap of 2-3 hours between the two attacks.

ii. *Cataplexy:* This is characterised by a loss of muscle tone in the various parts of body, e.g. jaw

Table 11.4: Causes of Hypersomnia

1. Medical illnesses
   - i. Narcolepsy (in about 25% of all patients with hypersomnia)
   - ii. Sleep apnoea (in about 50% of all patients with hypersomnia)
   - iii. Kleine-Levin syndrome
   - iv. Menstrual-associated somnolence
   - v. Sleep deprivation
   - vi. Following or with insomnia
   - vii. Encephalitis
   - viii. Hypothyroidism
   - ix. Head Injury
   - x. Cerebral tumours in the region of mid-brain
   - xi. Hypothalamic lesions
   - xii. Trypanosomiasis
   - xiii. PMS (Periodic movements in sleep); in about 10% of all patients with hypersomnia.
2. Alcohol and drug use
   - i. Stimulant withdrawal
   - ii. Alcohol intoxication
   - iii. Use of CNS depressant medications.
3. Psychiatric disorders
   - i. Dysthymia
   - ii. Atypical depression
   - iii. Seasonal mood disorder.
4. Idiopathic hypersomnia.

drop, or paresis of all skeletal muscles of body resulting in a fall. This may be precipitated by sudden emotion. The consciousness is usually clear and memory is normal, unless sleep attacks supervene.

iii. *Hypnagogic hallucinations:* These are vivid perceptions, usually dream-like, which occur at the onset of sleep and are associated with fearfulness. When these occur at awakening, they are called *hypnopompic hallucinations.*

iv. *Sleep paralysis* (least common)*:* This occurs either at awakening in the morning (usually) or at sleep onset. The person is conscious but unable to move his body. The episode may last from 30 seconds to a few minutes and may cause significant distress.

Not all symptoms of the tetrad are present in one person. The other associated symptoms are fugue states, blackouts and blurring of vision. Polysomnography helps in making a diagnosis in doubtful cases, showing a decreased REM latency.

The treatment consists of forced naps at regular times in the day, stimulant medication (such as amphetamines) or modafinil in some patients, and/or antidepressants (particularly when cataplexy is a prominent symptom).

2. Sleep Apnoea

This condition is characterised by presence of repeated episodes of apnoea during sleep. In this context, apnoea is defined as the cessation of airflow at the nostrils (and mouth) for 10 seconds or longer. The apnoea can be of central type, obstructive type or mixed type.

It is commoner in elderly and obese (*Pickwickian syndrome*). Typically, there are 5 or more apnoeic episodes per hour of sleep and the total number of apnoeic episodes exceeds 30 during one night's sleep. In severe cases, the number of episodes may be in hundreds. The patients are usually not aware of the occurrence of apnoea. Instead, they complain of an inability to stay awake in the day time and non-restorative sleep at night. The bed partner may report of loud snoring, restless sleep or of periodic absences of breathing.

The diagnosis can be established in doubtful cases using polysomnography, with the respiratory tracings included. Sleep apnoea can be a dangerous condition. It can cause cardiac arrhythmias, pulmonary and systemic hypertension, and death.

The treatment consists of avoidance of alcohol and depressant medications, use of stimulants such as caffeine, regular exercises, losing excess weight, teaching correct sleeping posture, and corrective procedures for obstructive sleep apnoea (e.g. mechanical tongue retaining device). Very severe obstructive sleep apnoea may necessitate tracheostomy (functional only at night), CPAP (continuous positive airway pressure) through nasal mesh, or even pharyngoplasty.

3. Kleine-Levin Syndrome

This is a rare syndrome characterised by:

1. Hypersomnia (always present), occurring recurrently for long periods of time.
2. Hyperphagia (usually present), with a voracious appetite.
3. Hypersexuality (associated at times), consisting of sexual disinhibition, masturbatory activity, exhibitionism, and/or inappropriate sexual advances.

The associated features include apathy, irritable behaviour, confusion, social withdrawal, bizarre behaviour, psychotic symptoms (such as delusions and hallucinations), and disorientation. One or more of these symptoms may occur during the episode. EEG abnormalities, usually showing intermittent non-specific slowing, are common but are not diagnostic.

A typical episode lasts for one to several weeks, followed usually by a complete remission. The common age of onset is the second decade of life. Apparently this disorder has a finite course with a large majority of patients recovering completely before the fifth decade of life. The disorder is almost always seen in males.

No specific treatment is available but Lithium and occasionally Carbamazepine have been reported to be successful.

Treatment

1. A thorough physical and psychiatric assessment.
2. Treatment of the underlying cause is the most important method.
3. Associated or underlying insomnia should be looked for and treated.
4. Withdrawal of current medication causing hypersomnia, especially depressant medication.
5. Benzodiazepines at night may paradoxically decrease hypersomnia by correcting night time insomnia.

Disorders of Sleep-wake Schedule

These are characterised by a disturbance in the timing of sleep. The person with this disorder is not able to sleep when he wishes to, although at other times he is able to sleep adequately. This is due to a mismatch between person's circadian rhythm and the normal sleep-wake schedule demanded by the environment.

Aetiology

The common causes of disorders of sleep-wake schedule are listed below:

1. 'Jet lag' or rapid change of time zone: This typically occurs during international flights crossing many 'time zones'. At the new place, the person's internal time of sleep and the sleep time of surroundings are different, leading to insomnia during the new sleep time and somnolescence in the new daytime, thus causing impairment of functioning.
2. 'Work-shift' from day to night or vice-versa.
3. Unusual sleep phases: Some persons are unable to sleep early. They typically sleep late at night and get up late in the morning. They are called as 'owls'. Others are similarly unable to remain awake at night. They typically sleep early at night and get up early in the morning. They are called as 'larks'. Some others have a longer-than 24 hour sleep-wake cycle (usually of 25 hours).

Treatment

No specific treatment is usually needed. Benzodiazepines may be needed for short-term correction of insomnia. Changes in 'work-shifts' may be needed for persons with unusual sleep phases. Exposure to sunlight during outdoor activity (instead of staying indoors) and adopting the local (new) hours for sleeping (and working) can help in combating jet lag.

Parasomnias

Parasomnias are dysfunctions or episodic nocturnal events occurring with sleep, sleep stages or partial arousals. Most parasomnias are common in childhood though they may persist into adulthood.

Stage 4 Sleep Disorders

These disorders occur during deep sleep, i.e. Stages 3 and 4 of NREM-sleep.

The common Stage 4 parasomnias are:

1. *Sleep-walking (somnambulism):* The patient carries out automatic motor activities that range from simple to complex. He may leave the bed, walk about or leave the house. Arousal is difficult and accidents may occur during sleep-walking.
2. *Sleep-terrors* or *night terrors (pavor nocturnus):* The patient suddenly gets up screaming with autonomic arousal (tachycardia, sweating and hyperventilation). He may be difficult to arouse and rarely recalls the episode on awakening. In contrast, *nightmares* (which occur during REM-sleep) are clearly remembered in the morning.
3. *Sleep-related enuresis* (bedwetting): This is discussed in detail in Chapter 14.
4. *Bruxism* (teeth-grinding): The patient has an involuntary and forceful grinding of teeth during sleep. Though the bed partner reports loud sounds produced by grinding of teeth and destruction of the tooth enamel is obvious, the patient remains completely unaware of the episode(s).
5. *Sleep-talking (somniloquy):* The patient talks during stages 3 and 4 of sleep but does not remember anything about it in the morning on awakening.

These disorders are often co-existent. As they occur during stage 4 (and 3) of NREM-sleep, they are more common during the first one-third of the night (There is more NREM-sleep in the first third of the night while the last third has more REM-sleep). Arousal is difficult and on waking-up, there is a complete amnesia for the event(s).

Treatment

Since benzodiazepines suppress stage 4 of NREM-sleep, a single dose at bedtime usually provides relief from stage 4 parasomnias.

Other Sleep Disorders

Nightmares (dream anxiety disorder) occur during the REM-sleep. They are characterised by fearful dreams occurring most commonly in the last one-third of night sleep. The person wakes up very frightened and remembers the dream vividly.

This is in contrast to night terrors which occur early in the night, are a stage 4 NREM disorder, and are characterised by complete amnesia. In both the conditions, the observer finds the person frightened during the episode.

Other sleep disorders include nocturnal angina, nocturnal asthma, nocturnal seizures, paroxysmal nocturnal haemoglobinuria, nocturnal head banging, and familial sleep paralysis.

Treatment

There is no specific treatment. Treatment of the underlying condition is the most important step. The treatment of nightmares is by suppression of REM-sleep, e.g. by bedtime dose of a benzodiazepine. However, on stopping the drug, a rebound increase in symptoms may occur.

Chapter 12

Behavioural Syndromes Associated with Psychological Disturbances and Physiological Factors

The disorders can broadly be classified into the following categories:
1. Eating Disorders
2. Sleep disorders
3. Sexual disorder and dysfunctions
4. Postpartum psychiatric disorders
5. Psychosomatic disorders

In addition to these, the chapter also describes briefly consultation liaison psychiatry and psychiatric aspects of grief and bereavement.

EATING DISORDERS

Eating disorders are characterised by clinical presentation primary focused on eating behaviour. The following disorders are briefly discussed in the chapter:
1. Anorexia nervosa
2. Bulimia nervosa
3. Obesity (associated with other psychological disturbances)
4. Binge-eating disorder
5. Psychogenic vomiting

Anorexia Nervosa

Anorexia nervosa is an eating disorder characterised by the following prominent clinical features:
1. It occurs much more often in females as compared to the males. The common age of onset is adolescence (13-19 years of age).

2. There is an intense fear of becoming obese. This fear does not decrease even if body becomes very thin and underweight.
3. There is often a body-image disturbance. The person is unable to perceive own body size accurately. However, body image disturbance may sometimes not be seen in patients from non-Western cultural settings and several such cases have been described from India.
4. There is a refusal to maintain the body weight above a minimum normal weight for that age, sex and height.
5. Significant weight loss occurs, usually more than 25% of the original weight. The final weight is usually 15% less than the minimum limit of normal weight (for that age, sex and height) or a Quetelet's body-mass index (BMI) of 17.5 or less (Quetelet's body-mass index = weight in kg divided by square of height in meters).
6. No known medical illness, which can account for the weight loss, is present.
7. Absence of any other primary psychiatric disorder.
8. Amenorrhoea, primary or secondary, is often present in females.

In addition to these typical clinical features, other associated features are often present. The patient imposes dietary restrictions on self; can have peculiar patterns of handling food, such as breaking food into small bits, hiding food; and can engage in vigorous exercises. 'Anorexia' is actually a misnomer as there is never really a decrease in appetite, initially; in fact patient is often preoccupied with food. A lot of time may be spent in collecting recipes and cooking food for significant others.

Depressive symptoms are common and so are obsessive-compulsive personality traits. Psychomotor activity is usually increased. In severe cases, fine *lanugo hair* may develop all over the body. Women with anorexia nervosa can present with poor sexual adjustment, with conflicts about being a woman and fear of pregnancy. Many patients are unconsciously unable to accept a 'female role'.

A large number (up to 50%) of patients with anorexia nervosa also have bulimic episodes. These are characterised by rapid consumption of large amounts of food in a relatively short period of time, occurring usually when alone. This is known as *eating binges* or *binge-eating*. These binges are followed by intense guilt and attempts to remove eaten food, for example, by self-induced vomiting, laxative abuse, and/or diuretic abuse.

If untreated, the weight loss can become marked. Death may occur due to hypokalaemia (caused by self-induced vomiting), dehydration, malnutrition or congestive cardiac failure (caused by anaemia).

Anorexia nervosa should be differentiated from other conditions capable of causing significant weight loss. These include medical illnesses (such as hypopituitarism, lateral hypothalamic lesion and debilitating systemic illnesses, e.g. disseminated tuberculosis) and psychiatric disorders (such as depressive disorder and schizophrenia).

Another important differential diagnosis is bulimia nervosa. Although bulimic episodes are common in anorexia nervosa (binge eating followed by vomiting), patients of bulimia nervosa usually maintain a near normal body weight (or are overweight), in sharp contrast to the patients with anorexia nervosa.

Treatment

The treatment of anorexia nervosa can be considered in two phases, which often merge into each other.

- Short-term treatment, to encourage weight gain and correct nutritional deficiencies, if any.
- Long-term treatment, aimed at maintaining the near normal weight achieved in short-term treatment and preventing relapses.

The various treatment modalities used can include:

1. Behaviour therapy (BT): Behavioural treatments are based on providing positive reinforcements (and at times, negative reinforcements) contingent on weight gain by the patient. See Chapter 18 for further details for BT.

   A too rapid weight gain is not desirable or safe. The weight gain should not exceed 1.5 to 2 kg in a fortnight. As patients are usually unable to eat a large meal, especially in the initial part of treatment, it is advisable to suggest more number of meals (about six) per day. Occasionally, forceful Ryle's tube feeding may be needed initially, in resistant patients.

2. Individual psychotherapy is often helpful in addition to supportive physical treatment. This could involve psychotherapy with a focus on cognitive behaviour therapy, psychodynamic principles or supportive measures. See Chapter 17 and 18 for more details.

3. Hospitalisation, with adequate nursing care for food intake and weight gain, can be helpful in short-term treatment as well as prevention and/or treatment of complications. However, hospitalisation does not necessarily ensure long-term improvement. It is important to keep a close eye on water and electrolyte balance, need for supplementation with vitamins and minerals, and prevent osteoporosis.

4. Drugs are an important adjunct to other modes of therapy. The drugs used can include:
   i. Antipsychotics: Chlorpromazine is rarely used these days. Olanzapine has efficacy in improving weight gain but it is important to be aware of possibility of prolongation of QTc particularly in patients with low BMI.
   ii. Antidepressants (such as fluoxetine, clomipramine) for treatment of anorexia nervosa and/or associated depression.

iii. Cyproheptadine: This is particularly helpful in inducing weight gain, decreasing depressive symptoms and increasing appetite, if anorexia is actually present. The usual dose is 8-32 mg/day, in divided doses. However, co-prescription with SSRIs can interfere with their effectiveness as Cyproheptadine is a serotonin antagonist.

5. Group therapy and family therapy can be helpful in psycho-education for the patient and carers/family about nature of anorexia nervosa and its treatment. Psycho-education may also include discussion of current social norms of slimming and fitness, since there is evidence to suggest that anorexia nervosa is far more common in countries with social pressures for slimming, such as USA and UK. India is indeed quite fast catching up with similar social pressures.

The prognosis is generally better if diagnosis is made early, absence of previous hospitalisations and absence of bulimic episodes. Weight gain and improvement in mental outlook often precede return of menstrual function.

Bulimia Nervosa

Bulimia nervosa is an eating disorder characterised by the following clinical features:
1. Bulimia nervosa usually has an onset in early teens or adolescence.
2. There is an intense fear of becoming obese. There may be an earlier history of anorexia nervosa.
3. There is usually body-image disturbance and the person is unable to perceive own body size accurately.
4. There is a persistent preoccupation with eating, and an irresistible craving for food. There are episodes of overeating in which large amounts of food are consumed within short periods of time (*eating binges*).
5. There are attempts to 'counteract' the effects of overeating by one or more of the following: self-induced vomiting, purgative abuse, periods of starvation, and/or use of drugs such as appetite suppressants.

6. No known medical illness is present which can account for the disorder.
7. Absence of any other primary psychiatric disorder.

Treatment

The various treatment modalities that can be used include:
1. Behaviour therapy: This is based on providing positive reinforcements (and at times negative reinforcements) contingent on the control of binge eating by the patient. See Chapter 18 for further details for BT.
2. Individual psychotherapy: See Chapters 17 and 18 for further details.
3. Antidepressant drugs are an important adjunct to other modes of therapy. A Selective serotonin uptake inhibitor (SSRI) such as Fluoxetine (in doses of 20-60 mg) is particularly useful as it can cause loss of appetite at least in the initial phase of treatment, along with its antidepressant effect. The drugs used in the past have included tricyclic antidepressants such as imipramine, though they are currently not widely used.
4. Group therapy and family therapy: These methods are used for psycho-education of patient and carers/family about nature of bulimia nervosa and its treatment.

Obesity (Overeating Associated with Other Psychological Disturbances)

Obesity caused by a reaction to distressing events is included here. Obesity caused by drugs or endocrinal factors, or due to constitutional factors is not considered a psychiatric disorder.

Treatment options depend on the underlying cause; for example, psychotherapy (for present or past psychological distress), antidepressants (for depression), advice from dietician, drug treatment, or even bariatric surgery.

Binge Eating Disorders

In binge eating disorder, large amounts of food are consumed in a relatively short period, followed by severe discomfort and feelings of self-denigration. There is a sense of lack of control over eating during the episode. Additionally, there also may be eating of large amounts of food throughout the day with no planned meal times, eating alone because of being embarrassed, and/or feeling guilty and depressed after overeating.

The disorder is not listed separately in ICD-10 and symptoms of binge eating are also seen in bulimia nervosa.

Treatment is similar to bulimia nervosa, though the role of drug treatment in binge eating disorder is not so clear.

Psychogenic Vomiting

This is a clinical syndrome in which biopsychosocial factors interact to produce symptoms which are often mistaken for upper gastrointestinal tract disease, anorexia nervosa, dissociative (conversion) disorder, somatization disorder, or malingering.

The characteristic clinical features include:

1. Repeated vomiting, which typically occurs soon after a meal has begun or just after it has been completed.
2. Vomiting often occurs in complete absence of nausea or retching (Patients say that food just seems to come back up).
3. Vomiting is often self-induced and can be suppressed, if necessary.
4. Despite repeated vomiting, weight loss is not usually significant.
5. The course of illness is usually chronic with frequent remissions and relapses.

Treatment

1. The first and most important step is correct diagnosis and exclusion of other physical and/or psychiatric causes.
2. Identification of psychosocial stressor.
3. Environmental manipulation and encouragement of coping strategies to deal with stress.
4. Psychotherapy of either cognitive behavioural or psychodynamic nature (see Chapters 17 and 18 for further details).

NON-ORGANIC SLEEP DISORDERS

Non-organic sleep disorders are discussed in Chapter 11.

SEXUAL DYSFUNCTIONS, NOT CAUSED BY ORGANIC DISORDERS OR DISEASE

Non-organic sexual dysfunctions are discussed in Chapter 10.

POSTPARTUM PSYCHIATRIC DISORDERS (MENTAL AND BEHAVIOURAL DISORDERS ASSOCIATED WITH PUERPERIUM, NOT CLASSIFIED ELSEWHERE)

Pregnancy and puerperium are highly stressful periods in a woman's life. The person is threatened by:

1. Physical, physiological and endocrinal changes occurring in one's body,
2. Reorganisation of psyche in accordance with the new 'mother-role' (in the first pregnancy),
3. Body image changes, and
4. Unconscious intrapsychic conflicts relating to pregnancy, childbirth and motherhood may become activated.

It is no surprise then that 25-50% of all women can develop psychological symptoms in the puerperal period. The commonest type of presentation is mild depression and irritability, often known as *post-natal blues*. These *'blues'* pass-off within a few days and usually need no active management except monitoring and support.

However, in 1.5-4.6/1,000 deliveries (average 2/1000 deliveries), the mother can develop severe psychiatric symptoms including psychotic symptoms. This is known as postpartum psychosis.

The postpartum psychosis can present with:

1. Depressive episode with psychotic symptoms (most common), or
2. Schizophrenia-like symptoms, or
3. Manic episode, or
4. Delirium (least common).

Typically, the onset of symptoms occurs 3-7 days after delivery. An onset before the 3rd day postpartum is rare. The symptoms usually peak by the end of 4th week, and may necessitate admission to a hospital setting. As the puerperium lasts for 6 weeks, the relevant postpartum period for psychiatric symptomatology to appear is 6 weeks (according to ICD-10). Hence, any psychiatric symptoms appearing within 6-week period after delivery are called as postpartum psychiatric disorder(s), if they do not fulfil the criteria of the major psychiatric disorders.

It was earlier believed that schizophreniform disorder is the commonest postpartum psychiatric disorder in developing countries (such as India), in contrast to developed countries where depression is usually more common. However, recent studies negate this hypothesis. Even in India, depressive episode is the most common type of postpartum psychiatric disorder encountered in routine clinical practice though psychotic symptoms are frequently present.

The factors involved in causation are both biological (changes in endocrine status especially steroid withdrawal, sleep disturbances, amine disturbances) and psychosocial (intrapsychic conflicts relating to motherhood, family and interpersonal conflicts in light of the new 'role').

Presently, it is believed that postpartum psychosis is not a special or separate category, but only a residual category in ICD-10. Depressive episode or schizophreniform disorder occurring separately or as a part of postpartum psychiatric disorder are very similar, except the presence of confusion as a prominent and common symptom in postpartum psychiatric disorders. Childbirth merely acts as a stressful event precipitating the illness.

Postpartum psychoses have a better prognosis as compared to similar disorders occurring in a non-postpartum setting; however 15-25% of these patients have a recurrence, usually of the same type, during the next puerperium. Patients with a history of postpartum or postnatal depression are also considered high risk for development of bipolar disorder. During an episode, presence of folate deficiency can prolong the duration of psychiatric disorder and may make it chronic.

Treatment

1. Treatment of the type of postpartum psychiatric disorder, such as antidepressants and/or ECTs for the depressive episode; antipsychotics and/or mood stabilisers for the manic episode; antipsychotics for the psychotic symptomatology.
2. Psychotherapy for psychological issues, especially after recovery from psychosis has occurred.
3. General supportive care during the puerperium.
4. Lithium, antipsychotics and antidepressants are excreted in milk and may be dangerous to the infant. A judicious decision has to be made regarding feeding of the infant, depending on the dose prescribed, social support available and risks of keeping the infant and mother separate.
5. As patients can lack insight, have poor judgement, may be unable to care for themselves and the baby, and are receiving psychotropic medication, it is not uncommon that the baby receives 'top feeds' (supplementary feeds). In that case, it may be necessary to extract milk from breast daily (or more often) either manually or with a breast-pump. It is more practical to give oral Stilboestrol, Pyridoxine (100 mg/day) or very rarely Bromocriptine to inhibit lactation. It is important to remember the risk of psychosis with Bromocriptine.

PSYCHOSOMATIC DISORDERS (PSYCHOLOGICAL OR BEHAVIOURAL FACTORS ASSOCIATED WITH DISORDERS OR DISEASES CLASSIFIED ELSEWHERE)

Psychosomatic disorders (a term coined by Heinroth in 1918) are those disorders in which psychosocial factors are very important in causation. Broadly applied, this term can encompass all physical illnesses. A narrow but more practical definition would include those physical disorders which are either initiated or exacerbated by the presence of meaningful psychosocial environmental stressors. ICD-10 lists these disorders under the category of Psychological or behavioural factors associated with disorders or diseases classified elsewhere.

Franz Alexander, the Father of Psychosomatic Medicine, initially described the seven classical psychosomatic illnesses (Table 12.1). His *specificity hypothesis* stated that if a specific environmental stressor or emotional conflict occurs, it results in a specific illness in a genetically predetermined organ.

George Engel in 1977, described a *biopsychosocial model* to explain the complex interaction between biological, psychological and social spheres resulting

Table 12.1: Classical Psychosomatic Disorders

The 7 classical psychosomatic disorders are:
1. Bronchial asthma
2. Ulcerative colitis
3. Peptic ulcer
4. Neurodermatitis
5. Thyrotoxicosis
6. Rheumatoid arthritis
7. Essential hypertension.

in a psychosomatic illness. This viewpoint has become very popular and is now almost integral to psychiatric teaching and practice throughout the World. It can be depicted in a diagram (Fig. 12.1).

Beginning from seven classical psychosomatic illnesses of Alexander, number of these illnesses continued to increase as their biopsychosocial causation became more evident and clear. At present, the list of psychosomatic illnesses is virtually endless as it is not difficult to imagine the effect of psychosocial factors on most illnesses. The important and common psychosomatic illnesses are mentioned in Table 12.2.

It is not the purpose of this book to go into the details of these physical disorders. However, certain important aspects and conditions are described, which are often not available in detail in most medical textbooks.

Type A Personality

When personality characteristics of a patient with coronary artery disease (CAD) are examined, there may be preponderance of a certain type of personality traits, collectively described as coronary prone

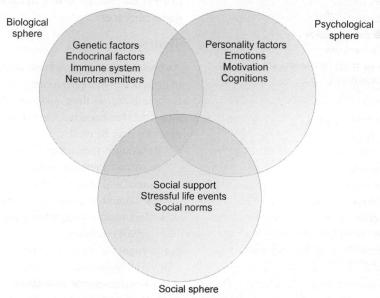

Fig. 12.1: A Biopsychosocial Model for Psychosomatic Illness

Table 12.2: Common Examples of Psychosomatic Disorders

I. Cardiovascular disorders
1. Essential hypertension
2. Coronary artery disease
3. CCU delirium or post-cardiac surgery delirium
4. Migraine
5. Cerebrovascular disease
6. Mitral valve prolapse syndrome (MVPS)

II. Endocrine disorders
1. Diabetes mellitus
2. Hyperthyroidism
3. Cushing's syndrome
4. Peri-menopausal syndrome
5. Amenorrhoea
6. Menorrhagia

III. Gastro-intestinal disorders
1. Oesophageal reflux
2. Peptic ulcer
3. Ulcerative colitis
4. Crohn's disease

IV. Immune disorders (These overlap with other disorders mentioned in this table)
1. Auto-immune disorders such as Ulcerative colitis, Systemic lupus erythematosus (SLE)
2. Allergic disorders such as Bronchial asthma, Hay fever
3. Viral infections

V. Musculo-skeletal disorders
1. Rheumatoid arthritis
2. Systemic lupus erythematosus (SLE)

VI. Respiratory disorders
1. Bronchial asthma
2. Hay fever
3. Vasomotor (allergic) rhinitis

VII. Skin disorders
1. Psoriasis
2. Pruritus
3. Urticaria
4. Alopecia areata
5. Acne vulgaris
6. Psychogenic purpura
7. Trichotillomania
8. Dermatitis artifacta
9. Lichen planus
10. Warts.

Type A behaviour by Friedman and Rosenman. This Type A behaviour is characterised by following features:

Time Urgency

There is always a hurry to finish the task at hand. This is extended even to day-to-day routine activities such as eating, bathing. Speech is usually hurried and the psychomotor activity is often increased.

Excessive Competitiveness and Hostility

There is a need to always win, with mistrust for other people's motives. Rage ensues, if the person is interrupted from achieving an objective.

Overall, there is a chronic struggle to achieve (or complete) a large number of tasks, working against the limits of time available and/or other people in the surrounding environment. In contrast, *Type B behaviour* is just the opposite, characterised by a relaxed unhurried attitude and less vigorous attempts to achieve a goal.

Some studies report that persons with Type B personality are paradoxically more successful than those with Type A personality. It is important to note that not all patients with CAD present with Type A personality traits.

Treatment

As persons with Type A behaviour are usually aware of presence of these personality traits, they may come for treatment on their own, or may need treatment after CAD has occurred. One or more of the following methods may be used.

1. Relaxation techniques: This is one of the most important methods aimed at reducing the basal generalised anxiety or inner sense of restlessness. The common techniques include:
   i. Jacobson's progressive muscular relaxation (PMR) technique
   ii. Yoga
   iii. Autohypnosis
   iv. Transcendental meditation
   v. Biofeedback.

2. Behaviour modification techniques.
3. Individual psychotherapy, usually cognitive behaviour therapy.
4. Group therapy.

Post-cardiac Surgery Delirium

This is a condition similar to ICU (Intensive care unit) syndrome. A fairly common disorder, its onset typically occurs after 24-48 hours of surgery. The patients, who develop post-surgery delirium, can sometimes be the ones who are most fearful before the surgery.

Many causes have been attributed for delirium, which include:

1. Cardiac status.
2. Presence of preoperative, subclinical organic brain disease.
3. Restrictive environment of the ICU/CCU, with isolation.
4. Electrolyte imbalance.
5. Preoperative anxiety, fearfulness, depression or denial.

Probably the condition is aetiologically multifactorial and should be treated as a type of delirium (see Chapter 4).

Treatment

1. Preoperative measures.
   i. Allaying the anxiety and fears of the patient.
   ii. Treatment of depression, if present.
   iii. Easy access to clocks and windows in ICU/CCU, to keep the patient oriented in time.
   iv. Allowing a family member to stay near the patient.
2. Treatment of delirium as described in Chapter 4.

Since delirium can be life threatening, as patients can take out IV lines, catheters or other 'life-lines' and can jump down from balcony or window, urgent treatment is often needed. Small doses of benzodiazepines (such as Diazepam or Lorazepam) or antipsychotics (such as Haloperidol or Risperidone) can be used orally or parenterally. Later the patient can be switched to low dose oral haloperidol or risperidone till recovery from delirium occurs.

Anticholinergic medication should not routinely be added to antipsychotics, as it may actually worsen the delirium. However, it may be needed if there are any significant extrapyramidal adverse effects present.

PSYCHIATRY IN MEDICINE

About one-third to two-third of medical outpatients may have primary or associated psychiatric disorders. If minor psychological and social problems are also taken into consideration, this number would be even larger. Since these patients may benefit from a psychiatric referral, psychiatrists are becoming increasingly involved in treatment of medical and surgical patients. In fact a whole new branch of consultation-liaison psychiatry has sprung up in the last few decades.

Consultation-liaison psychiatry is an area of clinical psychiatry which includes diagnostic, therapeutic, teaching and research activities of psychiatrists in the non-psychiatric parts of the hospital.

The common reasons for a psychiatric referral include:

1. Suicidal attempt, ideation or threat.
2. Grossly 'abnormal' behaviour disturbing the inpatient setting.
3. Presence of disorders related to alcohol or substance abuse/dependence such as severe withdrawal symptoms.
4. Organic brain syndromes.
5. Psychosomatic disorders.
6. Psychological reaction to medical illness.
7. Uncertain diagnosis (No medical illness can be found despite the presence of significant symptoms).
8. Manipulative or difficult or hostile patient.
9. Psychiatric side-effects of drugs.
10. Patient is unable to manage his or her own affairs.
11. Presence of severe primary psychiatric disorder(s).

A large number of medical illnesses can present with psychiatric symptomatology. It is important to keep in mind the possibility of a secondary mental disorder, i.e. a psychiatric disorder which is caused

Table 12.3: Physical Illness and Psychopathology

	Physical Illness	Psychiatric Symptomatology (Not all symptoms are present in one patient)
1.	Hyperthyroidism (Thyrotoxicosis)	Anxiety, depression (with apathetic hyperthyroidism), impairment of higher mental functions, paranoid disorder, delirium (with thyroid storm), mania, schizophreniform disorder, organic mental disorder
2.	Hypothyroidism (Myxoedema)	Apathy and lethargy, memory impairment, slow thinking, poor attention span, irritable mood, paranoid ideation, severe depressive episode, dementia, *myxoedema madness*
3.	Hyperadrenalism (Cushing's syndrome)	Depression, with paranoid ideation, generalised anxiety, psychosis with somatic delusions
4.	Adrenal cortical deficiency (Addison's disease)	Depression, with paranoid deficiency ideation, delirium (toxic psychosis), stupor
5.	Hyperpituitarism (Acromegaly)	Apathy, depression, anxiety
6.	Hypopituitarism (Simmond's disease)	Depression with memory disturbances, hypersomnia, delirium, stupor or coma
7.	Hyperparathyroidism	Depression, delirium (with *parathyroid crises*), coma (following recurrent seizures), early dementia
8.	Hypoparathyroidism	Delirium (particularly in postoperative cases), dementia (in idiopathic hypoparathyroidism), depression (with partial parathyroid insufficiency), mental retardation (especially in pseudo-hypoparathyroidism and pseudo-pseudo-hypoparathyroidism), 'pseudoneurosis'
9.	Phaeochromocytoma	Anxiety and panic attacks
10.	Acute intermittent porphyria	Acute anxiety, severe excitement or psychomotor withdrawal, conversion symptoms, schizophreniform disorder (rare), stupor or coma (rare)
11.	AIDS (Acquired immunodeficiency syndrome)	Anxiety, depression, delirium, dementia (AIDS-dementia complex), organic catatonia, adjustment disorder, suicidal behaviour, delusional disorder
12.	Systemic lupus erythematosus (SLE)	Depression, delirium (toxic psychosis), steroid psychosis (iatrogenic), schizophreniform disorder (uncommon)
13.	Hepatolenticular degeneration (Wilson's disease)	Personality changes (slow and insidious), mental retardation (in early onset), dementia (in late onset), schizophreniform disorder (can become chronic), antisocial behaviour, with rapid mood swings, poor impulse control and aggressive behaviour
14.	Multiple sclerosis	Euphoria or depression, histrionic personality traits, conversion and/or dissociation symptoms, dementia (if of long duration)
15.	Parkinsonism	Depression, dementia, paranoid features
16.	Pancreatic carcinoma	Severe depression
17.	Progressive supra-nuclear palsy (PSP)	Depression, dementia

by an underlying physical disease. Some important physical illnesses with their commonly presenting psychiatric symptoms are listed in Table 12.3.

In addition, a large number of physical disorders such as auto-immune disorders; infections; nutritional deficiencies (particularly pellagra, pernicious anaemia, beriberi); malignancies; alcohol and drug abuse; side-effects or toxicity of many medications; metabolic and water and electrolyte disturbances (and many others) may present with psychiatric symptomatology either alone (especially in initial stages) or with other physical signs and symptoms. Some of these have been mentioned under the causes of organic mental disorders.

GRIEF

Grief is the normal response of an individual to the loss of a loved object. An "object" (psychological speaking) can include a close relative or a friend, material values or non-material things such as reputation and self-esteem.

Grief is a universal phenomenon which is usually transient and self-limiting. Uncomplicated grief is not a psychiatric disorder and does not usually require any psychiatric treatment. However, as physicians (and psychiatrists) are sometimes called to intervene in severe cases with complications, the condition is discussed under this chapter.

Bowlby (1961) described three phases of the behaviour response to loss of a loved object:

i. protest,
ii. despair, and
iii. detachment.

Following the loss, there is often a state of shock. The grieved person feels a sense of bewilderment or numbness, or may completely deny the loss. Although most commonly this state lasts for a few hours, sometimes it may extend up to 2 weeks. This period may depend on individual characteristics such as meaning of loss, personality factors and suddenness of loss. When the full extent of loss is realised, various physical and mental symptoms appear. These include repeated sighing and crying, difficulty in breathing, choking sensation, weakness, poor concentration and poor appetite. These symptoms usually last for 4-6 weeks but may sometimes extend up to 6 months.

Preoccupation with the memory of the deceased is a characteristic feature. This is associated with vivid mental images, vivid dreams and idealisation of the deceased (often ignoring negative qualities). These preoccupations are usually of a comforting nature. This may be associated with a 'sense of presence' of the deceased in the surroundings and a misinterpretation of voices and faces of others as that of the lost person. Rarely, fleeting hallucinations may occur.

The grieved person often becomes depressed (Table 12.4) and may become somewhat withdrawn socially. Guilt feelings, hostility towards others, panic attacks, sense of futility, tiredness, neglect of work and self, insomnia and suicidal ideas may occur. The person may identify with the deceased, sometimes even taking on the deceased's qualities, mannerisms and characteristics. Finally, a period of reorganisation sets in and readjustment to the environment occurs.

Grief has been classified by Gurmeet Singh in to normal grief and morbid grief reaction. Morbid grief has been further divided in to pathological and complicated grief reactions.

Pathological Grief Reaction

When there is an exaggeration of one or more symptoms of normal grief, or the duration becomes prolonged beyond 6 months without spontaneous recovery, grief becomes *morbid*.

Table 12.4: Grief and Depression

Features		Grief	Severe Depression
1.	Identification with the deceased	Normal	Abnormal
2.	Ambivalence	Less	More
3.	Suicidal ideas	Rare	Common
4.	Global worthlessness	Rare	Common
5.	Self-blame for loss	Limited	Global
6.	Response evoked from others	Empathy; Sympathy	Annoyance; Irritation
7.	Self-limited	Usually	May not be
8.	Response to assurance	Usually good	Usually Not as good
9.	Vulnerability to physical illness	Increased	Increased
10.	Response to Antidepressants	Poor	Good

The various subtypes are:

i. chronic grief (duration more than 6 months);
ii. delayed grief (onset after 2 weeks of loss);
iii. inhibited grief (denial of loss);
iv. excessive anxiety, guilt, anger or religiosity grief;
v. identification with the deceased;
vi. over-idealisation of the deceased; and
vii. anniversary reactions (grief reaction on death anniversary).

Complicated Grief Reaction

Here, the grief is complicated by specific neurotic or psychotic illness, in addition to grief reaction symptoms. The various subtypes described include hysterical, phobic, obsessive-compulsive, manic or acute psychotic episode.

Treatment

1. Normal grief does not require any psychiatric treatment. Occasionally, mild anxiolytic or hypnotic may be needed for short-term use.

2. In morbid and (especially) complicated grief, medication may be needed depending on the presenting clinical features.

3. The emphasis should be on:

   i. Helping the person face the loss by counteracting denial.
   ii. Ventilation of feelings (catharsis).
   iii. Encouraging presence of significant others.
   iv. Bringing together similarly grieved persons, to encourage communication, share experiences of the loss and to offer companionship, and social and emotional support. In some countries (such as UK), referral to CRUSE counselling is often helpful. There are now some organisations providing help in some parts of India, for example, Sangath Bereavement Service (in Goa); Courage-India and Can-Support (for cancer related bereavement counselling).
   v. Encouragement of goal-directed activities, in a supportive manner.

Chapter 13

Mental Retardation

NORMAL CHILD DEVELOPMENT

For understanding behavioural and psychological problems of childhood, it is essential to know the normal patterns of child development. Although no two children are alike, there are general similarities in the mental and physical development of all normal children. A newborn human infant is probably the most helpless of all mammalian infants, and needs much more time to become self-dependent.

The normal development of a child can be divided into four major areas (these are modified after the Denver Development Screening Test, DDST).

1. Motor behaviour.
2. Adaptive behaviour.
3. Language, and
4. Personal and social behaviour.

As normal children cross these milestones or developmental levels at nearly expected age limits (within a few months' range) it is best to describe these developmental changes as milestones. In addition to these milestones, there are other developmental parameters such as height, weight, activity level and general health which have an important bearing on the development of a child. These milestones should not be seen as rigid set of dates and slight delays from these milestone dates is not abnormal. Statistically only those values, which are outside two standard deviations from the population mean are considered abnormal. However, *statistical abnormality* is not always the same as *clinical abnormality*.

INTELLECTUAL DEVELOPMENT

Intellectual development goes hand-in-hand with the development of physical and behavioural characteristics. According to Jean Piaget, it can be divided into the following stages.

Sensori-Motor Stage

This stage extends from birth to 2 years of age, and is characterised by:
  i. Actions related to sucking, orality and assimilation of objects.
 ii. Ability to think of only one thought at a time.
iii. Inanimate objects are given human qualities.
 iv. 'Out of sight' means ceasing to exist.

Concrete Thinking Stage

This stage lasts from 2 years to 7 years of life, and is characterised by:
  i. Egocentric thought with a unique logic of its own, involving a limited point of view and lacking introspection.
 ii. Inability to generalise from specific events and to specify from general events.

Abstract or Conceptual Thinking Stage

This stage begins at 7 years of age and lasts till 11 years of age, although it may be said to continue throughout life. This is characterised by:
  i. Ability to focus on several dimensions of a problem at one time, mentally.

Table 13.1: Normal Developmental Milestones

Age	Developmental Milestones	Age	Developmental Milestones
1. Motor Behaviour		1½ years	Makes a tower of 3-4 cubes; Scribbles spontaneously, imitating writing; Sometimes may draw a vertical line
< 4 weeks	Moves head laterally in prone position		
4 weeks	Momentarily lifts head when prone		
3 months	Head-holding; Lifts head to 90° when prone	2 years	Turns one page of a book at one time; Makes a tower of 6-7 cubes; Draws (copies) a horizontal line
5 months	Sits with support; Rolls over		
6 months	Lifts head and upper chest with support of extended arms	3 years	Makes a tower of 9-10 cubes; Makes a 3-cube bridge; Draws (copies) a circle.
8 months	Sits steadily with straight back; Crawls; Early stepping movements when feet are placed on ground, with support	4 years	Draws (copies) a cross.
		5 years	Draws (copies) a square; Draws (copies) a recognisable man
10 months	Pulls from supine to sitting and sitting to standing; Stands holding furniture; Cruises around; Stands without support momentarily; Creeps on ground without support of abdomen	6 years	Draws (copies) a triangle
		7 years	Draws (copies) a diamond (Fig. 13.1)
		8 years	Draws (copies) the following figures (Figs 13.2 and 13.3)
14-15 months	Walks well without support; Walks backwards and sideways	9 years	Draws (copies) the following figure (Fig. 13.4)
2 years	Runs well; Climbs stairs alone; Kicks a large ball; Throws a ball overhead	**3. Language**	
		4 weeks	Turns head and responds to sound of a bell; Vocalises (apart from crying)
2½ years	Walks on tip-toes		
3 years	Climbs stairs in a coordinated manner, with alternate feet going up the staircase; Rides a tricycle; Makes a broad jump; Jumps in place	3 months	Laughs aloud
4 years	Stands on one foot for 5 seconds		
5 years	Heel-to-toe walk; Jumps on one foot		
2. Adaptive Behaviour (includes fine motor movements)			
4 weeks	Momentarily regards close moving objects, close to mid-line		
3 months	Follows the moving objects, even away from mid-line; converges and focuses		
4-5 months	Grasps objects crudely; Reaches to grasp		
6 months	Transfer objects from one hand to other		
9-10 months	Claps hands and matches two hand-held objects in mid line; Thumb-finger grasp		
1 year	Gives hand-held objects to mother, when asked; Turns 2-3 pages of a book at one time		

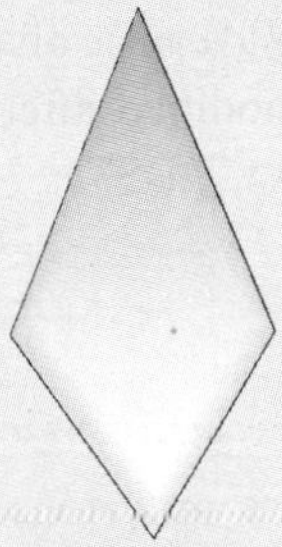

Fig. 13.1

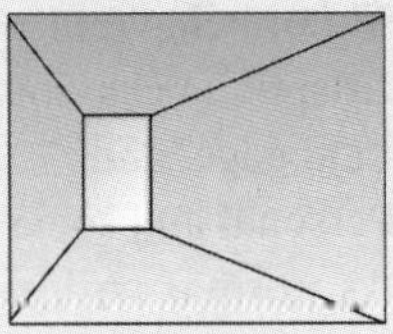

Fig. 13.2

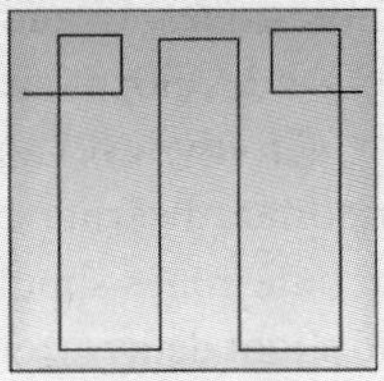

Fig. 13.3

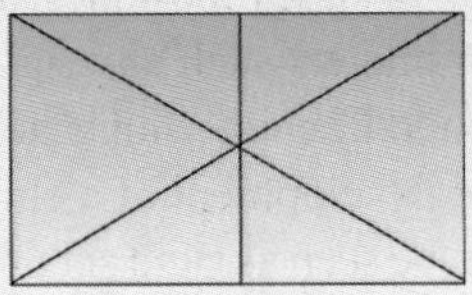

Fig. 13.4

Contd...

Contd...

9 months	Speaks mama, dada, m-m-m, ah (and other vowel sounds); Responds to name	3 months	Recognises mother
10 months	Understands spoken speech to some extent, e.g. where is 'mama'?	6 months	Takes foot to mouth; Smiles back at mirror-image of self
1-1¼ years	Uses 3-5 words meaningfully	9 months	Responds to social play; Resists pulling away of toy and tries to reach for it; Holds milk-bottle and eats a biscuit all by oneself
18 months	About 10 words spoken including name		
2 years	Combines 2 different words; Names at least one object in picture; Points to at least one named body part; Simple sentences made	1½ years	Feeds oneself with a spoon, with little spilling; Mimics actions of others; Pulls a toy with a string; Toilet training started
3 years	Uses plurals; Has a fairly good vocabulary	2 years	Wears simple garments, socks and shoes
		3 years	Unbuttons buttons; Buckles shoes; Can dress and undress, with help
5 years	Colour naming accurately (primary colours); Defines words		
4. Personal and Social Behaviour		4 years	Buttons the dress well; Washes own face; Plays with other children easily; Separates from mother with little difficulty.
4 weeks	Regards face intently		
2-3 months	Social smile	5 years	Dresses without supervision.

ii. The thought process is flexible and reversible.

iii. Ability of abstraction, i.e. ability to generalise from specific and ability to find similarities and differences among specific objects.

Adolescent Thinking or Formal Operational Stage

This stage begins at 11 years of age and continues life-long. This is characterised by:

i. Ability to imagine the possibilities inherent in a situation, thus making the thought comprehensive.

ii. Ability to develop complete abstract hypotheses and to test them.

By the end of adolescence, the individual's intellectual ability is nearly completely developed, although learning and intellectual growth go-on throughout the lifespan of individual.

MENTAL RETARDATION

One to three percent of the general population has mental retardation. In some countries (such as UK), the word *learning disability* is used instead to avoid the pejorative connotations associated with the word *mental retardation*. However, in this book, the term mental retardation is retained as it is the preferred term in both ICD-10 and DSM-IV-TR.

Mental retardation is defined as significantly sub-average general intellectual functioning, associated with significant deficit or impairment in adaptive functioning, which manifests during the developmental period (before 18 years of age). General intellectual functioning is usually assessed on a standardised intelligence test with significantly sub-average intelligence as two standard deviations below the mean (usually an IQ of below 70), whilst adaptive behaviour is the person's ability to meet responsibilities of social, personal, occupational and interpersonal areas of life, appropriate to age, sociocultural and educational background. Adaptive behaviour is measured by clinical interview and standardised assessment scales.

Very often, it is assumed that the persons with mental retardation constitute a homogenous group. This is however not true. Persons with mental retardation vary in their behavioural, psychological, physical and social characteristics as much as the so-called 'normal' general population does.

Another common error is taking the IQ score as the measure of someone's intelligence. It should be remembered that a person with mental retardation must have a deficit in both general intellectual functioning and adaptive behaviour.

A classification of mental retardation on the basis of IQ (Intelligence Quotient, which is equal to mental age, i.e. MA, divided by chronological age, i.e. CA, multiplied by 100; i.e. IQ = MA/CA × 100), is provided in Table 13.2.

Mild Mental Retardation

This is the commonest type of mental retardation, accounting for 85-90% of all cases. The diagnosis is made usually later than in other types of mental retardation.

In the preschool period (before 5 years of age), these children often develop like other normal children, with very little deficit. Later, they often progress up to the 6th class (grade) in school and can achieve vocational and social self-sufficiency with a little support. Only under stressful conditions or in the presence of an associated disease, supervised care may be needed.

This group has been referred to as 'educable' in a previous educational classification of mental retardation.

Moderate Mental Retardation

About 10% of all persons with mental retardation have an IQ between 35 and 50. In the educational classification, this group was earlier called as 'trainable', although many of these persons can also be educated.

In the early years, despite a poor social awareness, these children can learn to speak. Often, they drop out of school after the 2nd class (grade). They can be trained to support themselves by performing semi-skilled or unskilled work under supervision. A mild stress may destabilise them from their adaptation; thus they work best in supervised occupational settings.

Table 13.2: Classification of Mental Retardation by IQ

Mental Retardation Level	IQ Range
1. Mild	50-70*
2. Moderate	35-50*
3. Severe	20-35*
4. Profound	<20*

(*As intelligence tests employed to measure IQ generally have an error of measurement of about 5 points, each figure means ± 5 points, e.g. IQ of 50 means an IQ of 50 ± 5, depending on the adaptive behaviour).

Severe Mental Retardation

Severe mental retardation is often recognised early in life with poor motor development (significantly delayed developmental milestones) and absent or markedly delayed speech and other communication skills.

Later in life, elementary training in personal health care can be given and they can be taught to talk. At best, they can perform simple tasks under close supervision. In the earlier educational classification, they were called as 'dependent'.

Profound Mental Retardation

This group accounts for about 1-2% of all persons with mental retardation. The associated physical disorders, which often contribute to mental retardation, are common in this subtype.

The achievement of developmental milestones is markedly delayed. They often need nursing care or 'life support' under a carefully planned and structured environment (such as group homes or residential placements).

Aetiology

Mental retardation is a condition which is caused not only by biological factors but also by psychosocial factors. In more than one third of cases, no cause can be found despite an extensive search.

Some of the common causes of mental retardation are listed in Table 13.3. There appears to be a

Table 13.3: Some Causes of Mental Retardation

1. **Genetic (probably in 5% of cases)**
   i. Chromosomal abnormalities (such as Down's syndrome, Fragile-X syndrome, Turner's syndrome, Klinefelter's syndrome)
   ii. Inborn errors of metabolism, involving amino-acids (phenylketonuria, homo-cystinuria, Hartnup's disease), lipids (Tay-Sachs disease, Gaucher's disease, Niemann-Pick disease), carbohydrates (galactosaemia, glycogen storage diseases), purines (Lesch-Nyhan syndrome), and mucopolysaccharides (Hurler's disease, Hunter's disease, Sanfillipo's disease).
   iii. Single-gene disorders (such as tuberous sclerosis, neurofibromatosis, dystrophia myotonica)
   iv. Cranial anomalies (such as microcephaly)
2. **Perinatal causes (probably in 10% of cases)**
   i. Infections (such as rubella, syphilis, toxoplasmosis, cytomegalo-inclusion body disease)
   ii. Prematurity
   iii. Birth trauma
   iv. Hypoxia
   v. Intrauterine growth retardation (IUGR)
   vi. Kernicterus
   vii. Placental abnormalities
   viii. Drugs during first trimester.
3. **Acquired physical disorders in childhood** (probably in 2-5% of cases)
   i. Infections, especially encephalopathies
   ii. Cretinism
   iii. Trauma
   iv. Lead poisoning
   v. Cerebral palsy.
4. **Sociocultural causes** (probably in 15% of cases)
   i. Deprivation of sociocultural stimulation.
5. **Psychiatric disorders** (probably in 1-2% of cases)
   i. Pervasive developmental disorders (such as Infantile autism)
   ii. Childhood onset schizophrenia.

preponderance of males among people with mental retardation. Some important causes of mental retardation are discussed below.

Phenylketonuria

An inborn error of metabolism, it accounts for about 0.5-1% of all cases of mental retardation. It is an autosomal recessive (AR) disorder, most prevalent in North Europe. The basic defect is absence or inactivity of phenylalanine hydroxylase, a hepatic enzyme, responsible for catalysis of phenylalanine to paratyrosine conversion (Fig. 13.5). It results in marked increase in blood phenylalanine levels and its metabolites. There is also a decrease in 5-HT, epinephrine and norepinephrine levels in brain.

The majority of patients with phenylketonuria have severe mental retardation. The associated features may include short stature, fair complexion with coarse features, widely spaced upper incisors, eczematous dermatitis, epilepsy, hyperactivity, poor communication skills and poor motor coordination. EEG may be abnormal in up to 80% of cases.

However, the physical appearance may be normal and diagnosis made only after investigations, which include:

1. *Ferric chloride test:* Addition of $FeCl_3$ to urine gives a green colour in patients with phenylketonuria. This results from the presence of phenylpyruvic acid in urine. This test may be positive in other aminoacidurias as well.
2. *Guthrie's test:* This involves a bacteriological procedure for measurement of phenylalanine levels in blood.
3. *Chromatography:* An early diagnosis is clearly of paramount importance, since mental retardation of phenylketonuria is preventable, if diagnosis is made early in life. The treatment consists of a low phenylalanine diet, best started before the age of 6 months and usually continued up to 5-6 years of age. The diet should not be completely devoid of phenylalanine, as it is an essential amino-acid and its absence may itself be hazardous.

Other disorders which cause mental retardation and are preventable by dietary treatment, include:

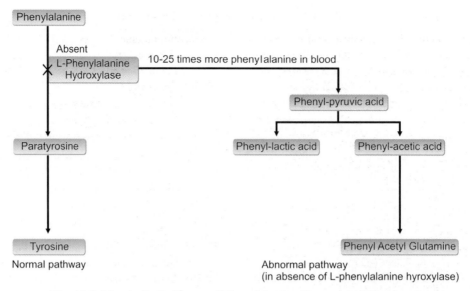

Fig. 13.5: Metabolic Pathways of Phenylalanine: Normal and Abnormal

1. Homocystinuria: The treatment is with methionine-free diet.
2. Galactosaemia: The treatment is with lactose and galactose-free diet.
3. Maple syrup urine disease (Menkes' disease): The treatment is with a diet low in leucine, iso-leucine and valine.
4. Hyperprolinaemia: The treatment is with low proline diet.
5. Leucine-sensitive hypoglycaemia: The treatment is with low-protein, leucine-deficient diet.
6. Fructose intolerance: Fructose, sucrose and other sugars should be replaced in diet.

Down's syndrome

Down's syndrome or mongolism occurs in 1 out of every 700 births. It accounts for about 10% of children with moderate to severe mental retardation.

There are three types of chromosomal aberrations in Down's syndrome:

1. Trisomy-21 is the commonest where karyotype of mother is normal.
2. Mosaicism, with both normal and trisomic cells present.
3. Translocation between chromosome 21 and 15. Thus, the total number of chromosomes is 46, in spite of 3 chromosomes at 21. The translocation is inherited, with asymptomatic carriers containing only 45 chromosomes.

The most important risk factor is higher maternal age (>35 years), with a risk of 1:50 after the age of 45. The clinical features may include generalised hypotonia, hyperflexibility, round face, oblique palpebral fissures, a flat nasal bridge, short ears, loose skin folds at the nape of neck, persistent epicanthic folds, single palmar crease, high arched palate, thick tongue, incurved little fingers and Brushfield spots on irides.

Congenital heart disease (in about 35% of cases), gastrointestinal anomalies (in about 10%), chronic serous otitis media (in >50%), hypothyroidism and Alzheimer's disease (in 30's and 40's), epilepsy (in about 10%), ocular disorders, reduced fertility and reduced life span (often due to antecedent complications like infections) are common.

The diagnosis is made by clinical assessment and chromosomal studies. At present, there is no effective pharmacological treatment available.

Tuberous Sclerosis

This is an autosomal dominant disorder, also known as *epiloia*. It occurs in about 1:15,000 persons in general population. The characteristic clinical features are known as Vogt's triad, which consist of:

i. Mental retardation, ranging from mild to severe.
ii. Convulsions.
iii. *Adenoma sebaceum*, present on the face (usually red) and also on the rest of the body (usually brownish white). The distribution on the face is usually of butterfly type.

Multiple glial nodules appear throughout the cerebral cortex and cerebellum. Tumours in the various other parts of the body (e.g. rhabdomyoma of heart, mixed tumours of kidney, retinal nerve tumours) may occur. In addition, periosteal thickening, pulmonary fibrosis, renal failure and cardiac failure can be manifested.

There is no effective treatment at present except symptomatic management of seizures and other systemic manifestations.

Fragile-X Syndrome

This is second commonest chromosomal aberration causing mental retardation. Occurring in about 1 out of 1000 live births, it is diagnosed on chromosomal studies. The characteristic presence of a fragile site at the tip of the long arm of X-chromosome appears as a constriction.

Clinically, the person may have a short stature, large head, large 'bat' ears, long face and big sized testes (in males after puberty). The associated psychiatric disorders, like attention deficit disorder, may be present.

Cretinism

Goitrous cretinism is a common cause of mental retardation in India. It is endemic in iodine-deficient areas such as the goitrous Himalayan belt. Early recognition and treatment is essential, as it is a preventable cause of mental retardation.

The clinical features include goitre, dwarfism, coarse skin, ossification delays, apathy, hoarseness of voice, large tongue, subnormal temperature, pot belly, anaemia, hypotonia of muscles, hypertelorism and mental retardation, which may be severe to profound.

Cerebral Palsy

This is a syndrome consisting of a conglomeration of perinatal disorders of various aetiologies, presenting with a common feature of paralysis of limbs. The paralysis may be monoplegia, hemiplegia, paraplegia, triplegia or quadriplegia. It is usually of upper motor neuron type, presenting with spasticity.

The extrapyramidal symptoms may be present and seizures may occur often. Mental retardation is present in about 70% of all cases, and ranges from mild to severe.

Diagnosis

The diagnosis is made by the following steps:

1. History.
2. General physical examination.
3. Detailed neurological examination.
4. Mental status examination, for the assessment of associated psychiatric disorders and the clinical assessment of the level of intelligence.
5. Investigations.
   i. Routine investigations.
   ii. Urine test, e.g. for phenylketonuria, maple syrup urine disease.
   iii. EEG, especially in presence of seizures.
   iv. Blood levels, for inborn errors of metabolism.
   v. Chromosomal studies, e.g. in Down's syndrome, prenatal (by amniocentesis or chorionic villus biopsy) and postnatal.
   vi. CT scan or MRI scan of brain, e.g. in tuberous sclerosis, focal seizures, unexplained neurological syndromes, anomalies of skull configuration, severe or profound mental retardation without any apparent cause, toxoplasmosis.
   vii. Thyroid function tests, particularly when cretinism is suspected.
   viii. Liver function tests, e.g. in mucopolysaccharidosis.
6. Psychological tests

The commonly used tests for measurement of intelligence include:

i. Seguin form board test.
ii. Stanford-Binet, Binet-Simon or Binet-Kamath tests.
iii. Wechsler Intelligence Scale for Children (WISC) for 6½ to 16 years of age.
iv. Wechsler's Preschool and Primary Scale of Intelligence (WPPSI) for 4 to 6½ years of age.
v. Bhatia's battery of performance tests.
vi. Raven's progressive matrices (coloured, standard and advanced).

The tests used for the assessment of adaptive behaviour include:

i. Vineland Social Maturity Scale (VSMS).
ii. Denver Development Screening Test (DDST).
iii. Gessell's Development Scale.

Differential Diagnosis

The diagnosis of mental retardation is usually simple. However, while making this diagnosis, the following conditions must be kept in mind, as they can be and are many times mistaken for mental retardation, with disastrous results.

1. Deaf and dumb (This possibility must always be ruled out either by clinical examination and/or by audiometry).
2. Deprived children, with inadequate social stimulation (Although this can also cause mental retardation, many children become 'normal' intellectually on providing adequate stimulation).
3. Isolated speech defects.
4. Psychiatric disorders (such as infantile autism, childhood onset schizophrenia).
5. Systemic disorders (without mental retardation but with physical debilitation).
6. Epilepsy.

Management

The management of mental retardation can be discussed under prevention at primary, secondary and tertiary levels.

Primary Prevention

This consists of:

1. Improvement in socioeconomic condition of society at large, aiming at elimination of under-stimulation, malnutrition, prematurity and perinatal factors.
2. Education of lay public, aiming at removal of the misconceptions about individuals with mental retardation.
3. Medical measures for good perinatal medical care to prevent infections, trauma, excessive use of medications, malnutrition, obstetric complications, and diseases of pregnancy.
4. Universal immunisation of children with BCG, polio, DPT, and MMR.
5. Facilitating research activities to study the causes of mental retardation and their treatment.
6. Genetic counselling in at-risk parents, e.g. in phenylketonuria, Down's syndrome.

Secondary Prevention

1. Early detection and treatment of preventable disorders, e.g. phenylketonuria (low phenylalanine diet), maple syrup urine disease (low branched amino-acid diet) and others as discussed earlier; hypothyroidism (thyroxine).
2. Early detection of handicaps in sensory, motor or behavioural areas with early remedial measures and treatment.
3. Early treatment of correctable disorders, e.g. infections (antibiotics), skull configuration anomalies (surgical correction).
4. Early recognition of presence of mental retardation. A delay in diagnosis may cause unfortunate delay in rehabilitation.
5. As far as possible, individuals with mental retardation should be integrated with normal individuals in society, and any kind of segregation or discrimination should be actively avoided. They should be provided with facilities to enable them to reach their own full potential. However, there is a role of special schools for those with more severe mental retardation.

Tertiary Prevention

1. Adequate treatment of psychological and behavioural problems.
2. Behaviour modification, using the principles of positive and negative reinforcement.
3. Rehabilitation in vocational, physical, and social areas, commensurate with the level of handicap.
4. Parental counselling is extremely important to lessen the levels of stress, teaching them to adapt to the situation, enlisting them (especially parents) as co-therapists, and encouraging formation of parents' or carers' organisation (s) and self-help groups.
5. Institutionalisation or residential care may be needed for individuals with profound mental retardation.

6. Legislation: In 1995, the 'Persons with Disability Act' came in to being in India. This act envisages mandatory support for prevention, early detection, education, employment, and other facilities for the welfare of persons with disabilities in general, and mental retardation in particular. This Act provides for affirmative action and non-discrimination of persons with disabilities.

In 1999, the 'National Trust Act' came in to force. This Act proposes to involve the parents of mentally challenged persons and voluntary organisations in setting up and running a variety of services and facilities with governmental funding.

Chapter 14

Child Psychiatry

CLASSIFICATION IN CHILD PSYCHIATRY

The various psychiatric disorders seen in childhood ('disorders of psychological development' and 'behavioural and emotional disorders with onset usually occurring in childhood and adolescence') are discussed under the following headings:

1. Mental retardation
2. Specific developmental disorders
3. Pervasive developmental disorders
4. Hyperkinetic disorders
5. Conduct disorders
6. Tic disorders
7. Enuresis and encopresis
8. Speech disorders
9. Habit disorders
10. Other disorders.

MENTAL RETARDATION

Mental retardation (or learning disability) has been discussed in Chapter 13.

SPECIFIC DEVELOPMENTAL DISORDERS

Mental retardation is a generalised impairment in nearly all areas of functioning. In contrast, specific developmental disorders are characterised by an inadequate development in usually one specific area of functioning.

The deficit in functioning may be in scholastic skills, speech and language, and motor skills. These may include reading (*developmental reading disorder*), language (*developmental language disorder*), arithmetic or mathematics (*developmental arithmetic or mathematics disorder*), articulation (*developmental articulation disorder* or *phonological disorder*), or coordination (*developmental coordination disorder*). Sometimes, more than one developmental disorder is present.

All developmental disorders either cause impairment in academic functioning at school, especially when language is affected, or impairment in the daily activities. A large majority of these children have an underlying cerebral disorder. Boys are usually more affected than girls.

Before making a diagnosis of specific developmental disorder, it is important to keep in mind the mental age, IQ, sociocultural background, schooling, impairment(s) in vision and hearing, or any neurological deficit.

Specific Reading Disorder

It is also called as *developmental reading disorder* or *dyslexia*.

The child presents with a serious delay in learning to read which is evident from the early years. The problems may include omissions, distortions, or substitutions of words, long hesitations, reversal of words, or simply slow reading.

Writing and spelling are also impaired. It is important to differentiate the disorder from scholastic backwardness; therefore a proper assessment is mandatory.

Specific Arithmetic Disorder

It is also called as *developmental arithmetic disorder* or *developmental mathematic disorder* or *dyscalculia*.

The child presents with arithmetic abilities well below the level expected for the mental age (below par). The problems may include failure to understand simple mathematical concepts, failure to recognise mathematical signs or numerical symbols, difficulty in carrying out mathematical manipulations, and difficulty in learning mathematical tables.

Specific Developmental Disorder of Speech and Language

It is also called as *developmental language disorder*, *developmental communication disorder*, or *dysphasia*.

There are three main types:

i. *Phonological disorder:* Also called as *dyslalia*, it is characterised by below par accuracy in the use of speech sounds despite normal language skills. The problems include severe articulation errors that make it difficult for others to understand the speech. Speech sounds or phonemes are omitted, distorted or substituted (e.g. wabbit for rabbit, ca for car, bu for blue).

ii. *Expressive language disorder:* It is characterised by a below par ability of using expressive speech. The problems include restricted vocabulary, difficulty in selecting appropriate words, and immature grammatical usage. Cluttering of speech may also be present.

iii. *Receptive language disorder:* The disorder often presents as a receptive-expressive language disorder and both receptive and expressive impairments are present together. The disorder is characterised by a below par understanding of language. Problems include failure to respond to simple instructions; it is obviously important to rule out deafness and pervasive developmental disorder.

Specific Developmental Disorder of Motor Function

It is also called as *motor skills disorder*, *developmental coordination disorder*, *clumsy child syndrome* or *motor dyspraxia*. It is characterised by poor coordination in daily activities of life, e.g. in dressing, walking, feeding, and playing. There is an inability to perform fine or gross motor tasks.

Treatment

The treatment of specific developmental disorders is based on learning theory principles and is behavioural in approach. It involves use of special remedial teaching, focusing on the underlying deficit (for example, perceptual motor training in motor skills disorder).

The treatment of common co-morbid emotional problems is often necessary. Parental education and counselling are important components of good management.

PERVASIVE DEVELOPMENTAL DISORDERS

Infantile autism was described for the first time by Leo Kanner in 1943 as 'autistic disturbance of affective contact'. This syndrome has variously been described as *autistic disorder*, *pervasive developmental disorder*, *childhood autism*, *childhood psychosis* and *pseudo-defective psychosis*.

This syndrome is more common (3-4 times) in males and has a prevalence rate of 0.4-0.5 per 1000 population. Although earlier it was thought to be commoner in upper socioeconomic classes, recent studies have failed to confirm this finding.

Typically, the onset occurs before the age of 2½ years though in some cases, the onset may occur later in childhood. Such cases are called as *childhood onset autism* or *childhood onset pervasive developmental disorder*. Autism occurring before or after 2½ years of age is not clinically very different.

Clinical Features

The characteristic features are:

1. *Autism* (marked impairment in reciprocal social and interpersonal interaction):
   i. Absent social smile.
   ii. Lack of eye-to-eye-contact.
   iii. Lack of awareness of others' existence or feelings; treats people as furniture.
   iv. Lack of attachment to parents and absence of separation anxiety.
   v. No or abnormal social play; prefers solitary games.
   vi. Marked impairment in making friends.
   vii. Lack of imitative behaviour.
   viii. Absence of fear in presence of danger.
2. *Marked impairment in language and non-verbal communication*
   i. Lack of verbal or facial response to sounds or voices; might be thought as deaf initially.
   ii. In infancy, absence of communicative sounds like babbling.
   iii. Absent or delayed speech (about half of autistic children never develop useful speech).
   iv. Abnormal speech patterns and content. Presence of echolalia, perseveration, poor articulation and pronominal reversal (I-You) is common.
   v. Rote memory is usually good.
   vi. Abstract thinking is impaired.
3. *Abnormal behavioural characteristics*
   i. Mannerisms.
   ii. Stereotyped behaviours such as head-banging, body-spinning, hand-flicking, lining-up objects, rocking, clapping, twirling, etc.
   iii. Ritualistic and compulsive behaviour.
   iv. Resistance to even the slightest change in the environment.
   v. Attachment may develop to inanimate objects.
   vi. Hyperkinesis is commonly associated.
4. *Mental retardation*
   Only about 25% of all children with autism have an IQ of more than 70. A large majority (more than 50%) of these children have moderate to profound mental retardation. There appears to be a correlation between severity of mental retardation, absence of speech and epilepsy in autism.
5. *Other features*
   i. Many children with autism particularly enjoy music.
   ii. In spite of the pervasive impairment of functions, certain islets of precocity or splinter functions may remain (called as *Idiot savant syndrome*). Examples of such splinter functions are prodigious rote memory or calculating ability, and musical abilities.
   iii. Epilepsy is common in children with an IQ of less than 50.

The course of infantile autism is usually chronic and only 1-2% become near normal in marital, social and occupational functioning. A large majority (about 70%) lead dependent lives.

Aetiology

Presently, the cause of infantile autism seems to be predominantly biological. Earlier reports of cold, 'refrigerator' mothers causing autism in their children have not been substantiated and have unnecessarily lead to undue distress to parents of children with autism.

The evidence for biological causation includes a higher than average history of perinatal CNS insult, EEG abnormalities, epilepsy, ventricular dilatation on brain imaging, increased serotonin (5-HT) levels in brain and/or neurophysiological abnormalities in some patients.

Treatment

The treatment consists of three modes of intervention which are often used together.

1. *Behaviour Therapy*
   i. Development of a regular routine with as few changes as possible.
   ii. Structured class room training, aiming at learning new material and maintenance of acquired learning.
   iii. Positive reinforcements to teach self-care skills.

iv. Speech therapy and/or sign language teaching.

v. Behavioural techniques to encourage interpersonal interactions.

2. *Psychotherapy*

Parental counselling and supportive psychotherapy can be very useful in allaying parental anxiety and guilt, and helping their active involvement in therapy. However, overstimulation of child should be avoided during treatment.

3. *Pharmacotherapy*

Drug treatment can be used for treatment of autism as well as for treatment of co-morbid epilepsy.

i. Haloperidol decreases dopamine levels in brain. It is believed to decrease hyperactivity and behavioural symptoms. Risperidone, an atypical antipsychotic, is helpful in some patients and is licensed in some countries for treatment of autism in children aged 5 and above. Both haloperidol and risperidone can cause extrapyramidal side-effects (EPSE), though usually more with haloperidol.

The starting dose for Risperidone is usually 0.25-0.5 mg (based on body weight), with a dose range of 0.02-0.06 mg/kg/day.

ii. Other drugs such as SSRIs, chlorpromazine, amphetamines, methysergide, imipramine, multi-vitamins and triiodothyronine have been tried with limited success and should be used only by the experts in the field.

iii. Anticonvulsant medication is used for the treatment of generalised or other seizures, if present.

OTHER PERVASIVE DEVELOPMENTAL DISORDERS

Childhood psychosis is a vague term which includes all psychotic illnesses occurring in childhood, such as infantile and childhood onset autism, childhood schizophrenia, mood disorders, and organic psychiatric disorders. This term has frequently been misused in the past, also meaning at times infantile autism alone. This is a term which is probably best dispensed with.

Schizophrenia, mood disorders and organic psychiatric disorders have a nearly similar picture in children as in adulthood. Sometimes, childhood onset schizophrenia may be mistaken for autism. The most important differentiating features are:

1. Delusions, formal thought disorder and hallucinations may be present in childhood-onset schizophrenia while they are always absent in infantile autism.

2. Typical age of onset of symptoms is before 2½ years in infantile autism while it is after 5-6 years in childhood onset schizophrenia.

3. Moderate to severe mental retardation and epilepsy are common in infantile autism while they are rare in childhood-onset schizophrenia. Mental retardation, if ever present, is usually of mild type.

Another type of childhood psychosis, called *Heller's syndrome* or *disintegrative psychosis*, has often been described in literature. Typically, the age of onset is between 3 to 5 years and the syndrome is characterised by a rapid downhill course, leading to deterioration and development of neurological deficits. This is really a 'rag-bag' category containing diverse organic brain syndromes of varying aetiologies (For example, some are caused by lipoid degeneration of ganglia in central nervous system). Prognosis is usually poor in this condition.

Two other syndromes with autistic features have been described; namely, Asperger's syndrome and Rett's syndrome.

Asperger's syndrome is characterised by autism without any significant delay in language or cognitive development (including intelligence). This syndrome occurs predominantly in boys (male : female ratio = 8:1). It probably represents mild cases of autism and has been also called as *high functioning autism*.

Rett's syndrome is a disorder which is only reported in girls so far. After an apparently normal early development and normal head circumference at birth, there is a deceleration of head growth between the age of 5 months and 30 months. There is also a loss of purposive hand movements and acquired fine motor manipulative skills between the same ages, with the subsequent development of stereotyped movements of hands (e.g. hand-wringing). Later, other movement disorders also develop and severe mental handicap is invariable.

ATTENTION DEFICIT DISORDER (HYPERKINETIC DISORDER)

This is a syndrome first described by Heinrich Hoff in 1854. Since then, it has been known by a variety of names such as *minimal brain dysfunction (MBD), hyperkinetic syndrome, Strauss syndrome, organic drivenness* and *minimal brain damage*.

A relatively common disorder, it occurs in about 3% of school age children. Males are 6-8 times more often affected. The onset occurs before the age of 7 years and a large majority of patients exhibit symptoms by the 4th year of age.

Attention deficit disorder (ADD) is of four clinical types: with hyperactivity, without hyperactivity, residual type, and with conduct disorder.

1. **Attention deficit disorder with hyperactivity (Hyperkinetic disorder):** This is the commonest type. The characteristic clinical features are:
   Poor attention span with distractibility
       i. Fails to finish the things started.
       ii. Shifts from one uncompleted activity to another.
       iii. Doesn't seem to listen.
       iv. Easily distracted by external stimuli.
       v. Often loses things.
   Hyperactivity
       i. Fidgety.
       ii. Difficulty in sitting still at one place for long.
       iii. Moving about here and there.
       iv. Talks excessively.
       v. Interference in other people's activities.
   Impulsivity
       i. Acts before thinking, on the spur of the moment.
       ii. Difficulty in waiting for turn at work or play.

2. **Attention deficit disorder without hyperactivity:** It is a rare disorder with similar clinical features, except hyperactivity.
3. **Residual type:** It is usually diagnosed in a patient in adulthood, with a past history of ADD and presence of a few residual features in adult life.
4. **Hyperkinetic disorder with conduct disorder (Hyperkinetic conduct disorder).**

Diagnosis

The diagnosis can be made on the basis of:
1. Teacher's school report (often the most reliable).
2. Parent's report.
3. Clinical examination (many children with hyperactivity may be able to sit still in the new setting of the hospital and thus the diagnosis may be missed).

Hyperactivity is also a common clinical symptom in mental retardation. Thus, mental retardation should always be excluded, before making a diagnosis of ADD.

Aetiology

Many factors, such as minimal brain damage, maturational lag, genetics, neurotransmitters (norepinephrine and dopamine) and early developmental psychodynamic factors have been incriminated. The cause is not yet known but it is more likely to be a biological factor than a purely psychosocial one, though a focus on both factors is important in the management of an individual patient.

Course

A large majority (about 80%) of patients improve on their own by the time of puberty, though a few (15-20%) may have persistent symptoms even in adulthood. Impulsivity and inattention are usually the most common residual features after puberty while hyperactivity often tends to remit.

ADD can also present in adulthood and Adult ADD is recognised by both ICD-10 and DSM-IV-TR. These includes graduates of childhood onset ADD which continue to have symptoms in adulthood and those who begin with symptoms for the first time in adulthood.

Treatment

The management of ADD consists of the following methods:

Pharmacotherapy

1. Stimulant medication: Dextro-amphetamine or dexamphetamine (2.5-20 mg/day) and methyl-phenidate (5-60 mg/day) have been traditionally used. Currently, Methylphenidate is the drug of choice in the treatment of ADD, with a high response rate. Methylphenidate is also available in sustained release formulations which are preferable due to improved treatment concordance and convenience of once a day dose.

   Both dexamphetamine and methylphenidate act on the reticular activating system, causing stimulation of the inhibitory influences on the cerebral cortex, thus decreasing hyperactivity and/or distractibility.

2. Others: When stimulant medication is not available or is not effective, other drugs can be used after careful individual consideration of the risks and benefits in the individual patient. These include clonidine, tricyclic antidepressants (such as imipramine), bupropion, venlafaxine, chlorpromazine, thioridazine, and lithium carbonate.

   Atomoxetine, a norepinephrine reuptake inhibitor, may be an alternative for children who do not respond to stimulants. The usual dose range is 0.5-1.2 mg/kg/day. Atomoxetine appears to be the drug of choice in adult ADD.

   Barbiturates are contraindicated in ADD as they increase hyperactivity.

Behaviour Modification

Counselling and Supportive Psychotherapy

Behaviour modification and counselling are very important in the successful management of ADD and can be used along with drug therapy.

CONDUCT DISORDERS

Conduct disorder is characterised by a persistent and significant pattern of conduct, in which the basic rights of others are violated or rules of society are not followed. The diagnosis is only made when the conduct is far in excess of the routine mischief of children and adolescents. The onset occurs much before 18 years of age, usually even before puberty.

The disorder is much more (about 5-10 times) common in males. In United States of America, about 10% of all male children under the age of 18 have conduct disorder.

According to ICD-10, there are four subtypes of conduct disorder:

1. Conduct disorder confined to the family context.
2. Unsocialised conduct disorder.
3. Socialised conduct disorder.
4. Oppositional defiant disorder.

   The characteristic clinical features include:

1. Frequent lying.
2. Stealing or robbery.
3. Running away from home and school.
4. Physical violence such as rape, fire-setting, assault or breaking-in, use of weapons.
5. Cruelty towards other people and animals.

   In the more common socialised (group) type of conduct disorder, the person claims loyalty to his or her group. The unsocialised (solitary) type is a more serious disorder with usually a severe underlying psychopathology. Earlier, the patients with conduct disorder were called as *juvenile delinquents*.

   Many patients of conduct disorder, especially socialised (group) type, go on to improve markedly and may lead well adjusted lives. Some others, especially those with severe symptomatology, have a more chronic course and may be diagnosed with *antisocial personality disorder* (or traits) after 18 years of age.

   In addition to the typical symptoms of conduct disorder, secondary complications often develop such as substance misuse or dependence, unwanted pregnancies, criminal record, suicidal and homicidal behaviour.

The treatment of conduct disorder is usually difficult. The most frequent mode of management is placement in a corrective institution, often after the child has had legal difficulties. Behavioural, educational and psychotherapeutic measures are usually employed for the behaviour modification.

Drug treatment may be needed in presence of epilepsy (anticonvulsants), hyperactivity (stimulant medication), impulse control disorder and episodic aggressive behaviour (lithium, carbamazepine), and psychotic symptoms (antipsychotics).

TIC DISORDERS

Tic disorders are characterised by the presence of tics. Tic is an abnormal involuntary movement (AIM) which occurs suddenly, repetitively, rapidly and is purposeless in nature. It is of two types:

1. Motor tic, characterised by repetitive motor movements.
2. Vocal tic, characterised by repetitive vocalisations.

Tic disorders can be either transient or chronic. Transient tic disorders are more common in boys and can occur in 5-20% of children. Tics are easily worsened by stressful life situations, fatigue and/or use stimulants such as caffeine and nicotine. A vast majority of these disappear by adulthood.

A special type of chronic tic disorder is *Gilles de la Tourette's syndrome* or *Tourette's disorder*.

Tourette's Disorder

Tourette's disorder is typically characterised by:

1. Multiple motor tics.
2. Multiple vocal tics.
3. Duration of more than 1 year.
4. Onset usually before 11 years of age and almost always before 21 years of age.

The disorder is usually more common (about three times) in males and has a prevalence rate of about 0.5 per 1000 people.

Motor Tics

The motor tics in Tourette's disorder can be simple or complex.

i. Simple motor tics: These may include eye-blinking, grimacing, shrugging of shoulders, tongue protrusion.
ii. Complex motor tics: These are facial gestures, stamping, jumping, hitting self, squatting, twirling, echokinesis (repetition of observed acts), copropraxia (obscene acts).

Motor tics are often the earliest to appear, beginning in the head region and then progressing downwards. These are later followed by the vocal tics.

Vocal Tics

The vocal tics in Tourette's disorder can also be simple or complex.

i. Simple vocal tics: Simple vocal tics include coughing, barking, throat-clearing, sniffing, and clicking.
ii. Complex vocal tics: These include some very characteristic, though not always present, symptoms of Tourette syndrome; for example, echolalia (repetition of heard phrases), palilalia (repetition of heard words), coprolalia (use of obscene words), and mental coprolalia (thinking of obscene words).

Obsessions and Compulsions are often the associated symptoms. These are usually the last symptoms to appear.

Aetiology

The aetiology of Tourette syndrome is not known but the presence of learning difficulties, neurological soft signs, hyperactivity, abnormal EEG record, abnormal evoked potentials, and abnormal CT Brain findings in some patients, point towards a biological basis.

There is some evidence to suggest that Tourette syndrome may be inherited as autosomal dominant disorder with variable penetrance.

Treatment

Pharmacotherapy is usually the preferred mode of treatment though there is lack of clear evidence of efficacy. Antipsychotics are often helpful in small doses and several drugs have been tried including haloperidol, risperidone, olanzapine, aripiprazole, ziprasidone, quetiapine, and sulpiride. Treatment options are often chosen based on adverse effect profile of each drug (which adverse effects to avoid). SSRIs (such as fluoxetine) have been used for the treatment of co-morbid obsessive compulsive symptoms.

In the resistant cases or in case of severe side-effects, pimozide or clonidine can be used under expert supervision. Behaviour therapy can sometimes be used, as an adjunct.

NON-ORGANIC ENURESIS

Enuresis is repetitive voiding of urine, either during the day or night, at inappropriate places. This state of affairs is normal in infancy.

Most children achieve bladder control by the age of three years. By the age of 5 years, there are still about 7% of children who wet their bed. Technically, enuresis is diagnosed only after 5 years of age (and at least 4 years of mental age).

Enuresis can be either of:

1. Primary type, where bladder control has never been achieved, or
2. Secondary type, where enuresis emerges after a period of bladder control (at least one year).

The majority (about 80%) of children with enuresis have nocturnal bed wetting only. Non-organic enuresis is more common (about two times) in males.

Aetiology

The exact cause of enuresis is not known. A variety of factors, which are implicated in its causation, are largely biopsychosocial. About 75% of children with enuresis have a first degree relative with history of enuresis.

The most commonly occurring factors, however, are psychosocial, such as emotional disturbances, insecurity, sibling rivalry, death of a parent. An organic cause must be looked for in children with diurnal enuresis (15% of all cases of diurnal enuresis) and adolescents with enuresis. The organic causes are present in about 5% of cases and include worm infes-

tation, spina bifida, neurogenic bladder, urinary tract infection, diabetes mellitus, and seizure disorder.

In secondary enuresis, the age of onset is usually 5-8 years. Enuresis tends to remit spontaneously and only 1% of children with enuresis continue to have the disorder in adulthood.

Treatment

The management consists of one or more of the following measures:

1. Restriction of fluid intake after 8 PM, in nocturnal enuresis.
2. Bladder training during daytime, aimed at increasing the holding-time of bladder. This is carried out in a step-by-step manner using positive reinforcements.
3. Interruption of sleep before the expected time of bed wetting. The child should be fully woken up and made aware of passing of urine.
4. Conditioning devices, which cause an alarm to sound as soon as the voided urine touches the bed-sheet. It is important to check the child's hearing before starting treatment. The alarm causes inhibition of further micturition and the child awakens. If properly used, it is an effective method of therapy.
5. Supportive psychotherapy for the child, parents and the whole family is often needed.
6. Pharmacotherapy: Drug treatment is usually not a preferred option for the treatment of enuresis.

The drug of choice in those who need pharmacotherapy has traditionally been a tricyclic antidepressant, usually imipramine (25-75 mg/day). It probably acts by its anticholinergic effect as well as by decreasing the deep sleep (stage 4 NREM-sleep) period. However, there is a risk of sudden death in some children with the use of tricyclic antidepressants. It should never be used for children under the age of 6 years.

Intranasal desmopressin has been found useful in some patients and is a good alternative. The other drugs that have been used for this purpose include diazepam, anticholinergics, amphetamines, placebos, but none have shown a good therapeutic response.

NON-ORGANIC ENCOPRESIS

Encopresis is repetitive passage of faeces at inappropriate time and/or place, after bowel control is physiologically possible. This is not due to the presence of any organic cause, which is called as faecal incontinence. Normally, toilet training is achieved between the ages of 2 and 3. Encopresis is defined as occurring after the age of 4 years.

Encopresis can be either of:

1. Primary type, where toilet training has never been achieved, or
2. Secondary type, where encopresis emerges after a period of faecal continence. This type typically occurs between the ages of 4 and 8.

Encopresis is more common (about 3-4 times) in males. By the age of 5 years, 1-1.5% of children suffer from encopresis. It tends to remit spontaneously with increasing age and by the age of 16 there are virtually no adolescents with encopresis. About 25% of these patients have associated enuresis.

Aetiology

The factors implicated in causation of encopresis include:

1. Inadequate, inconsistent toilet training.
2. Sibling rivalry.
3. Maturational lag.
4. Underlying hyperkinetic disorder.
5. Emotional disturbances.
6. Mental retardation.
7. Childhood schizophrenia.
8. Autistic disorder.

Whenever presented with a patient of encopresis, organic causes (faecal incontinence) must be ruled out (such as Hirschsprung's disease, overflow diarrhoea with constipation, hypothyroidism, inflammatory bowel disease and neurological lesions).

Treatment

The best treatment of encopresis is preventive. The toilet training period should be made as consistent and smooth as possible. The family environment should be warm and understanding. The emotional disturbances of the child should not be ignored and should be dealt with at the earliest. The communication between the family members should be direct.

After encopresis has developed, the treatment of choice is behaviour therapy, using reinforcements (both positive and negative). The other treatments include psychotherapy, biofeedback and imipramine (in non-retentive encopresis).

SPEECH DISORDERS

Stuttering is a disorder of speech, characterised by the following features:

1. Disturbed fluency and rhythm of speech.
2. Intermittent blocking.
3. Repetition of words rapidly.
4. Prolongation of sounds.
5. Associated anxiety or distress.

Earlier stammering and stuttering were differentiated on the basis of minor differences. At present, they are thought to be synonymous. The disorder is a fairly common one, affecting 2-5% of all children and 0.5-1% of all adults. Males are more commonly (about three times) affected.

Differential diagnosis is from cluttering, which is characterised by an erratic and dysarrhythmic pattern of speech, with jerky and rapid spurting of words. Unlike in stuttering where the person is aware of the difficulty in speech, the affected person in cluttering is usually unaware of the abnormal speech pattern.

Treatment

The treatment is by behaviour modification techniques such as desensitisation, biofeedback and stammer suppresser; and by techniques to diminish anxiety like relaxation therapy, drug therapy, or individual or group psychotherapy.

HABIT DISORDERS

These are stereotyped disorders which are intentionally and repetitively produced but serve no constructive or socially acceptable function.

The common habit disorders include thumb sucking, nail biting, pulling out of hair (*trichotillomania*), head banging, masturbation, teeth grinding, picking of nose, biting parts of the body, skin-scratching, body rocking, breath-holding, and swallowing of air (*aerophagia*).

These habits range from normal to abnormal, depending on the severity of occurrence and the time of presentation during the developmental period (what is normal in infancy, may be abnormal in later childhood). Many of habit disorders, particularly those which are self-stimulating in nature, are called as *gratification habits*. These have been considered by some as *masturbatory equivalents*. These habit disorders tend to be commoner in individuals with mental retardation or learning disability.

Treatment

The treatment is by behaviour modification techniques and treatment of underlying psychopathology, if present.

ELECTIVE (SELECTIVE) MUTISM

Elective mutism is characterised by the presence of marked, emotionally determined, selectivity in speaking, despite the presence of language competence in at least some situations.

Typically, it is first manifested in early childhood and is seen more often in girls. It is estimated to be present in 3-8/10,000 children. It may be associated with temperamental traits involving social anxiety, withdrawal, sensitivity or resistance. The child is often mute in front of strangers or at school. Other socio-emotional disturbances may also be present.

Elective mutism should be differentiated from shyness in normal children, mental retardation, pervasive developmental disorder, expressive language disorder, and conversion disorder. Most cases improve with the passage of time, though some children may require pharmacotherapy (such as with fluoxetine) and/or psychosocial management.

OTHER DISORDERS

The other childhood psychiatric disorders include separation anxiety disorder, phobic anxiety disorder of childhood, social anxiety disorder of childhood, sibling rivalry disorder, mixed disorders of conduct and emotions, and reactive attachment disorder of childhood.

HISTORY OF TREATMENT IN PSYCHIATRY

The treatment of psychiatric disorders in past had often constituted of merely institutionalisation (i.e. admission in an asylum or mental hospital), sometimes along with the use of treatment which now seems either ridiculous or fantastic or mostly both. The advent of psychopharmacology in the last six decades has brought treatment of psychiatric disorders within the realm of scientific medicine.

Some important milestones in the treatment of psychiatric disorders are summarised in Table 15.1.

CLASSIFICATION OF PSYCHOTROPIC DRUGS

The drugs which have a significant effect on higher mental functions are called as *psychoactive* or *psychotropic drugs*. These psychotropic drugs can be broadly classified as follows:

1. Antipsychotics
2. Antidepressants
3. Mood stabilising drugs (or drugs for maintenance treatment of bipolar disorder)
4. Anti-anxiety and hypnosedatives
5. Anticonvulsants (or anti-epileptics)
6. Alcohol and drugs of dependence (discussed in Chapter 4)
7. Antiparkinsonian drugs

8. Miscellaneous drugs, such as stimulants, drugs used in treatment of eating disorders, drugs used in treatment of alcohol and drug dependence, anaesthetics, drugs used in treatment of dementia, drugs used in child psychiatry, vitamins, calcium channel blockers, and other drugs.

An Ideal Psychotropic Drug

An ideal psychotropic drug should have the following characteristics (modified after Hollister, 1983):

1. It should cure the underlying pathology causing the disorder or symptom(s) under focus, so that the drug can be stopped after sometime.
2. It should benefit all the patients suffering from that disorder.
3. It should have no side-effects or toxicity in the therapeutic range.
4. It should have rapid onset of action.
5. There should be no dependence on the drug and no withdrawal symptoms on stopping the drug.
6. There should be no tolerance to the drug so that same dose is effective for long duration of time.
7. It should not be lethal in overdoses.
8. It can be given in both inpatient and outpatient settings.

Although psychotropic drugs available at present are far from ideal, they are still helpful in alleviation of symptoms and suffering of patients. With increasing research, new emerging products appear to be better in efficacy and have fewer, though newer, side-effects.

Table 15.1: A Brief History of Psychopharmacology

< 4000 BC	Ayurveda describes treatment of psychiatric patients with sympathy and kindness. The methods of treatment included *dhatura* and roots of *serpentina* plant mixed with oil (*ghee*).
1853	Bromide used as a sedative-hypnotic.
1869	Chloral hydrate used in the treatment of melancholia and mania.
1882	Paraldehyde used as a hypnotic.
1883	Phenothiazines synthesised during synthesis of methylene blue (Bernthsen).
1903	Barbiturates (barbital) used for sedation in 1903; phenobarbital introduced in 1912.
1917	Malarial treatment for General Paralysis of Insane (GPI) received a Nobel prize (Julius von Wagner Jauregg).
1922	Barbiturate-induced coma introduced for the treatment of psychoses (Jacob Klaesi).
1927	Insulin-shock treatment introduced for schizophrenia (Manfred Sakel).
1931	First report of successful treatment of psychoses (Ganesh Sen and Kartik Bose from India); using Rauwolfia serpentina extract (reserpine). Report ignored till Nathan Kline (1958) confirmed the finding.
1934	Metrazol-induced convulsions used for the treatment of psychoses (Laszlo von Meduna).
1936	Frontal lobotomy advocated for treatment of psychiatric disorders (Egas Moniz and Almenda Lima).
1937	Amphetamines used in the treatment of behaviour disorders of children (C Bradley).
1938	Electroconvulsive therapy used for the treatment of psychoses (Ugo Cerletti and Lucio Bini).
1940	Phenytoin used as an anticonvulsant (Tracy Putnam).
1943	LSD synthesised (Albert Hofmann).
1949	Lithium used in mania (John F Cade); did not receive much attention even in Australia.
1950	Chlorpromazine synthesised while making a better antihistaminic than promethazine (Charpentier).
1950	Methylphenidate used in treatment of ADHD, then known as Minimal Brain Dysfunction (MBD).
1951	Lytic cocktail used (Laborit); Chlorpromazine earlier used (as '456 ORP') in artificial hibernation.
1951	Isoniazid (INH) found to have mood elevating properties in patients with tuberculosis. Iproniazid, a MAOI and a derivative of INH, was later (1958) introduced for treatment of depression.
1952	The revolution in psychopharmacology came with introduction of chlorpromazine (Jean Delay and Pierre Deniker). The number of admissions in mental hospitals show a sudden decrease after introduction of chlorpromazine.
1955	Meprobamate was introduced as an anti-anxiety agent.
1958	Imipramine, a tricyclic antidepressant (TCA) synthesised by Haflinger and Schindler in the late 1940's, was introduced for treatment of depression in 1958 (Thomas Kuhn).
1958	MAOIs (e.g. iproniazid) introduced for treatment of depression (Nathan Kline).
1958	Haloperidol synthesised in Belgium (Janssen).
1960	Chlordiazepoxide used as an anti-anxiety agent in 1960-1961 (Sternbach; Synthesised in 1957).
1966	Valpromide (Valproate) used in bipolar disorder (Lambert).
1968	Pimozide used for treatment of schizophrenia (Janssen).
1967	Clomipramine used in OCD (Fernandez and Lopez-Ibor).
1971	Carbamazepine used in bipolar disorder (Takezaki and Hanoaka) (Synthesized in 1953 by Schindler).
1986	Buspirone introduced in US market as a non-benzodiazepine anti-anxiety agent.
1988	Clozapine re-discovered in US as an effective treatment for refractory schizophrenia (Kane et al) (Synthesised in 1959). Approved by US FDA in 1990 and introduced in Indian market in 1995.
1990s	Second Generation Antipsychotics introduced in market starting with Risperidone.

The information in this chapter is necessarily very brief and introductory in nature. A much more detailed reading is definitely recommended before prescribing any psychotropic medication to a patient with consultation of local formularies and guidelines. This information should not be used to make any treatment decisions without further reading.

ANTIPSYCHOTIC DRUGS

Antipsychotics are psychotropic drugs which are used in the treatment of psychotic disorders and psychotic symptoms. These are also known as major tranquilisers, neuroleptics, ataractics, anti-schizophrenic drugs and D_2-receptor (dopamine receptor) blockers; however, the term *antipsychotic* appears to be the most appropriate and the most widely used term.

Indications

Antipsychotics have previously been used as urinary antiseptics and anti-helminthic; however, their use stopped was due to toxicity and lack of efficacy. Although they have been used in a wide variety of conditions in the past their current use includes the following conditions.

Organic Psychiatric Disorders
1. Delirium (in small doses; e.g. haloperidol, risperidone)
2. Dementia (careful and considered use for psychotic features, and severe agitation)
3. Delirium tremens (and psychoses occurring in drug and alcohol withdrawal states; e.g. haloperidol, risperidone)
4. Drug induced psychosis (e.g. haloperidol in amphetamine-induced psychosis)
5. Other organic mental disorders (e.g. organic hallucinosis; organic delusional disorder; secondary mania)

Non-organic Psychotic Disorders
1. Schizophrenia
2. Schizo-affective disorder
3. Acute psychoses

4. Mania (with or without mood stabilisers)
5. Maintenance treatment of bipolar disorders (e.g. olanzapine, quetiapine)
6. Major depression (for psychotic features, agitation, and melancholic features; along with antidepressants)
7. Delusional disorders

Neurotic and Other Psychiatric Disorders
1. Severe, intractable, and disabling anxiety (rarely used and not recommended)
2. Treatment refractory obsessive compulsive disorder (as an adjunct)
3. Anorexia nervosa (rarely used and not widely recommended)

Medical Disorders
1. Huntington's chorea (e.g. haloperidol)
2. Intractable hiccups (e.g. chlorpromazine in low doses) (rarely used)
3. Nausea and vomiting (rarely, in low doses); ondansetron, an anti-emetic drug, is a weak antipsychotic
4. Tic disorders, e.g. Gilles de la Tourette syndrome (e.g. haloperidol, risperidone)

Pharmacokinetics

The orally administered antipsychotics are absorbed erratically and variably from gastrointestinal tract, with uneven blood levels. Intramuscular and intravenous administration provides much more reliable blood levels. On an average, the oral liquid dose produces a peak level at 1½ hours and the intramuscular dose peaks at 30 minutes.

The antipsychotics are highly lipophilic and highly protein-bound. They easily enter areas with good blood supply such as brain, lung, kidneys and foetus, and accumulate there. They are not dialysable. The half-lives of most antipsychotics are long and theoretically a single daily dose is sufficient to produce sustained therapeutic blood levels. However in practice, divided doses are administered, at least initially, to decrease adverse effects. Later an attempt can be made to give the whole dose or a major part of total daily dose at night.

Steady state plasma levels are usually reached in 5-10 days. Once the drug is withdrawn, it may remain in body for many days to many months. The main metabolic pathway is through liver (hepatic microsomal enzymes). Oxidation and conjugation are the most important methods of metabolism for phenothiazines. Many of the metabolites, such as mesoridazine (for thioridazine), reduced haloperidol (for haloperidol) and 9-hydroxy-risperidone (for risperidone), are also active compounds. Chlorpromazine has more than 150 metabolites, some of which are active. The excretion of the metabolites is through kidneys and liver (enterohepatic circulation).

Most of the antipsychotics tend to have a therapeutic window. If the blood level is below this 'window', the drug is ineffective. If the blood level is higher than the upper limit of the 'window', there is toxicity or the drug is again ineffective.

Classification

A classification of currently available antipsychotic drugs is presented in Table 15.2.

Mechanism of Action

The exact mechanism of action of antipsychotics is unknown. However, one of the major mechanisms appears to be *antidopaminergic activity* of these drugs. Antipsychotic drugs block D_2-receptors, which are mainly present in mesolimbic-mesocortical system (mesolimbic system is concerned with emotional reactions), nigro-striatal system and tubero-infundibular system. The relative potencies of these drugs in competing for D_2-receptors parallel quite closely their clinical potencies.

It is currently believed that antipsychotic drugs are effective in treating psychosis due to their action on the D_2-receptors located in the mesolimbic system whilst extrapyramidal side-effects (EPSE) are caused by blockade of D_2-receptors situated in nigro-striatal system and hyperprolactinaemia is caused by D_2-blockade in tubero-infundibular system. However, other neurotransmitters (such as 5-HT, acetylcholine) are clearly implicated (see below; atypical antipsychotics). Sedation is caused by histaminergic

blockade which is usually highest for drugs such as chlorpromazine and thioridazine.

Second Generation Antipsychotics

A search for an antipsychotic drug which acts only on the mesolimbic system but has no effect on nigro-striatal or tubero-infundibular systems, has led to the development of a heterogeneous group of drugs collectively known as atypical or newer antipsychotics. These are also known as second generation antipsychotics (SGAs) or serotonin-dopamine antagonists or (SDAs). These include risperidone, quetiapine, olanzapine, amisulpride, paliperidone, zotepine, ziprasidone and aripiprazole.

By definition these drugs are effective antipsychotics without theoretically producing undesirable extrapyramidal side-effects (i.e. antipsychotics without neuroleptic effect), or causing elevation of serum prolactin levels. These are characterised by a selective limbic dopamine blockade, D_4-receptor blockade, or a combination of potent 5-HT$_2$ and weak D_2 antagonism. These drugs should theoretically be safer with lesser incidence of serious side-effects such as tardive dyskinesia and neuroleptic malignant syndrome.

Clozapine is one such drug but it can cause agranulocytosis and seizures. Risperidone, olanzapine, quetiapine, aripiprazole, amisulpride and ziprasidone are currently being used widely as atypical antipsychotics, while paliperidone and zotepine are also available in the international market.

Atypical antipsychotics, in addition to their effect on positive symptoms, are believed to be effective in treatment of negative symptoms (such as apathy, decreased sociality, anhedonia) of chronic schizophrenia. Clozapine in particular is effective in management of treatment-resistant schizophrenia. However, there is need for close haematological monitoring for neutropenia or agranulocytosis as suggested in SPC of the drug.

Side Effects

The antipsychotics are safe drugs with a high therapeutic index and wide margin of safety in routine clinical dosages. In spite of this safety, a wide range

Table 15.2: Classification and Properties of Antipsychotics

Drugs	Oral Dose (mg/d)	Parenteral Dose (mg)	#Some Common Adverse Effects**				
			Sedation	Hypotension	EPSE*	Weight Gain	Increased Prolactin
I. Phenothiazines							
A. Aliphatics							
1. Chlorpromazine (CPZ)	300-1000	50-100 IM	+++	+++	+	++	++
2. Triflupromazine	100-400	30-60 IM	++	++	++	++	++
B. Piperidines							
1. Mesoridazine	100-400	____	++	+	+	++	+
2. Thioridazine	300-600	____	+++	++	+	++	+
C. Piperazines							
1. Fluphenazine	2-20	____	+	+	+++	+	+++
2. Prochlorperazine	45-150	40-80 IM	+	+	+++	+	+++
3. Trifluoperazine	15-50	1-5 IM	+	+	+++	+	+++
II. Thioxanthenes							
A. Aliphatics							
1. Chlorprothixene	75-600	25-75 IM	+++	++	++	++	++
B. Piperazines							
1. Flupentixol	3-18	____	+	+	++	++	++
2. Thiothixene	6-60	2-6 IM	+	++	++	++	++
3. Zuclopenthixol	25-150	50-100 IM	++	++	++	++	+++
III. Butyrophenones							
1. Haloperidol	5-30	5-10 IM	+	+	+++	+	+++
2. Trifluperidol	0.5-8.0	2.5-5.0 IM	±	±	+++	+	++
IV. Diphenylbutylpiperidines							
1. Penfluridol	20-60 mg weekly	____	+	+	++	+	++
2. Pimozide	4-20	____	+	+	++	+	+++
V. Indolic Derivatives (Dihydroindolones)							
1. Molindone	50-225	____	++	0	+	±	±
VI. Dibenzoxapines							
1. Loxapine	25-250	____	++	++	++	+	+++
VII. Atypical or Second Generation Antipsychotics							
A. Dibenzodiazepines							
1. Clozapine	50-900	____	+++	+++	0	+++	0
B. Substituted Benzamides							
1. Amisulpride	400-1200	____	±	+	+	+	+++
2. Sulpiride (not called atypical usually)	400-2400	____	±	+	+	+	+++

Contd...

Contd...

Drugs	Oral Dose (mg/d)	Parenteral Dose (mg)	#Some Common Adverse Effects**				
			Sedation	Hypotension	EPSE*	Weight Gain	Increased Prolactin
C. *Benzisoxales*							
1. Iloperidone	4-24	———	0	+	+	+ +	0
2. Paliperidone	3-12	———	+	+ +	+	+ +	+ + +
3. Risperidone	2-8	———	+	+ +	+	+ +	+ + +
D. *Benzisothiazolyl*							
1. Ziprasidone	40-160	———	±	+	0	±	±
E. *Thienobenzodiazepine*							
1. Olanzapine	5-20	2.5-10 IM	+ +	+	±	+ + +	+
F. *Dibenzothiazepine*							
1. Quetiapine	150-750	———	+ +	±	0	+ +	0
G. *Partial Agonists*							
1. Aripiprazole	5-30	———	0	0	0	±	0
2. Bifeprunox	20	———	0	0	0	±	0
H. *Dibenzothiepin*							
1. Zotepine	75-300	———	+ +	±	+	+ +	+ +
I. *Dibenzooxepinopyrrole*							
1. Asenapine	5-10	———	0	±	0	±	0

\#   The estimate of common adverse effects in this table is a very rough and empirical guideline to the clinical use of antipsychotics. The drug dosage in each patient needs to be individualised based on the clinical symptoms, their severity, response to treatment and several other clinical factors.

*   EPSE means Extrapyramidal side effects.

**   0 = Absent; ± = Probable/Very little; + = Mild; + + = Moderate; + + + = Severe

of side-effects do occur with the use of antipsychotics even in the therapeutic doses.

The common side-effects are listed in Table 15.3 with their mechanisms of causation and management. Some of newer antipsychotics appear to have a higher association with metabolic syndrome (see Chapter 5 and Table 15.3).

It is important to monitor physical health whilst prescribing antipsychotics and the following are the most commonly recommended minimum suggestions. Other investigations may also be indicated (such as ECG, HbA_{1c}) based on clinical opinion.

Baseline (before prescribing): Obtaining detailed personal and family history, Weight, BMI, Waist circumference, Blood pressure, WBC and Neutrophil count, Fasting blood sugar, Serum lipids, and LFTs.

After 1 month: Weight, BMI, Blood pressure, Waist circumference, and Fasting blood sugar.

After 3 months: Weight, BMI, Blood pressure, Waist circumference, and Fasting blood sugar.

After 6 months: Weight, BMI, Blood pressure, Waist circumference, Fasting blood sugar, Serum lipids, and LFTs.

After 12 months: Weight, BMI, Blood pressure, Waist circumference, Fasting blood sugar, and Serum lipids.

Several antipsychotics can increase QTc interval (QT interval corrected for heart rate). These include sertindole, haloperidol, pimozide, ziprasidone, zotepine, quetiapine, or any intravenously administered antipsychotic. A similar effect is seen with administration of TCAs. QTc prolongation can be made worse with co-prescribed medications (e.g. anti-arrhythmics

Table 15.3: Side Effects of Antipsychotics

Category and Side Effect	Probable Cause	Maximum with (For example)	Minimum with (For example)	Management
A. Autonomic Side Effects				
1. Dry mouth	Muscarinic Cholinergic blockade	Chlorpromazine	Haloperidol Risperidone	Usually none; Tolerance develops; Occasionally Pilocarpine 2%
2. Constipation	–do–	Chlorpromazine	Haloperidol Risperidone	Usually none; Tolerance develops; Bulk (or sometimes other) laxatives
3. Cycloplegia	–do–	Chlorpromazine	Haloperidol Risperidone	Usually none; Tolerance develops; Occasionally Pilocarpine 2%
4. Mydriasis	–do–	Thioridazine; miosis with Chlorpromazine)	Haloperidol Risperidone	Usually none; Tolerance develops; Occasionally Pilocarpine 2%
5. Urinary Retention	–do–	Chlorpromazine	Haloperidol Risperidone	Usually none if only hesitancy occurs. Tolerance develops; Rule out BHP; Bethanethol or catheterisation for retention
6. Delirium (central anticholinergic syndrome)	–do–	Chlorpromazine	Haloperidol Risperidone	Physostigmine (neostigmine does not enter CNS); Diazepam sometimes supportive care
7. Orthostatic hypotension	α_1 Adrenergic blockade	Chlorpromazine	Haloperidol Aripiprazole	Usually none; Tolerance develops; change in posture slowly. When severe, use plasma expanders, raise leg, supportive measures.
8. Impotence	–do–	Chlorpromazine	Haloperidol	Decrease dose. If severe, change medication.
9. Impaired ejaculation	–do–	Thioridazine	Haloperidol	Decrease dose. If severe, change medication.
B. Extra-pyramidal Side Effects (EPSE)				
1. Parkinsonian syndrome (esp. tremor)	Dopaminergic (D_2) receptor blockade in striatal areas	Haloperidol	Clozapine Quetiapine Aripiprazole	Antiparkisonian medication for treatment; also for prevention if needed.
2. Akathisia (motor restlessness)	–do–	–do–	Clozapine Quetiapine	Change of medication or reduction; Beta-blockers such as Propranolol; Benzodiazepines

Contd...

Contd...

Category and Side Effect	Probable Cause	Maximum with (For example)	Minimum with (For example)	Management
3. Acute Dystonia	—do—	—do—	—do—	Antiparkinsonian medication; Rule out hypercalcaemia
4. Rabbit Syndrome (Peri-oral tremor)	—do—	—do—	—do—	Antiparkinsonian medication
5. Tardive Dyskinesia (late onset oro-facial dyskinesia)	Dopaminergic (D_2) receptor super-sensitivity	Not known	Clozapine	Treatment unsatisfactory, though several drugs are available. Prevention best.
6. Neuroleptic Malignant Syndrome (Fever, EPS, High CPK, catatonic symptoms and autonomic dysfunction)	Not known	Probably haloperidol	Not known	Bromocriptine, Dantrolene, Baclofen, General supportive care. Add-on lorazepam, Occasionally ECT

C. Other Central Nervous System Effects

Category and Side Effect	Probable Cause	Maximum with (For example)	Minimum with (For example)	Management
1. Seizures	Decreased seizure threshold	Clozapine Chlorpromazine (High doses)	Trifluoperazine	Decrease dose. Change to a safer antipsychotic
2. Sedation	Histaminergic blockade	—do—	Haloperidol Aripiprazole	This side effect may be beneficial. Otherwise decrease dose. Change drug. Give single dose only at night
3. Depression or Pseudo-depression	Decreased catecholamine levels in brain	Not known	SDAs (e.g. Ziprasidone)	Decrease dose. Change drug. Occasionally antidepressants or ECT.

D. Metabolic and Endocrine Side Effects

Category and Side Effect	Probable Cause	Maximum with (For example)	Minimum with (For example)	Management
1. Weight gain	H_1 blockade	Almost all antipsychotics esp. Clozapine and Olanzapine	Aripiprazole Haloperidol	Change drug. Dietary control. Exercises.
2. Diabetes	Not known	Clozapine Olanzapine	Ziprasidone Aripiprazole	Change drug. Dietary control.
3. Galactorrhoea with/without amenorrhoea	Increased Prolactin released due to dopaminergic blockade in hypothalamus	Haloperidol Risperidone	Aripiprazole Quetiapine	None. Change drug.

Contd...

Contd...

Category and Side Effect	Probable Cause	Maximum with (For example)	Minimum with (For example)	Management
E. Allergic Side Effects				
1. Cholestatic Jaundice	Hypersensitivity reaction	Chlorpromazine	Haloperidol	Change drug. Benign course. Supportive care.
2. Agranulocytosis (very rare)	—do—	Clozapine	—do—	Stop drug immediately. Treat infection. Isolation. General supportive care. Figastrim may be useful
F. Cardiac Side Effects				
1. ECG Changes (e.g. QTc prolongation)	Anticholinergic effect Calcium channel blocking effect	Thioridazine Pimozide	Aripiprazole	Change drug, if severe.
2. Sudden Death (very rare)	Probably ventricular fibrillation	Not known	Not known	None
G. Ocular Side Effects				
1. Granular deposits in cornea and lens	Not known (Probably photosensitivity	Chlorpromazine (High doses for long duration)	Haloperidol	Change drug.
2. Pigmentary retinopathy resembling retinitis pigmentosa	Not known	Thioridazine only (Dose-related)	All other antipsy-chotics	Never give more than 800 mg/day of thioridazine. Prevention only
H. Dermatological Side Effects				
1. Contact dermatitis	Allergic	Chlorpromazine (By handling)	—do—	Avoid handling. Symptomatic treatment
2. Photosensitive reaction	Probably photosensitive	—do— (High doses)	—do—	Avoid sunlight. Use sunscreen.
3. Blue-gray metallic discolouration	—do—	—do— (High doses for long duration)	—do—	Change drug.

such as quinidine, anti-malarials such as quinine, and antibiotics such as erythromycin) and/or medical conditions (such as ischaemic heart disease, extremes of ages).

This list of side-effects is necessarily incomplete and it is important to read the SPC of any drug before prescribing it in a patient.

Treatment Adherence

Many patients with schizophrenia can be unco-operative, with a poor treatment adherence (see Table 15.4). Therefore, it may at times be difficult to ensure adequate administration of antipsychotics on an outpatient basis.

Table 15.4: Some Factors in Poor Drug Concordance

1. **Drug Related Factors**
   i. Adverse effects (particularly their early appearance and persistence)
   ii. Slow onset of desirable effects
   iii. Complexity of regimen (e.g. several doses/day)
   iv. Route of administration (IM/IV as opposed to oral)
2. **Patient Related Factors**
   i. Poor education regarding illness and medication
   ii. Denial of illness/absent insight
   iii. Perceived stigma of mental disorder, medication, or visible side effects (e.g. dystonia)
   iv. Treatment access problems (e.g. poverty, cost of medications, distance from hospital)
   v. Low IQ and/or low educational level
   vi. Poor social support
   vii. Specific psychopathology, e.g. persecutory ideation, hopelessness
   viii. Poor doctor-patient relationship.

Table 15.5: Some Antipsychotic Depot Preparations*

1. Flupentixol decanoate 20-300 mg IM every 2-4 weeks (40 mg IM every 2 weeks roughly equivalent to 25 mg of fluphenazine decanoate IM every 2 weeks)
2. Fluphenazine decanoate 12.5-100 mg IM every 2-4 weeks (25 mg IM every 2 weeks roughly equivalent to 300 mg of oral Chlorpromazine per day)
3. Haloperidol decanoate 25-250 mg IM every 4 weeks (100 mg IM every 4 weeks roughly equivalent to 5 mg/day of oral haloperidol)
4. Olanzapine pamoate 150-300 mg IM every 2 weeks or 300-405 mg IM every 4 weeks (Note risk of post-injection syndrome; Also note dose escalation chart in SPC)
5. Pipotiazine palmitate 25-100 mg IM every 4 weeks
6. Risperidone Consta 25-50 mg IM every 2 weeks (Note delay in onset of action by 2-3 weeks and need for refrigeration)
7. Zuclopenthixol decanoate 200-400 mg IM every 2-4 weeks (200 mg IM every 2 weeks roughly equivalent to 25 mg/day of oral Zuclopenthixol)

*Check SPC (Summary of Product Characteristics) before prescribing any medicines

Since discontinuation of antipsychotic medication often leads to relapse, long-acting preparations of antipsychotics are valuable in the treatment. They may be given in a depot form, either intramuscularly or administered orally. There are several different preparations available in the international market but the preparations summarised in Table 15.5 are used most often.

Clinical Use

Some general principles regarding routine clinical use of antipsychotics include:

1. Although atypical antipsychotics are usually preferred, the choice of antipsychotic medication should be individualised in a particular patient. The recent evidence shows more differences in adverse effect profiles but not in efficacy between older and newer antipsychotics.
2. Whenever possible the lowest effective dose should be used.
3. Routinely only one antipsychotic should be used at one time. Rational polypharmacy should be reserved only for judicious treatment after non-response to single antipsychotics.
4. High doses of antipsychotics should be avoided.
5. Whenever appropriate, psychosocial management should be combined with antipsychotic treatment.
6. It is really important to monitor physical health on a regular basis whilst the patient receives antipsychotic medication (see above).
7. Do not use rapid neuroleptisation (parenteral use of a loading dose of antipsychotic medication), if possible.

ANTIDEPRESSANT DRUGS

Antidepressants are those psychotropic drugs which are used for treatment of depressive disorders. These have also been called as mood-elevators and *thymoleptics.*

Isoniazid (INH) was found to have mood elevating properties in some patients suffering from tuberculosis in 1951. Iproniazid, a MAO inhibitor and a derivative of INH, was later (1958) introduced for the treatment of depression. The first tricyclic antidepressant (TCA) *imipramine* was used in 1958 by Thomas Kuhn. It was different from phenothiazines by only a replacement of sulphur with an ethylene linkage. With this small structural difference (discovered by chance), imipramine was found not effective as an antipsychotic but instead quite beneficial in depressed patients. Since 1958, the number of antidepressants has been gradually increasing.

Antidepressants have no euphoriant effect when administered to normal, non-depressed individuals.

Indications

Presently, the indications for the use of antidepressants include:

Depression
1. Depressive episode (also called major depression, endogenous depression)
2. Depressive episode with melancholia (with or without ECTs)
3. Depressive episode with psychotic features (with antipsychotics or ECTs)
4. Dysthymia (with psychotherapy)
5. Reactive depression (with psychotherapy)
6. Depressive equivalents and masked depression (sometimes)
7. Atypical depression (e.g. MAO inhibitors)
8. Secondary depression (e.g. in hypothyroidism, Cushing's syndrome)
9. Abnormal grief reaction

Child Psychiatric Disorders
1. Enuresis (with or without behaviour therapy)
2. Attention deficit disorder with hyperactivity (in low doses, after 6 years of age, when stimulant medication is not available)
3. School phobia (sometimes, in low doses)
4. Separation anxiety disorder (in children)
5. Somnambulism
6. Night terrors

Other Psychiatric Disorders
1. Panic attacks (e.g. SSRIs)
2. Agoraphobia and social phobia
3. Obsessive compulsive disorder with or without depression (e.g. clomipramine, SSRIs)
4. Cataplexy (associated with narcolepsy)
5. Aggression in elderly (e.g. trazodone)
6. Eating disorders (e.g. fluoxetine in bulimia nervosa)
7. Borderline personality disorder (for treatment of depressive symptoms)
8. Trichotillomania (e.g. clomipramine; fluoxetine)
9. Depersonalisation syndrome
10. Post-traumatic stress disorder (PTSD)
11. Generalised anxiety disorder (e.g. SSRIs)
12. Nicotine dependence (e.g. bupropion is used for treatment of craving)
13. Alcohol dependence (e.g. fluoxetine sometimes used for treatment of craving)

Medical Disorders
1. Chronic pain (in low doses, e.g. amitriptyline, duloxetine)
2. Migraine (as an adjuvant)

Classification

Classification and properties of antidepressants (Table 15.6).

Pharmacokinetics

The oral dose of TCAs is incompletely though adequately absorbed. As they are highly anticholinergic in nature, they delay gastric emptying and slow gastrointestinal motility. SSRIs are well absorbed from the gastrointestinal tract.

These antidepressants, much like antipsychotics, are highly lipophilic and are highly protein bound. Thus they have a large volume of distribution and tend to accumulate in areas with good blood supply. Like antipsychotics, they are also not dialysable.

Their other pharmacokinetic properties of TCAs are similar to those of phenothiazines. The half-life is long, usually more than 24 hours. Although TCAs can be administered in a single night-time dose, the routine clinical practice is to prescribe divided doses, at least in the initial days of treatment, to prevent accumulated side-effects. The metabolism of TCAs is by oxidation (hepatic microsomal enzymes) followed by conjugation (glucoronic acid). The major metabolites of imipramine and amitriptyline (desipramine and

Table 15.6: Classification and Properties of Antidepressants

Drugs	Oral Dose (mg/d)	Some Common Adverse Effects[#]		
		Sedation*	Orthostatic Hypotension*	Anticholinergic*
I. Cyclic Antidepressants				
A. Tricyclic Tertiary Amines				
1. Amitriptyline	75-300	+ + +	+ + +	+ + +
2. Clomipramine	75-250	+ +	+ +	+ +
3. Dosulepin (Dotheipin)	75-300	+ + +	+ + +	+ +
4. Doxepine	75-300	+ + +	+ + +	+
5. Imipramine	75-300	+ +	+ +	+ +
6. Lofepramine	70-210	+	+	+
7. Tri-imipramine	75-300	+ + +	+ +	+ +
B. Tricyclic Secondary Amines				
1. Desipramine	75-300	±	+	+ +
2. Nortriptyline	75-200	+	+ +	+
3. Protriptyline	15-60	0	+ +	+ +
C. Tetracyclic Antidepressants				
1. Amoxapine	150-400	+	+	+ +
2. Maprotiline	75-225	+ +	+ +	+ +
3. Mianserin	30-120	+ + +	±	±
D. Bicyclic Antidepressants				
1. Viloxazine	100-300	±	±	±
II. Selective Serotonin Reuptake Inhibitors (SSRIs)				
1. Citalopram	20-40	±	±	0
2. Escitalopram	10-20	±	±	0
3. Fluoxetine	20-60	±	0	0
4. Fluvoxamine	50-300	±	±	±
5. Paroxetine	20-40	+	0	±
6. Sertraline	50-200	±	±	0
III. Serotonin Norepinephrine Reuptake Inhibitors (SNRIs)				
1. Duloxetine	60	±	±	±
2. Venlafaxine	75-375	+	±	±
IV. Norepinephrine Serotonin Reuptake Enhancers (NSREs)				
1. Tianeptin	37.5	+	0	±
V. Noradrenergic and Specific Serotonergic Antagonists (NaSSAs)				
1. Mirtazapine	15-45	+ + +	+	±
VI. Norepinephrine Dopamine Reuptake Inhibitors (NDRIs)				
1. Bupropion	150-450	Activating	0	0
VII. Serotonin Antagonists and Reuptake Inhibitors (SARIs)				
1. Nefazodone (withdrawn from market)	200-600	+ +	+	±
2. Trazodone	150-400	+ + +	±	±

Contd...

Contd...

Drugs	Oral Dose (mg/d)	Some Common Adverse Effects[#]		
		Sedation*	Orthostatic Hypotension*	Anticholinergic*
VIII. Noradrenergic Reuptake Inhibitors (NARIs)				
1. Reboxetine	8-10	±	±	±
IX. Mono-amine Oxidase Inhibitors (MAOIs)				
A. Irreversible Non-selective and Selective MAOIs				
Not available in India				
B. Reversible Selective MAO-B Inhibitors				
1. Selegiline	5-10	Useful in Parkinsonism		
C. Reversible Selective MAO-A Inhibitors (RIMAs)				
1. Moclobemide	300-600	Activating	0	0
X. Melatonin receptor agonist and 5-HT$_{2C}$ antagonist				
1. Agomelatin	25-50	+	0	0

The estimate of common adverse effects in this table is a very rough and empirical guideline to the clinical use of antidepressants. The drug dosage in each patient needs to be individualised based on the clinical symptoms, their severity, response to treatment and several other clinical factors.

* 0 = Absent; ± = Probable/Very little; + = Mild; + + = Moderate; + + + = Severe

nortriptyline respectively) are active antidepressants themselves. Fluoxetine is demethylated in liver to norfluoxetine.

With the regular administration of TCAs, a constant blood level is achieved usually by the end of two weeks. Although routine monitoring of blood levels is not indicated, it may become important in cases of toxicity. Also, some antidepressants such as nortriptyline and protriptyline have a *therapeutic window.*

Antidepressants (especially SSRIs, e.g. fluoxetine) also cause inhibition of cytochrome P450 enzymes in liver (e.g. CYP P450 2D6 and CYP P450 3A4).

The MAO inhibitors are absorbed well by oral route, and are predominantly metabolised in liver by acetylation.

Mechanism of Action

The exact mechanism of action is not clearly known. It appears from clinical studies that the predominant action of antidepressants is to increase the catecholamine levels in brain (*Amine hypothesis*).

Tricyclic antidepressants are also called as *Mono-amine reuptake inhibitors* (MARIs). Their main modes of action include:

1. Blocking reuptake of norepinephrine (NE), serotonin (5HT) and/or dopamine (DA) at the nerve terminals, thus increasing NE, 5HT and/or DA levels at the receptor site.
2. Down-regulation of the β-adrenergic receptors.

The *Mono-amine oxidase inhibitors* (MAOIs) instead act on mono-amine oxidase (MAO) which is responsible for degradation of catecholamines following their reuptake. The final effect is the same, i.e. a functional increase in the NE and/or 5HT levels at receptor site.

Another important clinical point is that it takes 5-10 days before a MAOI, and 2-3 weeks before a non-MAOI antidepressant, has any evident action on depression (although sleep, anxiety and agitation may respond earlier). The reason for this is not fully clear though an increase in brain amine levels is possibly responsible for antidepressant action. However, postsynaptic events (such as down-regulation of postsynaptic receptors) are probably more important and they take longer than an increase in amine levels. Therefore, it is of no benefit to prescribe antidepressants on an SOS or PRN (as needed) basis. They must be administered regularly in appropriate doses to achieve the desired effect.

It is essential to continue the antidepressant for a period of further 6 months after reaching remission, in the first episode of depressive disorder (and for longer duration in subsequent episodes) to prevent recurrence of symptoms. It is important to prescribe the antidepressant in the same dose as used for treatment unless there are adverse effects requiring a decrease in dose.

Only when adequate doses (150-300 mg imipramine equivalent) have been administered for an adequate period (at least 6 weeks) without a clinical response then the drug can be called ineffective for that patient. Another drug, usually from a different class or group, or ECT may then be used.

Side Effects and Toxicity

The common side effects of antidepressants with their management are summarised in Table 15.7.

TCAs are dangerous in overdose; amitriptyline and dosulepin (dotheipin) are particularly cardiotoxic whilst lofepramine is the safest amongst TCAs. Clinical features of overdose include agitation, delirium, paralytic ileus, urinary retention, coma, respiratory depression, seizures, hyperpyrexia, cardiac arrhythmias, conduction defects, mydriasis, and death. The lethal dose of imipramine is 1-2 g. (40-80 tabs. of 25 mg imipramine equivalence).

The treatment options in overdose include gastric lavage/induction of vomiting, activated charcoal for adsorption, cardio-respiratory resuscitation, treatment of seizures (if they occur), general supportive care and symptomatic management. Quinidine-like drugs are contraindicated whilst antiarrhythmics such as lignocaine can be helpful. Physostigmine 0.5 mg IV/IM bolus repeated to a total of 3-4 mg/day may be used under careful supervision. Coma often reverts in less than 24 hours, although toxicity lasts for 5-6 days.

Co-prescription of serotonergic drugs (such as SSRIs) with other serotonergic agents and especially MAOIs can lead to *serotonin syndrome*. It is characterised by a classic triad of mental status changes, neuromuscular abnormalities and autonomic hyper-

activity. These include anxiety, agitation, confusion, clonus (e.g. ankle clonus, ocular clonus), hyperreflexia, myoclonus, rigidity, increased heart rate, tremor, flushing, hyperthermia and excessive sweating. Death can occur in severe serotonin syndrome.

Treatment includes discontinuation of the offending drug(s), supportive management and (sometimes) use of serotonin and histamine antagonist cyproheptadine.

Refractory Depression

About 20-35% of patients do not respond to the antidepressant therapy. The chief reasons for this non-response include:

1. Poor drug concordance.
2. Inadequate dosage.
3. Insufficient treatment duration.
4. Low plasma antidepressant levels.
5. Incorrect diagnosis.

Even when these important reasons are excluded, there still remains a group (15-20%) of depressed patients who are non-responders or poor-responders. Such patients should receive a trial of another antidepressant preferably from a different group (e.g. SNRI) for adequate duration. In case the patient still does not respond, the treatment of choice of refractory depression is electroconvulsive therapy (ECT), though other treatment choices (such as lithium augmentation) are also available.

MOOD STABILISING DRUGS (DRUGS USED IN PROPHYLAXIS OF BIPOLAR DISORDER)

These drugs are usually effective in treatment of mania and therefore the word *antimanic* is often used to describe them. But as they are effective in preventing mood swings in bipolar disorder, the better term is *mood-stabilising agent* or a *prophylactic agent*. The most commonly used mood-stabilising agents include lithium, valproate, carbamazepine, and lamotrigine, though there are several other experimental mood stabilisers such as oxcarbazepine.

Table 15.7: Side Effects of Antidepressants

Category and Side Effect	Probable Cause	Maximum with (For example)	Minimum with (For example)	Management
A. Autonomic Side Effects				
1. Dry mouth	Muscarinic Cholinergic blockade	Amitriptyline	Fluoxetine	See table for side effects of antipsychotics (Table 15.3)
2. Constipation	–do–	Amitriptyline	Fluoxetine	
3. Cycloplegia	–do–	Amitriptyline	Fluoxetine	
4. Mydriasis	–do–	Amitriptyline	Fluoxetine	
5. Urinary retention	–do–	Amitriptyline	Fluoxetine	
6. Delirium	–do–	Amitriptyline	Fluoxetine	
7. Aggravation of narrow angle glaucoma	–do–	Amitriptyline	Fluoxetine	Do not use in elderly and in patients with past history. Change or stop drug.
8. Orthostatic hypotension	α_1 Adrenergic blockade	Amitriptyline	Fluoxetine	See table for side effects of antipsychotics (Table 15.3)
B. Sexual Side Effects				
1. Impotence	α_1 Adrenergic blockade	Amitriptyline	Mirtazapine Bupropion	
2. Impaired/ retarded ejaculation	α_1 Adrenergic blockade	Amitriptyline Paroxetine	Mirtazapine Bupropion	Cyproheptadine given 1 hour before, can reverse anorgasmia and retarded ejaculation caused by SSRIs.
3. Anorgasmia	5-HT blockade	SSRIs TCAs	Mirtazapine Bupropion	
4. Priapism	Not known	Trazodone	Not known	Stop drug; muscular relaxation; sometimes surgical procedure needed
C. CNS Effects				
1. Sedation	α Adrenergic blockade	Amitriptyline	Protriptyline Fluoxetine	This side effect may be beneficial; Otherwise decrease dose. Change drug. Give single dose only at night.
2. Tremor and Other EPSE	Serotonergic	Amoxapine	Not known	Decrease dose. Change drug.
3. Jitteriness syndrome	Adrenergic; Serotonergic	Imipramine Fluoxetine	MAOI	This is very common in first week of therapy. Add diazepam for first 1-2 weeks. Tolerance occurs.
4. Withdrawal syndrome (mild)	Dependence	Imipramine Paroxetine	Protriptyline Fluoxetine	Slow withdrawal of drug.
5. Seizures	Decreased threshold	Bupropion Amitriptyline	Nomifensine Fluoxetine	Decrease dose. Change drug.

Contd...

Contd...

Category and Side Effect	Probable Cause	Maximum with (For example)	Minimum with (For example)	Management
6. Aggravation of psychosis	Sympathomimetic	Not known	Amoxapine	Stop drug. Re-evaluate.
7. Precipitation of mania	Sympathomimetic	Tricyclics	Not known	Stop drug. Use mood stabilisers.
D. Cardiac Side Effects				
1. Tachycardia	Anticholinergic	Amitriptyline	Trazodone	Decrease dosage. Use safer drugs in elderly and those with past history or co-existing heart disease
2. Quinidine-like action (decreased conduction time)	Cardiotoxic	Amitriptyline	Fluoxetine	
3. ECG changes	Cardiotoxic	Amitriptyline	Fluoxetine	
4. Arrhythmias (in overdoses)	Cardiotoxic	Dosulepin Amitriptyline	Fluoxetine	
5. Direct myocardial depression (in overdoses)	Cardiotoxic	Amitriptyline	Fluoxetine	
6. Hypertension	Noradrenegic	Venlafaxine Duloxetine	SSRIs	Close monitoring; ECG and BP check before start (especially on higher doses); treat hypertension
E. Allergic Side Effects				
1. Agranulocytosis (very rare)	Hypersensitivity	Mianserin Mirtazapine	Not known	See table for side effects of antipsychotics (Table 15.3)
2. Cholestatic jaundice (very rare)	Hypersensitivity	Not known	Not known	
3. Skin rashes	Hypersensitivity	Not known	Not known	
4. Systemic vasculitis	Not known	Not known	Not known	
F. Metabolic and Endocrine Side Effects				
1. Weight gain	Not known	Mirtazapine Amitriptyline	Bupropion Fluoxetine can cause weight loss	Change drug. Exercise. Diet control.
G. Miscellaneous Side Effects				
1. Hypertensive crises	Interaction with tyramine in foods (cheese, red wine, chicken liver) and/or sympatho-mimetic drugs (e.g. ampheta-mine)	Tranylcypromine	Non-MAOIs	Prevent use of such agents with MAOI. Carry 'warning cards'. When crisis occurs, use alpha (α) blockers like phentolamine.

Contd...

Contd...

Category and Side Effect	Probable Cause	Maximum with (For example)	Minimum with (For example)	Management
2. Severe hepatic necrosis (rare)	Toxic or Hypersensitive	Iproniazid	Tranylcypromine	Stop/change drug. Supportive care; Death rate high.
3. Hyperpyrexia	Interaction with tricyclics or meperidine	Not known	Not known	Stop drug. Keep a gap of 1 week between imipramine and MAOI. Supportive care.
4. Bleeding	Decreased platelet serotonin	SSRIs	Not known	Change drug. Do not co-prescribe other drugs that increase risk of bleeding; Gastro-protective drugs such as PPIs can decrease risk to some extent in high-risk patients
5. Hyponatraemia	Probably SIADH	SSRIs SNRIs	Not known; Probably MAOIs	Risk higher in elderly; Avoid co-prescribing other drugs that cause hyponatraemia (such as diuretics); monitor closely

Recently, several atypical antipsychotics such as olanzapine, quetiapine and aripiprazole have been added to list of drugs used in *maintenance treatment* of bipolar disorder. In addition, other antipsychotics such as risperidone (and the others mentioned above) are also used as antimanic agents.

Lamotrigine and Quetiapine (and its metabolite norquetiapine) appear to have particular efficacy for treatment of bipolar depression. There is a risk of skin rash with lamotrigine particularly early in treatment and the risk appears higher with faster escalation of dose as well as with co-prescription of valproate. It is therefore important to increase the dose of lamotrigine very gradually as suggested in the summary of product characteristics (SPC) and the dose prescribed depends on other co-prescribed drugs (such as carbamazepine and valproate).

LITHIUM

Lithium (Li) is an element (Atomic number 3 and Atomic weight 7) which is the smallest alkali ion.

The element was discovered in 1817 by Arfuedson. Since then, it has been used for treatment of gout and for salt replacement in cardiac disease, but its use was restricted due to fatal toxicity.

It was rediscovered in 1949 by John Cade, for use in treatment of mania but its potential went unrecognised as it was discovered in Australia. Mogen Schou in 1957, had to rediscover it yet again before it became popular as a treatment of mania.

Indications

Although lithium salts are used in treatment of a myriad of psychiatric and non-psychiatric disorders, the established *indications* are only the following ones:
1. Treatment of acute mania
2. Prophylaxis of bipolar mood disorder.
   In addition, the following may also constitute *possible clinical indications* of lithium use:
3. Treatment of schizo-affective disorder
4. Prophylaxis of unipolar mood disorder
5. Treatment of cyclothymia

6. Treatment of acute depression (as an adjuvant for refractory depression)
7. Treatment of chronic alcoholism (in presence of significant depressive symptoms) and psychoactive use disorders (e.g. cocaine dependence)
8. Treatment of impulsive aggression
9. Treatment of Kleine-Levin syndrome.

Pharmacokinetics

Lithium is very rapidly absorbed from the gastrointestinal tract. The peak serum levels occur between 30 minutes to 3 hours. The absorption is virtually complete in about 8 hours.

The distribution is in total body water with a slow entry into the intracellular compartment. Lithium is not protein bound. The maximum levels occur in thyroid (3-5 times serum level), saliva (two times), milk (0.3-1.0 times) and CSF (0.4 times). The steady state levels are achieved in about 7 days. There is no metabolism of lithium in body and it is excreted almost entirely by the kidneys. Proximal reabsorption is influenced by the sodium balance, and depletion of sodium results in retention, causing higher blood levels of lithium.

Mechanism of Action

Lithium's mechanism of action is not known; however, the following mechanisms have been hypothesised:
1. It affects the Na^+-K^+ ATP-ase and accumulates intracellularly as a substitute of Na^+.
2. It inhibits the adenylate cyclase and thus decreases cAMP (II messenger) intracellularly.
3. It accelerates the presynaptic reuptake and destruction of catecholamines, like norepinephrine.
4. It inhibits the release of catecholamines at the synapse.
5. It decreases the postsynaptic serotonin 5-HT_2 receptor sensitivity.
6. It stabilizes the cell membrane, along with Ca^{++} and Mg^{++}.
7. It decreases the Ca^{++} mobilisation from the intracellular pools by ITP (inositol-triphosphate)-dependent Ca^{++} channels (*II messenger system*).

8. It interferes with the phosphatidyl-inositol cycle by blocking the conversion of IMP (inositol monophosphate) to inositol, by inositol monophosphate phosphatase. The muscarinic acetylcholine (Ach) receptor is among one of the neurotransmitter receptors linked to this system in brain. The antimanic effects of lithium may be attributed to this effect on Ach, thus affecting the cholinergic-adrenergic balance.

All these actions result in a decreased catecholamine activity, thus ameliorating mania. However, these mechanisms do not explain the antidepressant effect and the prophylactic effect in bipolar mood disorder. It is also described to possess NMDA (n-methyl d-aspartate) mediated neuroprotective properties.

There is a lag period of 7-10 days before the onset of action occurs, which is probably due to the time taken to achieve steady state levels.

Clinical Use

Lithium is available in market in the form of the following preparations.
1. Lithium carbonate (300 mg tablets; 400 mg sustained-release tablets)
2. Lithium citrate (300 mg/5 ml liquid; not available in India)

Before starting treatment, it is essential to ensure normal functioning of kidneys (one of the most important), thyroid, heart and central nervous system. After starting lithium, it is necessary to investigate these systems at repeated intervals.

The usual profile of investigations is as follows:
1. Routine general and systemic physical examination.
2. Routine blood counts (Hb, TC, DC).
3. Urine: routine and microscopic examination.
4. ECG.
5. Renal function tests (blood urea, serum creatinine, 24 hour urine volume, urine specific gravity). eGFR with creatinine clearance test, if indicated.
6. Thyroid function tests (TSH, T_3, T_4).

The initial daily starting dose of lithium for treatment of acute mania is usually 900-2100 mg/day,

Table 15.8: Blood Lithium Levels
(in treatment of bipolar disorder)

- Therapeutic levels = 0.6-1.2 mEq/L (For the treatment of acute mania)
- Prophylactic levels = 0.6-1.0 mEq/L (For relapse prevention in bipolar disorder)
- Toxic lithium levels > 2.0 mEq/L

given in 1-3 doses. Ideally, the treatment is started after serial lithium estimation, conducted after a loading dose of 600 mg or 900 mg of lithium carbonate, to determine pharmacokinetics. However, this method is much less frequently practiced these days.

During treatment it is essential to estimate blood lithium levels at regular intervals (usually 3 monthly) (Table 15.8). The blood sample for estimation is taken 12 hours after the last lithium dose. If any changes are made in lithium dosage, the next blood level is estimated after at least 5-7 days of the last change.

When stopping lithium treatment (except in cases of lithium toxicity), it is desirable to gradually taper the dose of lithium over several days or weeks in order to minimise the risk of early relapse on discontinuation.

There is evidence from several studies that lithium substantially reduces the risk of suicide in bipolar disorder; however, it has a narrow margin of safety and it is important to remember this particularly in patient with active ideas or plans of suicide.

Side Effects

Adverse effects are common and toxicity can occur easily, if blood levels reach about 2.0 mEq/L; life-threatening intoxication occurs, if levels reach about 3.5 mEq/L. In acute administration, toxicity is primarily neurological whilst during maintenance therapy renal side effects are the commonest.

The common side effects are listed below:

I. Neurological
1. Tremor: This is the commonest side effect, occurring in up to 50% of patients. Treatment is

by decreasing the dose of lithium or by adding propranolol.
2. Muscular weakness.
3. Cogwheel rigidity (mild).
4. Seizures (decreased threshold).
5. Neurotoxicity: The important features include delirium, cerebellar signs, abnormal involuntary movements, seizures, and later coma. In some individuals, toxicity may occur even within the therapeutic range. The treatment of choice for acute toxicity is haemodialysis.

II. Renal
The renal side effects occur in about 10-50% of all patients on maintenance lithium therapy. Some of the features include:
1. Polyuria, polydipsia.
2. Tubular changes.
3. Nephrogenic diabetes insipidus.
4. Nephrotic syndrome.

III. Cardiovascular
The effects on heart are similar to those of hypokalaemia. The commonest ECG change is T-wave depression.

IV. Endocrine
1. Goitre.
2. Hypothyroidism.
3. Abnormal thyroid function (30-40%).
4. Weight gain (pedal oedema is also common).

V. Gastrointestinal
These side effects include nausea, vomiting, diarrhoea, metallic taste and abdominal pain.

VI. Dermatological
These dermatological side effects include acneiform eruptions, papular eruptions and exacerbation of psoriasis.

VII. Side effects during pregnancy and lactation
1. Teratogenic (possibly).
2. Increased incidence of Ebstein's anomaly (distortion and downward displacement of tricuspid valve in the right ventricle), when taken in the first trimester.
3. Secreted in milk with 30-100% of the maternal blood lithium levels. Lithium can therefore cause toxicity in the infant.

Contraindications of Lithium Use

1. Presence of clear evidence of cardiac, renal, thyroid or neurological dysfunction
2. Presence of blood dyscrasia
3. During pregnancy and lactation
4. Concomitant administration of thiazide diuretics, tetracyclines or anaesthetics

ACE inhibitors (such as captopril), Angiotensin II receptor antagonists (such as losartan), NSAIDs (nonsteroidal anti-inflammatory drugs) and COX-2 inhibitors (such as celecoxib) can increase the risk of lithium toxicity in an unpredictable manner, especially in elderly.

VALPROATE

Valproate and lithium have been widely used as first line drugs for treatment of mania as well as for prophylaxis of bipolar mood disorder.

Valproic acid was first synthesised by Burton and used as an organic solvent. In 1963, Meunier serendipitously discovered the antiepileptic properties of valproic acid, while Lambert reported in 1966 that valpromide (a valproic acid analogue) might be effective as an antimanic. It was approved by the US FDA as an antiepileptic drug for absence seizures in 1978 and for the treatment of acute mania (and for migraine headache prophylaxis) in 1996.

Although its mechanism of action is not clearly understood, it increases GABA though other non-GABAergic mechanisms have been proposed.

The term *valproate* is often used to denote all commercial preparations, since the common entity in blood is valproic acid. The following preparations of valproate are available in India:

  i. Valproate sodium
 ii. Divalproex (Enteric-coated stable coordination compound composed of sodium valproate and valproic acid in a 1:1 molar relationship)
iii. Chrono preparations (Enteric-coated compound composed of sodium valproate and valproic acid in a 3:2 ratio).

It is rapidly and completely absorbed after oral administration. The peak plasma levels are reached at 1-4 hours after a single oral dose. The half-life of valproate is 8-17 hours.

The usual dose of valproate is 1000-3000 mg/day orally in divided doses. The therapeutic blood level is 50-125 mg/ml. Oral loading strategies (20-30 mg/kg/day) are rapidly effective in the management of acute mania.

Indications

In addition to its primary indication as an anticonvulsant, Valproate has several other indications in various psychiatric and neuropsychiatric disorders.

Bipolar Disorders

Acute Mania (as a first-line agent for the treatment of acute mania in oral and IV forms): Several factors associated with a favourable antimanic response to valproate (as well as carbamazepine) include:

a. Co-morbid substance abuse or other psychiatric disorders
b. Later age at onset and/or shorter duration of illness
c. History of poor response to lithium
d. Dysphoric mania, mixed affective episodes, or rapid cycling
e. Organic/complicated mania associated with seizure disorder, history of head trauma, or EEG abnormalities
f. D-M-I (Depression-Mania-Well Interval) pattern of illness, as opposed to the M-D-I pattern

There is some suggestion that patients non-responsive to valproate may respond well to carbamazepine.

Prophylaxis: Valproate is probably less effective in maintenance treatment of bipolar disorder than in treatment of acute mania. It has been used alone, as well as along with lithium and other mood stabilisers in the maintenance treatment.

The addition of valproate to lithium has been recognised as a useful treatment for mania refractory to lithium monotherapy.

Rapid cycling bipolar disorder and mixed (or dysphoric) mania: The patients with rapid cycling, mixed affective episodes, or dysphoric mania are often resistant to lithium treatment and respond better to valproate. Valproate is also effective in management of ultra-rapid cycling mood disorders.

Bipolar depression: Valproate appears to be generally more effective in the treatment of acute mania than in bipolar depression.

Neurological Disorders

Migraine and Pain syndromes: Valproate has been used for prophylaxis of migraine headaches, as well as for aborting an acute attack (IV route). Valproate has also been used in treatment of trigeminal neuralgia and neuropathic pain.

Seizure disorders: Valproate is primarily indicated for treatment of absence seizures (both simple and complex), complex partial seizures, myoclonic seizures, and generalised tonic-clonic seizures, as monotherapy as well as adjunct therapy.

Other Disorders

Valproate has also been used at times in several other conditions, including behavioural agitation in dementia, severe behavioural symptoms in mental retardation, ADHD and conduct disorder, schizoaffective disorder (bipolar type), alcohol withdrawal, tardive dyskinesia, impulse control disorder, panic disorder and borderline personality disorder.

Side Effects

Adverse effects are more common with valproate concentrations above 100 mg/ml.

The common side effects are nausea, sedation, tremor, flushing, weight gain, thrombocytopenia, menstrual disturbances (in women) and hair loss. There are some reports of polycystic ovaries and hyperandrogenism in young women with epilepsy.

The most serious, though relatively uncommon, side effects include hepatic toxicity (especially in young children), acute haemorrhagic pancreatitis, and Steven-Johnson syndrome.

The use of valproate in pregnancy and lactation should be best avoided. The NICE guidelines for treatment of bipolar disorder recommend that valproate is best avoided in women of childbearing potential (see Further Reading List).

In overdose, the amount of drug, that is not protein bound, is high. Therefore, dialysis is useful in the management of an overdose with valproate.

Drug Interactions

Certain drug may *increase* (such as aspirin, cimetidine, ibuprofen, erythromycin, fluoxetine, fluvoxamine, phenothiazines) or *decrease* (such as carbamazepine, phenytoin, phenobarbital, ethosuximide, rifampicin, mefloquine) the serum levels of valproate.

In addition, valproate *increases* serum levels of other drugs (such as lamotrigine, tricyclic antidepressants, zidovudine, tolbutamide).

CARBAMAZEPINE

Like lithium and valproate, carbamazepine too has been used as an antimanic and for prophylaxis of bipolar disorder. It is a tricyclic compound synthesised in 1953 by Schindler. It has a structure similar to TCAs. The onset of action can be faster as compared to lithium, but slower compared to valproate.

The usual dose is 600-1600 mg/day orally, in divided doses. The treatment is best monitored with repeated blood levels. The therapeutic blood levels are 4-12 µg/ml and the toxic blood levels are usually reached at >15 µg/ml.

Indications

The *indications* for use of carbamazepine include:
1. Seizures
   i. Complex partial seizures (CPS)
   ii. Generalised tonic clonic seizures
   iii. Alcohol withdrawal seizures (*rum fits*), if persistent (also used sometimes for treatment of simple alcohol withdrawal syndrome)
2. Psychiatric disorders
   i. Bipolar mood disorder (especially for rapid cyclers; lithium-refractory patients; lithium-

intolerant patients; for prophylaxis in some patients; for treatment of acute mania, especially severe and dysphoric mania)

   ii. Impulse control disorder and aggression (in some cases)

   iii. Psychosis (especially mania) with epilepsy

   iv. Borderline personality disorder (for treatment of mood swings)

   v. Cocaine withdrawal syndrome

3. Paroxysmal pain syndromes

   i. Trigeminal neuralgia

   ii. Phantom limb pain

   iii. Other paroxysmal pain syndromes (neuralgias).

Side Effects

The major side effects include diplopia, drowsiness, dizziness, nausea, vomiting, ataxia, skin rash, Steven-Johnson syndrome (erythema multiforme major), photosensitivity, cholestatic jaundice, acute oliguria with hypertension, leucopenia and thrombocytopenic purpura. The most dangerous side effects include bone marrow depression (causing aplastic anaemia), agranulocytosis and cardiovascular collapse.

Therefore, it is essential to monitor cardiac, renal, hepatic and bone-marrow functions during carbamazepine treatment. The use of carbamazepine in pregnancy and lactation should be best avoided.

The use of carbamazepine in management of bipolar disorder appears to be recently declining.

ANTI-ANXIETY DRUGS

Anti-anxiety drugs, also known as minor tranquilisers and anxiolytics, can be classified as follows:

Classification

Barbiturates

Barbiturates can be divided into four main types:

Long Acting

The duration of action is more than 8 hours. Examples include phenobarbital.

Intermediate Acting

The duration of action is 5-8 hours. Examples include amobarbital and pentobarbital.

Short Acting

The duration of action is 1-5 hours. Examples include secobarbital.

Ultra-Short Acting

The duration of action is less than 1 hour. Examples include thiopentone and methohexital.

Barbiturates are no longer used or recommended as anti-anxiety agents. They produce multiple side effects such as excessive sedation, respiratory and circulatory depression, hepatic enzyme induction, dependence, withdrawal symptoms, rebound increase in REM-sleep on withdrawal, and potential for use in suicide.

Non-barbiturate, Non-benzodiazepine Anti-anxiety Agents

These can be further divided into the following categories:

Carbamates

The common examples are meprobamate, tybamate and carisoprodol. These are not used commonly due to the potential for abuse and dependence.

Piperidinediones

An example is glutethimide. This drug too is not used now-a-days due to its dependence potential.

Alcohols

The examples include ethanol, chloral hydrate and ethchlorvynol. These drugs are highly dependence producing and clearly not recommended.

Quinazoline Derivatives

An example is methaqualone. Methaqualone had become a street drug (i.e. a drug of abuse) and its use was discontinued as an anti-anxiety agent and a hypnotic.

Anti-histaminics

The common examples include diphenhydramine, hydroxyzine and promethazine. In past, diphenhydramine was usually combined with methaqualone or diazepam. They may be used as hypnotic-sedatives, but their use as anti-anxiety agents is minimal and probably not safe.

Cyclic Ethers
An example is paraldehyde. It is not used commonly as it is not very effective and is also dependence producing.

Others
Antipsychotics (such as thioridazine, flupentixol, olanzapine, quetiapine) and antidepressants (such as doxepine) have sometimes been used for the treatment of severe, intractable anxiety. However, antipsychotics are not the drugs of first choice and should be used with extreme discretion (with balancing of risks and benefits) when all other drugs have failed to benefit.

Antidepressants (such as SSRIs, SNRIs and Mirtazapine) have recently emerged as treatments of choice in several anxiety disorders including generalised anxiety disorder, obsessive compulsive disorder, panic disorder and obsessive compulsive disorder. There is some data to support that smaller starting doses are better as anxiety symptoms may worsen initially in treatment.

Beta (β) Blockers
An example is propranolol which is particularly effective in treatment of peripheral somatic manifestations of anxiety. It is also helpful in treatment of anticipatory anxiety and situational anxiety. Propranolol can be used either alone or along with benzodiazepines. β-blockers are not treatments of first choice in the treatment of psychic or psychological manifestations of anxiety.

Propranolol is contraindicated in patients with bronchial asthma and cardiac conditions. It should be used with caution in patients of age 40 and above. The usual dose is 40-240 mg/day, administered in divided doses.

Benzodiazepines

Since the discovery of chlordiazepoxide in 1957 by Sternbach, benzodiazepines have replaced other antianxiety drugs and hypnotics though SSRIs are now gradually becoming drugs of first choice in management of anxiety disorders.

The benzodiazepines can be classified according to their elimination half-lives (Table 15.9).

Indications
The *indications* for use of benzodiazepines include the following:
1. Generalised anxiety disorder; adjustment disorder with anxious mood (Short-term use)
2. Panic disorder, agoraphobia, and school phobia (particularly alprazolam and clonazepam; short-term use, along with antidepressants)
3. Agitated depression (short-term use, along with antidepressants, for first 1-2 weeks)
4. Short-term treatment of insomnia
5. Stage 4 NREM-sleep disorders such as enuresis, somnambulism (diazepam reduces duration of Stage 4 NREM-sleep)
6. Nightmares (diazepam also reduces the REM-sleep duration).
7. Pre-medication in anaesthesia (intravenous lorazepam, midazolam, or diazepam)
8. Anticonvulsant use (drugs of choice for status epilepticus, myoclonic seizures and certain infantile spasms)
9. To produce skeletal muscle relaxation (e.g. in tetanus, cerebral palsy)
10. Treatment of alcohol and other drug withdrawal syndromes
11. For minor surgical, endoscopic or obstetric procedures
12. Acute mania (lorazepam, usually with lithium or atypical antipsychotics).
13. Antipsychotic-induced akathisia
14. Emergency management of acute psychoses (IV lorazepam, along with parenteral antipsychotics).
15. Narcoanalysis or abreaction (IV diazepam)

Whenever administered, benzodiazepines should not be *ordinarily* used for more than 2-4 weeks at a time; otherwise risk of dependence is quite high and tolerance occurs.

Mechanism of Action
The exact mechanism of action of benzodiazepines is not clear. The discovery of the benzodiazepine receptors in 1977 shed some light on the mode of action (Fig. 15.1).

Table 15.9: Classification and Properties of Benzodiazepines

Class and Drug	Elimination Half-life (Hours)	Usual Hypnotic Dose (mg HS/Nocte)	Oral Dose (mg/day)	Parenteral Dose (mg)	Active Metabolites	Other Comments
I. Very Short Acting Drugs						
1. *Midazolam*	2-5 hours	—	—	—	—	Used for anaesthesia
2. *Triazolam*	2-5 hours	0.125-0.25 mg	—	—	α-hydroxy-triazolam	Rapid oral absorption; Marketed as hypnotic
II. Short Acting Drugs						
1. *Alprazolam*	6-20 hours	—	0.5-6.0 mg	—	α-hydroxy-alprazolam	—
2. *Estazolam*	8-24 hours	1-2 mg	1-2 mg	—	—	—
3. *Loprazolam*	6-12 hours	1-2 mg	—	—	Piperazine N-oxide	—
4. *Lormetazepam*	10-12 hours	0.5-1.5 mg	—	—	Lorazepam	—
5. *Lorazepam*	10-20 hours	0.5-2.0 mg	2-6 mg	2-4 mg	None	High dependence potential
6. *Oxazepam*	5-15 hours	15-30 mg	15-120 mg	—	None	Slow oral absorption
7. *Temazepam*	10-20 hours	10-20 mg	10-20 mg	—	Oxazepam	Slow oral absorption
III. Long Acting Drugs						
1. *Chlorazepate*	30-100 hours	7.5-30 mg	7.5-60 mg	—	Nordiazepam	Hydrolysed to active form in stomach
2. *Chlordiazepoxide*	25-48 hours	10-25 mg	15-100 mg	50-100 mg	Desmethyl-demoxepam	Erratic absorption after IM injection
3. *Clonazepam*	20-40 hours	—	0.5-20 mg	2-5 mg	—	Also used in treatment of epilepsy
4. *Diazepam*	14-90 hours	2-10 mg	2-30 mg	2-20 mg	Nordiazepam	Erratic absorption after IM injection
5. *Flurazepam*	30-100 hours	15-30 mg	15-60 mg	—	Desmethyl-hydroxy-ethyl-flurazepam	Marketed as a hypnotic
6. *Halazepam*	30-60 hours	20-40 mg	40-160 mg	—	Nordiazepam	—
7. *Nitrazepam*	20-60 hours	5-10 mg	5-20 mg	—	Nordiazepam	Marketed as a hypnotic

Contd...

Contd...

Class and Drug	Elimination Half-life (Hours)	Usual Hypnotic Dose (mg HS/Nocte)	Oral Dose (mg/day)	Parenteral Dose (mg)	Active Metabolites	Other Comments
8. Prazepam	30-60 hours	10-20 mg	20-60 mg	—	Nordiazepam and Diazepam	Slow oral absorption
9. Quazepam	40-160 hours	7.5-15 mg	7.5-30 mg		—	Probably selective for benzodiazepine receptor I; may cause less cognitive/motor disturbances.

Each drug is described under the headings of elimination half-life (hours); usual hypnotic dose (mg nocte/HS); usual oral dose (mg/day; if applicable); usual parenteral dose (mg; if applicable); active metabolites and other comments.

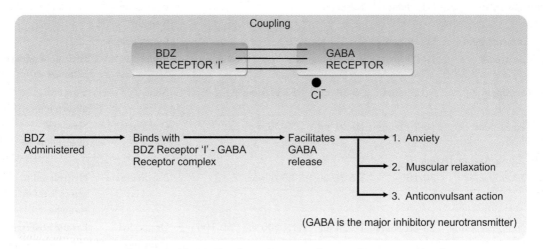

Fig. 15.1: Probable Mechanism of Action of Benzodiazepines (BDZ)

There are, presently, two known benzodiazepine (BDZ) receptors.
1. BDZ Receptor I, which is linked with the GABA (Gamma-Aminobutyric acid) receptor and is involved in mediation of sleep.
2. BDZ Receptor II, which is alone and is involved in cognition and motor control.

Thus, benzodiazepines act by enhancing GABA transmission in the brain.

Benzodiazepine receptor antagonists (such as flumazenil) are anxiety-provoking agents. Flumazenil has a half-life of 60 minutes and administered in a parenteral dose of 0.2-1.0 mg IV given over 1-2 minutes in treatment of benzodiazepine toxicity.

Classification of Benzodiazepines

Each drug is described in Table 15.9 under the headings of elimination half-life (hours); usual hypnotic dose (mg nocte/HS); usual oral dose (mg/day; if applicable); usual parenteral dose (mg; if applicable); active metabolites and other comments.

Side Effects

The side effects of benzodiazepines include nausea, vomiting, weakness, epigastric pain, diarrhoea, vertigo, blurring of vision, body aches, urinary incontinence (rare), impotence, sedation, lassitude, increased reaction time, ataxia (in high doses), dry mouth, retrograde amnesia (rare), impairment of driving skills, severe effects when administered with alcohol, irritability, disinhibited behaviour, dependence and withdrawal symptoms (on stopping the drug).

Cross-tolerance occurs with barbiturates, methaqualone and ethyl alcohol. A worsening of depression and pre-existing psychosis with use of benzodiazepines has been reported.

Since withdrawal symptoms usually occur after long-term use, benzodiazepines should be withdrawn slowly.

Newer Drugs

1. Buspirone

Buspirone is a non-benzodiazepine, anti-anxiety drug. It is an azaspiro decanedione (azapirone) derivative. Buspirone is a 5-HT$_{1A}$ partial agonist and a selective DA autoreceptor antagonist. It also inhibits the spontaneous firing of 5-HT neurons.

It does not seem to act on the benzodiazepine receptors. It is anxioselective, with no sedative action, and no anticonvulsant or muscle-relaxant properties.

It is administered in a dose of 15-30 mg/day, in a thrice daily schedule due to a short half-life. As it has a slower and more gradual onset of action, it usually takes about two weeks before its anti-anxiety effects are evident. Buspirone is not useful in treatment of panic disorder. The common side effects include dizziness, headache, lightheadedness and diarrhoea.

As it is an anxio-selective and lacks any risk of dependence, it was hoped that it might replace the benzodiazepines as the drug of choice in treatment of generalised anxiety disorders. However, it is not as widely used as it was once expected.

2. Zopiclone

Zopiclone belongs to a new class of non-benzodiazepine drugs, the cyclopyrrolones. Cyclopyrrolone derivatives also act on the GABA receptors, but at a site distinct from that of benzodiazepines. Zopiclone has a short duration of action as well as shorter onset. After oral administration, it is absorbed rapidly, with peak plasma concentration occurring in about 60 minute. The elimination half-life is 4-6 hours.

The usual dose of zopiclone is 3.75-7.5 mg at bedtime (lower dose in elderly patients and in patients with severe hepatic failure). The side effects include bitter taste, dry mouth, drowsiness, nausea and headache. Its safety in children, in pregnancy and lactation is not proven. It is clinically superior to benzodiazepines in subjective awakening quality, well-being, and attention span in the morning.

3. Zolpidem

Zolpidem is an imidazopyridine derivative which is marketed as a hypnotic. It is administered in a dose of 5-10 mg for hypnotic use. It has a half-life of 2-3 hours; therefore it is useful in the treatment of difficulty in initiation of sleep (initial insomnia).

The side effects include drowsiness, dizziness, headache, depression, nausea, dry mouth, and myalgia. It should not be used for more than two weeks at one time. Its safety in children, in pregnancy and lactation is not proven.

4. Zalpelon

Zalpelon is a pyrazolo-pyrimidine derivative which is marketed as a hypnotic. Although a non-benzodiazepine drug, it acts on the omega-1 benzodiazepine receptor located on the alpha sub-unit of the GABA-A receptor complex (causing sedation), with very little effect on omega-2 and omega-3 receptors.

It is administered in a dose of 5-10 mg for hypnotic use. It has a half-life of one hour with a rapid onset of effect. Therefore, it is useful in treatment of difficulty in initiation of sleep (initial insomnia). It can be taken again at night if there is more than 4 hours of sleep time remaining. Because of the very short half-life, there is virtually no hangover in the morning.

The side effects include headache, drowsiness, dizziness, nausea, and myalgia. It should not be used for more than 2 weeks at one time. Its safety in children, in pregnancy and lactation is not proven.

5. Other Drugs

The other newer hypnosedative and anti-anxiety drugs include *suriclone* (a cyclopyrrolone derivative; a hypnotic), *bretazenil* and *imidazenil* (partial benzodiazepine agonists; anxiolytic without sedation; rapid onset of action), *abecarnil* (β-carboline partial agonist at benzodiazepine receptor; anxiolytic and anticonvulsant), *tiagabine*, *riluzole*, and *alpidem* (anxiolytic).

Pregabalin is licensed for treatment of anxiety in some countries. Cognitive behaviour therapy with or without medication is helpful in treatment of several anxiety disorders.

Chapter 16

Other Biological Methods of Treatment

The last 75 years have seen the development of several biological methods of treatment for treatment of psychiatric disorders. The earlier modes of treatment, such as malarial treatment for general paralysis of insane (GPI), insulin coma therapy, atropine coma therapy, continuous sleep treatment, sub-convulsive ECT, chemical convulsive therapy, sleep deprivation, mega-vitamin therapy and hallucinogens (to name a few important methods) are no longer used in routine clinical practice.

Although there are other new biological methods recently introduced for the treatment of psychiatric disorders, such as *vagal nerve stimulation* (VNS), *transcranial magnetic stimulation* (TMS) and *deep brain stimulation* (DBS), these are not discussed in this book.

There are two methods which though introduced at the same time have been revised extensively and are still in use presently. These methods are electroconvulsive therapy and psychosurgery.

ELECTROCONVULSIVE THERAPY

Brief History

Von Meduna, in 1934, used 25% camphor in oil intramuscularly to produce convulsions for the first time for therapeutic purposes. Later, he used pentylenetetrazol (metrazol) for the same purpose.

A much safer form of convulsive therapy was used by Cerletti and Bini in 1938 (Table 16.1). They called it EST or electroshock therapy. Later, this method of treatment came to be known as ECT or electroconvulsive therapy. The 1970s saw widespread criticism of ECT, with many legislations passed in the US states (e.g. in California, 1975), restricting the use of ECT. Following this, widespread modifications in the ECT technique made it even safer mode of treatment.

In 1974, the American Psychiatric Association's (APA's) Council on Research and Development appointed a Task Force on ECT. *The APA Task Force on ECT*, in 1976, gave its report which provided clear guidelines for use of ECT and declared it to be a safe and effective method of treatment when used by professionals trained in the technique. The 1990 APA Task Force Report on ECT redefined the indications, gave guidelines for obtaining consent and set standards for training, treatment and privileging of ECT. The most recent version of this task force report became available in 2001.

Indications

The indications for electroconvulsive therapy are:
1. Major severe depression
    i. With suicidal risk (This is the first and most important indication for ECT)
    ii. With stupor
    iii. With poor intake of food and fluids

Table 16.1: A Brief Early History of Biological Treatments in Psychiatry

Year	Treatment	Started by
1785	Camphor-induced seizures	W Oliver
1917	Malarial treatment of GPI	Julius Wagner von Jauregg
1922	Barbiturate coma therapy	Jacob Klaesi
1931	Reserpine (1st drug treatment in psychosis)	Ganesh Sen, Kartik Bose
1933	Insulin coma therapy	Manfred Sakel
1934	Cardiazol (metrazol) induced seizures	LLJ von Meduna
1936	Psychosurgery (prefrontal leucotomy)	Egas Moniz, Almenda Lima
1938	Electroshock (electroconvulsive therapy)	Ugo Cerletti, Lucio Bini
1949	Lithium (for mania)	John F Cade
1952	Chlorpromazine (1st antipsychotic)	Jean PL Delay, Pierre Deniker
1954	Meprobamate	FM Berger
1958	Iproniazid (1st MAO inhibitor)	Nathan Kline
1958	Imipramine (1st tricyclic antidepressant)	Thomas Kuhn
1958	Haloperidol (1st non-phenothiazine antipsychotic)	Janssen
1960	Chlordiazepoxide (1st benzodiazepine)	Hugo Sternbach

   iv. With melancholia

   v. With psychotic features

   vi. With unsatisfactory response to drug therapy

   vii. Where drugs are contraindicated, or have serious side effects

   viii. Where speedier recovery is needed.

2. Severe catatonia (non-organic)

   i. With stupor

   ii. With poor intake of food and fluids

   iii. With unsatisfactory response to drug therapy

   iv. Where drugs are contraindicated, or have serious side-effects.

   v. Where speedier recovery is needed.

3. Severe psychoses (schizophrenia or mania)

   i. With risk of suicide, homicide or danger of physical assault

   ii. With unsatisfactory response to drug therapy

   iii. Where drugs are contraindicated, or have serious side effects

   iv. With very prominent depressive features (e.g. schizo-affective disorder).

The use of ECT in mania and schizophrenia is not a treatment of first choice and is employed only in the above-mentioned conditions. A history of good response with ECT and patient preference for ECT also determine the use of ECT.

The 1990 APA Task Force on ECT also defined as *suggestive indications* (for occasional use) the following disorders:

1. Organic mental disorders (e.g. organic mood syndrome, organic hallucinosis, organic delusional disorder, and delirium).

2. Medical disorders (e.g. organic catatonia, neuroleptic malignant syndrome and parkinsonism).

Pre-treatment Evaluation

The pre-treatment evaluation consists of the following steps:

1. An *informed consent*, taken from the patient. If the patient does not have capacity or competence to give consent, consideration must be given to the most recent legal guidelines and local procedures which can include the best interest decision with consent of guardian/family and additional opinion from another professional.

2. Detailed medical and psychiatric history taking, which includes the current and past treatment history.

3. General and systemic physical examination.
4. Routine laboratory investigations, such as Hb, TC, DC, ESR, urinary examination, ECG, X-ray chest, and any other investigations in the light of history and examination. Other optional investigations, which are not done routinely, include EEG and estimation of plasma pseudocholinesterase activity (for patients who would receive succinylcholine for general anaesthesia).
5. Examination of fundus oculi to rule out papilloedema.

Contraindications

Absolute

The only absolute contraindication is the presence of *raised intracranial tension* (so an examination of the fundus oculi is an essential step). However, the APA Task Force Report on ECT recognises this too as a relative contraindication.

Relative

These include:
1. Recent myocardial infarction (MI)
2. Severe hypertension
3. Cerebrovascular accident (CVA)
4. Severe pulmonary disease
5. Retinal detachment, and
6. Pheochromocytoma.

Technique

The techniques used for ECT administration are of two types:
   i. ***Direct ECT*** is administered in the absence of muscular relaxation and general anaesthesia. All the other steps are the same as in modified ECT. This method of treatment is nowadays very infrequently used and not understandably encouraged by most guidelines.
   ii. ***Modified ECT*** is modified by drug-induced muscular relaxation and general anaesthesia administered by an anaesthetist.

ECT is usually administered in the morning after an overnight fast. If given at any other time during the day, the patient should be *empty stomach* for at least 4 hours. No oral medication should be given in the morning. The *bladder* (and bowel) should be emptied just before the treatment, as incontinence can occur during the induced seizure. Dentures, if present, should be removed, and the presence of loose teeth should be ruled out. Tight clothing, and metallic and sharp objects (if any) should be removed from the person's body.

The usual anaesthetic precautions are taken. The patient is placed on a hard bed which is well insulated. A slow intravenous drip may be started (though not needed in all patients). Atropine (0.6 mg) is given IV just before the treatment or else is given IM or SC 30 minutes before treatment. Atropine is given to decrease the oral secretions and to prevent vagal stimulation during ECT which can cause cardiac arrest. However, this method is not followed at many centres these days.

This step is followed by administration of an anaesthetic agent such as propofol (0.75–2.5 mg/kg) or thiopentone (2-5 mg/kg, usually individualised dose for each patient) and a muscle relaxant like succinylcholine (0.5-1.5 mg/kg). An anaesthetic mask is placed on the face and ventilation with 100% oxygen is given. As succinylcholine is a depolarising blocking agent, its administration is followed by muscular fasciculations which move from above downwards. When the fine twitching movements disappear from the lower extremities, it is the time of complete muscular relaxation.

Now a mouth gag is inserted between teeth, to prevent tongue bite during convulsion and pressure is applied on mandible to approximate upper and lower teeth till convulsions stop. The electrodes (usually U-shaped) are moistened with saline or 25% bicarbonate solution and are applied on head. According to the position of application of electrodes, ECT is of two types:
   i. *Bilateral ECT:* This is the standard form of ECT used most commonly. Each electrode is placed 2.5-4.0 cm (1-1½") above the midpoint, on a line joining the tragus of the ear and the lateral canthus of the eye.

ii. *Unilateral ECT:* In this type, electrodes are placed only on one side of head, usually the non-dominant side (right side of head in right-handed individual). There are various positions described for the electrode placement.

The unilateral ECT is safer, with much fewer side effects, particularly those of memory impairment. However, according to the APA ECT Task Force Report, bilateral ECT is superior to unilateral ECT in effectiveness.

The electrode placement sites are cleaned with normal saline or 25% bicarbonate solution, or a conducting gel is applied. One attendant places one hand each on both thighs near the knee joint, while another attendant holds the shoulders. This is usually a must in direct ECT, but may also be done in modified ECT. This is to prevent falls from the bed and causation of fracture or dislocation due to muscular contractions (which may occasionally occur even in modified ECT).

The therapeutic adequacy of the treatment is usually gauzed by the occurrence of a generalized tonic-clonic seizure lasting for not less than 25-30 seconds. This is ensured by:

1. Observing the seizure (in direct ECT).
2. EEG recording during ECT (in modified ECT).
3. Occluding the circulation of one extremity with a BP apparatus cuff, before giving succinyl-choline. Thus, the whole body is paralyzed but one extremity convulses and can be directly observed.
4. Observing plantar extension and eyelid contractions which may be seen despite the muscular relaxation (not a very reliable method).

Most guidelines recommended that seizure activity by EEG of at least 25 seconds and observed convulsion of at least 15 seconds was needed for the seizure to be classified as adequate. However, the recent (Third) Report of the Royal College of Psychiatrists' Special Committee on ECT (2004) recommended that there is not enough evidence to suggest that the observed seizure duration is important. According to this report, a bilateral generalized seizure is more important.

The usual dose for obtaining an adequate seizure response is 90-150 volts (average 110 volts) for 0.1-1.0 seconds (average 0.6 seconds). The usual amount of current passed in an ECT session is 200-1600 mA.

Earlier, the ECT machines used a *sine wave* to deliver the current (with a positive and a negative wave constituting a cycle). However, with *sine wave*, unnecessarily excessive and inefficient electrical stimulus is delivered. The newer ECT machines instead use a *brief pulse* wave form that delivers the electrical stimulus, usually in a 1-2 msec time period at a rate of 30-100 pulses/second. Therefore, the *brief pulse* current is more efficacious and safer than the *sine wave* current. There are clear guidelines available regarding the procedure with the new machines.

The stimulus dosing protocols have two principles, namely *calculation of the seizure threshold* (the minimum stimulus that induces an adequate seizure) and *calculation of the treatment stimulus* (usually 1.5 times supra-threshold for the bilateral and 2.5 times for the unilateral ECT). So, the patient is stimulated at higher stimulus levels during the treatment than the seizure threshold (therefore, suprathreshold).

After seizure has occurred, the mouth gag is removed, secretions are removed by a suction machine from the oral cavity, and oxygen mask is applied. Till consciousness is regained, the patient is turned to one side to prevent aspiration. The vital parameters are constantly monitored till recovery occurs. The patient is made to rest, for about 30 minutes to 1 hour, on bed after the treatment is over.

Duration of Therapy

The total duration and number of treatments given depends on the diagnosis, presence of side effects, and the response to treatment. Usually 6-10 treatments are sufficient, although up to 15 treatments can be given if needed. The treatments should be spaced, so that no more than 3 ECTs are given per week.

Although ECT is very effective in severe depressive disorder (for example), the benefit lasts only till the ECTs are given. There is no residual benefit after the treatment is over. Hence, the patient needs antidepressants (for example) during and after the ECTs are over.

Mechanism of Action

The efficacy of ECT is linked with production of generalised tonic-clonic seizures though, as stated above, there is some recent doubt about the need for a seizure duration of 25-30 sec. Although the exact mechanism is unclear, one hypothesis states that ECT possibly affects the catecholamine pathways between diencephalon (from where seizure generalisation occurs) and limbic system (which may be responsible for mood disorders), also involving hypothalamus.

As ECT increases the threshold for further seizures, it may paradoxically act as an anticonvulsant. ECT also causes down-regulation of β_1 receptors in cortex and hippocampus.

Side Effects

1. Side effects associated with general anaesthesia: *Deaths* during ECT are usually due to the general anaesthesia, succinylcholine (in patients with deficiency of pseudo-cholinesterase) or drug-interactions. According to the APA Task Force Report (2001), the approximate mortality rate is 1:10,000 patients (or 1:80,000 treatments), which is similar to any operative procedure under anaesthesia.

2. *Memory disturbances* (both anterograde and retrograde) are very common. These are usually mild and recovery occurs within 1-6 months after treatment. Unilateral ECTs cause much less memory disturbance than bilateral ECTs.

3. *Confusion* may occur in the postictal period. Like memory disturbances, confusion is much commoner with bilateral ECTs. Usually, no treatment is needed. Parenteral diazepam may be given for excitement during this period.

4. *Other side effects* include headache, prolonged apnoea, prolonged seizure, cardiovascular dysfunction, emergent mania, muscle aches and apprehension.

ECT does *not* cause any brain damage.

PSYCHOSURGERY

Definition

Psychosurgery is defined (by APA's Task Force) as, a surgical intervention, to sever fibres connecting one part of brain with another, or to remove, destroy or stimulate brain tissue, with the intent of modifying behaviour, thought or mood disturbances, for which there is no underlying organic pathology (i.e. the disturbance is 'functional').

Brief History

Although surgery on skull (such as trephining) was done for mental illnesses even in 'primitive' times, psychosurgery was introduced as *leucotomy* by Egas Moniz and Almenda Lima in 1936. Egaz Moniz later even received a Noble prize. Freeman and Watts later introduced *prefrontal lobotomy* in 1937, while in India, Govindaswami and Rao performed the first leucotomies in 1944.

Psychosurgery came in for a severe public criticism in the 1950s when its use decreased substantially. In the last few decades, several better methods of treatment have been developed which are safer and more specific. In addition, careful guidelines for the use of psychosurgery have also been laid down.

Anatomical Basis

It is believed that limbic system is closely linked with normal and abnormal emotional reactions. The limbic system (Fig. 16.1) consists mainly of cingulum (cingulate gyrus and cingulate bundle), hippocampus, parahippocampal gyri, fornix, amygdala, parts of thalamus, parts of hypothalamus and posterior part of orbital frontal cortex.

The limbic system is closely connected with the frontal and temporal lobes, midbrain and other parts of brain, by many connecting fibres. The aim of psychosurgery is to produce surgical lesions in carefully selected parts of limbic system and/or its connecting fibres. One major part of limbic system, believed to be important in emotional experiences, is *Papez circuit*. This important circuit, which lies within the limbic

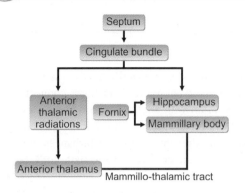

Fig. 16.1: Papez Circuit

system, connects cingulate bundle, hippocampus, anterior thalamus, mammillary bodies, fornix and septum (Fig. 16.1).

Indications

The current indications for psychosurgery include the following:

1. Chronic, severe, incapacitating depression, which has not responded to all available treatments.
2. Chronic, severe, incapacitating obsessive-compulsive disorder (OCD), which has not responded to all available treatments.
3. Chronic, severe, incapacitating anxiety disorder, which has not responded to all available treatments.
4. Schizophrenia with severe depressive component, which has not responded to all available treatments.
5. Severe, pathological and uncontrolled aggressive behaviour associated with a psychiatric or neurological illness (e.g. temporal lobe epilepsy).

It is believed that the maximum improvement occurs in distress, tension, anxiety and agitation rather than in other symptoms. An intact, well-maintained premorbid personality is a good prognostic sign.

Techniques

Before any procedure, an *informed consent* must be obtained by the neurosurgeon and the treating team. Currently, all techniques use *stereotactic methods* so that the lesion made is precise and side effects produced are few. The available procedures include bimedial leucotomy, orbital undercutting, rostral leucotomy, prefrontal leucotomy, anterior or posterior cingulumectomy and stereotactic tractotomy (in addition to those mentioned below).

The lesion is produced by electrocoagulation, freezing, thermocoagulation, ultrasonic method, Yttrium-90 seeds, or laser.

The currently employed procedures include:

1. ***Stereotactic Subcaudate Tractotomy:*** A large subcaudate lesion is produced. It is recommended for severe depression, severe anxiety, severe obsessive-compulsive disorder and schizo-affective disorder.
2. ***Stereotactic Limbic Leucotomy:*** A small subcaudate lesion is made, in addition to a lesion in cingulate bundle. It is used for treatment of intractable obsessive-compulsive disorder and schizophrenia.
3. ***Amygdalotomy:*** This is used for severe, pathological, uncontrolled and intractable aggression associated with neuropsychiatric disorders.

Side Effects

With the use of stereotactic procedures, side effects are very rare. These include a less than 1% risk of seizures, a very uncommon risk of personality change (which used to be frequent with earlier procedures) and a 1:1,000 to 1:10,000 mortality risk.

Comments

It must be remembered that at present, psychosurgery is an extremely uncommon procedure in the routine psychiatric practice in India and most of the world. Most psychiatrists would have never referred any patient for the procedure.

Chapter 17   Psychoanalysis

The term *psychoanalysis* can denote one or more of the following:
1. A psychological theory of mind and personality development based primarily on the concept of intrapsychic 'conflict'.
2. A procedure for investigation of unconscious psychical processes, otherwise inaccessible.
3. A therapeutic technique of treating psychiatric disorders by psychological means.

HISTORICAL OVERVIEW

Although the credit for 'invention' of psychoanalysis belongs to Sigmund Freud (1856-1939), he drew heavily from the work of several prominent researchers including Jean-Martin Charcot (hypnosis), Theodor Meynert (neuroanatomy and psychiatry), Ernst Brucke (physiology and physiochemistry), Hippolyte Bernheim (hypnosis) and Josef Breuer (hysteria), among others.

Although there were several changes in psychoanalysis, some of them even fundamental, as Freud's thinking evolved over the years, an attempt is made here to illustrate the basic concepts of psychoanalysis as it existed near the end of Freud's career.

BASIC CONCEPTS

Topographic Theory of Mind

This theory was advanced by Freud in the year 1900, in the book called *The Interpretation of Dreams.*

Although it was later almost replaced by the *structural theory*, it is still useful in understanding the mental mechanisms.

The tripartite division of mind included the unconscious, the preconscious and the conscious.

The Unconscious

Much of the mental activity lies outside the sphere of consciousness. However, this unconscious mental activity influences the conscious thought and behaviour even if it is not available to voluntary recall.

The unconscious contains those ideas and affects which have been repressed (by the censor, as *repression* is known). This repressed material can only reach consciousness through *preconscious* when the censor is relaxed (for example, in dreams or abreaction) or overpowered (for example, in slips of tongue or free association).

The unconscious mental activity is characterised by *primary process thinking* which is typically found in young children, severe psychosis, mental retardation and dreams. It is different from normal thinking (*secondary process thinking*) in that it strives for immediate discharge of drive energy, lacks contact with reality, is full of contradictions, lacks organisation and logical connections, and is based on the *pleasure principle.*

The Preconscious

This region of mind lies between the unconscious and the conscious, with access to both. The unconscious mental contents can reach the conscious only through the preconscious. It is not present at birth but develops in childhood, paralleling the ego development. The *censor* lies here, maintaining the repressive barrier.

The preconscious mental contents can easily become conscious with *focusing of attention.*

The Conscious

If mind can be divided in portions, the conscious constitutes only a tiny part of it. Freud conceptualised conscious as a type of special sense organ of attention concerned with registration of stimuli from both within and without. The conscious mental contents are characterised by *secondary process thinking* based on the *reality principle.*

In addition to the topographic model of mind, Freud also theorised the concept of *psychic determinism* which means that *all* mental activity is meaningful and purposeful, though unconscious, and is linked with the previous life experiences. Hence, according to this principle, no mental activity can be accidental or purposeless.

Structural Theory of Mind

In 1923, in 'The Ego and The Id', Freud divided the mental apparatus into three dynamic structures: the id, the ego and the super-ego (Fig. 17.1).

The Id

The id is theorised to be the original state of human mental apparatus with which a newborn baby is born. It is totally unconscious, containing the basic drives and instincts concerned with survival, sexual drive and aggression. It is characterised by *primary process thinking* and is based on *pleasure principle*, lacking any direct link with reality. The only urge of these drives is immediate gratification.

The Ego

The ego is primarily determined by the experience of reality and is, therefore, guided by the *reality principle.* It is predominantly conscious though some parts (such as ego defense mechanisms) are unconscious. Ego maintains a balance between the id and the super-ego on one hand and the reality on the other.

For example, the individual observes a pleasurable object surrounded by a barrier. The id wants immediate gratification by obtaining the object, without seeing the reality of a barrier around it. The super-ego, on the other hand, proclaims that it is sinful to derive pleasure from an object surrounded by barrier. The ego strikes a balance between the two, as well as the real world, and decides to wait and find a way to 'climb' the barrier and derive pleasure. Although simplistic, the example illustrates the ego's function of delaying gratification in view of the reality.

The ego is the seat of conscious, intellectual, self-preservative and defensive functions of mental apparatus.

The Super-ego

The super-ego is predominantly an unconscious subdivision of mental apparatus that develops from the ego. It is especially concerned with moral standards and has two parts: a punitive conscience and a non-punitive ego ideal.

Both derive from the effect of parental influence on the ego. This parental influence not only includes the effect of actual parents but also of the important family members, religion and important people in the surrounding environment (such as celebrities). The criticisms, prohibitions, guilt-arousing statements and punishments are introjected as *conscience*

On the other hand, the approvals and rewards become introjected as the *ego ideal.* The ego ideal is later involved in the setting of personal goals and aspirations.

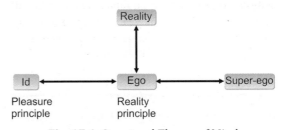

Fig. 17.1: Structural Theory of Mind

Ego Defense Mechanisms

The term *ego defense mechanism* refers to the automatic, involuntary, and unconsciously instituted psychological activity by which the unacceptable urges or impulses are excluded from the conscious awareness. These defense mechanisms are a function of ego.

The defense mechanisms usually operate on an unconscious level (except, for example, *suppression* which is a voluntary defense mechanism). In contrast, *coping mechanisms* are voluntary and conscious mechanisms of defense which an individual employs to deal with day-to-day external and conscious fears and conflicts.

There is no 'standard' list of defense mechanisms; however, a few commonly used ego defense mechanisms are listed in Table 17.1, along with definitions, clinical illustrations and examples in normal situations.

No ego defense mechanism is by itself psychotic, neurotic, immature, mature or normal. Almost all mechanisms of defense can be used in normal individuals. It is an exclusive or abnormally excessive use that makes a defense mechanism neurotic or psychotic.

The Theory of Psychosexual Development

In 1905, in 'Three essays on the theory of sexuality', Freud enunciated his theory of infantile sexuality and described the psychosexual stages of development (Table 17.2 for a very brief summary).

Table 17.1: Commonly used Ego Defense Mechanisms

Defense Mechanism	Definition	Example(s) in Normal life	Illustration(s) from Clinical Situations
A. Primary			
1. Repression	Unconsciously excluding from conscious awareness of anxiety provoking ideas and/or feelings	1. 'Forgetting' 2. Slips of the tongue	Psychogenic amnesia
B. Psychotic/Narcissistic			
1. Regression	Reversion to modes of psychological functioning that are characteristic of earlier life stages, especially childhood years	1. Dreams 2. *Regression in the service of ego* (ability of a mature adult to appropriately indulge periodically in playful childlike activities)	1. Neuroses (mild regression) 2. Psychoses (more pervasive regression) 3. Severe, prolonged physical illness
2. Denial	Involuntary exclusion of unpleasant or painful reality from conscious awareness	1. Grief 2. Children (3-6 year olds)	1. Psychoses 2. Alcohol dependence
3. Projection	Unconscious attribution of one's own attitudes and urges to other person(s), because of intolerance or painful affect aroused by those attitudes and urges	A universal phenomenon though occurs more commonly in children	Persecutory delusions and hallucinations
4. Distortion	Unconscious gross 'reshaping' of external reality to satisfy inner needs	—	1. Hallucinations 2. Delusions, especially of grandiosity

Contd...

Contd...

Defense Mechanism	Definition	Example(s) in Normal life	Illustration(s) from Clinical Situations
C. Neurotic/Immature			
1. Conversion	A repressed, forbidden urge is simultaneously kept out of awareness and also expressed in symbolic/ disguised form of some somatic conversion 'reaction' (usually either motor or sensory)	Sometimes seen in normal individuals when exposed to catastrophic stress; otherwise presence always implies psychopathology	Conversion disorder (Hysteria)
2. Dissociation	Involuntary splitting or suppression of a mental function or a group of mental functions from rest of the personality in a manner that allows expression of forbidden unconscious impulses without having any sense of responsibility for actions	Near death experience	Dissociative disorders, e.g. psychogenic amnesia, psychogenic fugue, multiple personality, somnambulism, possession syndrome
3. Displacement	Unconscious shifting of emotions, usually aroused by perceived threat, from an unconscious impulse to a less threatening external object which is then felt to be the source of threat	Normal, day-to-day deflection of 'anger' on a substitute target	1. Phobia (especially in children) 2. OCD
4. Isolation (Isolation of affect)	Separation of the idea of an unconscious impulse from its appropriate affect, thus allowing only the idea and not the associated affect to enter awareness	1. Grief 2. Ability to discuss traumatic events without the associated disturbing emotions, with passage of time	Obsessional thoughts
5. Reaction formation	Unconscious transformation of unacceptable impulses into exactly opposite attitudes, impulses, feelings or behaviours	Normal character formation in childhood (from 3 years onwards)	Obsessive compulsive personality traits and disorder
6. Undoing	Unconsciously motivated acts which magically/symbolically counteract unacceptable thoughts, impulses or acts	1. Checking of gas knobs or locks to ensure safety 2. Automatically saying 'I am sorry' on bumping into somebody	1. Compulsive acts in OCD 2. Compulsive rituals

Contd...

Contd...

Defense Mechanism	Definition	Example(s) in Normal life	Illustration(s) from Clinical Situations
7. Rationalisation	Providing 'logical' explanations for irrational behaviour motivated by unacceptable unconscious wishes	A universal phenomenon	Usually used to explain behaviours resulting from other defense mechanisms
8. Intellectualisation	Excessive use of intellectual processes (logic) to avoid affective expression (emotion)	When faced with stressful situation, use of logic to focus closely on external reality and avoiding expression of inner feelings (e.g. fear)	—
9. Acting out	Expression of an unconscious impulse, through action, thereby gratifying the impulse	Destruction of any object in a 'fit of rage'	Impulse control disorders
10. Schizoid fantasy	Withdrawal into self to gratify frustrated wishes by fantasy	Seen in adolescence (wish fulfilling daydreams)	Schizoid and schizotypal personality disorder
11. Turning against the self (Retroflexion)	Unconscious deflection of hostility towards another person onto oneself resulting in lowered self-esteem, self-criticism and at times injury to self	1. Head banging in children 2. Destruction of property or self in a fit of rage	1. Suicide 2. Severe depression 3. Any form of deliberate self harm (DSH)
12. Introjection	Unconscious internalisation of the qualities of an object or person	1. Identification with the aggressor (e.g. sometimes seen in victims kidnapped by terrorists; also known as *Stockholm syndrome*) 2. Grief reaction	Depression
13. Hypochondriasis	Unconscious transformation of unacceptable impulses into inappropriate somatic concern	Abnormal illness behaviour in physically disordered or normal individuals	Hypochondriasis
14. Inhibition	Involuntary decrease or loss of motivation to engage in some goal-directed activity to prevent anxiety arising out of conflicts with unacceptable impulses	1. Writing 'blocks' or work 'blocks' '2. Social shyness	1. OCD 2. Phobias

Contd...

Contd...

Defense Mechanism	Definition	Example(s) in Normal life	Illustration(s) from Clinical Situations
15. Compensation (Counter-phobic defense)	Unconscious tendency to deal with a fear or conflict by unusual degree of effort in the opposite direction	1. Involvement in dare-devil activities (e.g. sky diving to counter fear of heights) 2. Excessive pre-occupation with body building to counter feelings of inferiority	1. Nymphomania (to counter a sense of sexual inadequacy) 2. Keeping excessive details in a diary in patients suffering from dementia
16. Splitting	Unconscious viewing of self or others as either good or bad without considering the whole range of qualities	Believing personalities to be either 'black' or 'white' without the shades of 'grey' (e.g. in a 'typical' Bollywood movie, the Hero often is all good and the Villain all bad)	Borderline personality disorder
D. Mature			
1. Sublimation	Unconscious gradual channelisation of unacceptable infantile impulses into personally satisfying and socially valuable behaviour patterns	Channelisation of sexual or aggressive impulses into creative activities (e.g. diverting forbidden sexual impulses into artistic paintings)	—
2. Suppression (Voluntary)	Voluntary postponement of focusing of attention on an impulse which has reached conscious awareness	Voluntary decision not to think about an argument with a close friend while going for an interview	—
3. Anticipation	Realistic thinking and planning about future unpleasurable events	Anticipation is a universal phenomenon occurring in all intelligent individuals	—
4. Humour	Overt expression of unacceptable impulses using humour in a manner which does not produce unpleasantness in self or others	A universal phenomenon	—

No ego defense mechanism is psychotic, neurotic, immature, mature or normal per se. Almost all mechanisms of defense are sometimes used in normal individuals. It is an exclusive or abnormally excessive use that makes a defense mechanism neurotic or psychotic.

Table 17.2: Psychosexual Stages of Development (Sigmund Freud)

	Phase	Age Range	Normal Development	Psychiatric syndromes theorised to result from fixation (and regression) to this stage
1	Oral phase	Birth to 1-1½ years	Major site of gratification is the oral region. It consists of 2 phases: i. Oral erotic phase (sucking) ii. Oral sadistic phase (biting)	1. Dependent personality traits and disorder 2. Schizophrenia (oral and pre-oral phase) 3. Severe mood disorder 4. Alcohol dependence syndrome and drug dependence
2	Anal phase	1-1½ years to 3 years	Major site of gratification is the anal and perianal area; major achievement is toilet training (sphincter control). It consists of 2 phases: i. Anal erotic phase (excretion) ii. Anal sadistic phase ('holding' and 'letting go' at will)	1. Obsessive compulsive personality traits and disorder 2. OCD (Anal sadistic phase)
3	Phallic (Oedipal) phase	3 to 5 years	Major site of gratification is the genital area; genital masturbation is common at this stage. According to Freud, this development is different in both sexes. *Male development* The boy develops *castration anxiety* (fear of castration at the hand of his father in retaliation for the boy's desire to replace his father in his mother's affections). This leads to formation of the *Oedipus complex* (aggressive impulses directed towards the father; named after the Greek tragedy *Oedipus rex* in which Oedipus unknowingly kills his father and marries his mother, unaware of their true identities). Oedipus complex is usually resolves by identification with father, attempting to adopt his characteristics. *Female development* The girl develops *penis envy* (discontent with female genitalia following a fantasy that they result from loss of penis). This is theorised by Freud to lead to a wish to 'receive' the penis and to bear a child. Resolution occurs by identification with the mother. This phase has been called *as Electra complex.*	1. Sexual deviations 2. Sexual dysfunctions 3. Neurotic disorders

Contd...

Contd...

	Phase	Age Range	Normal Development	Psychiatric syndromes theorised to result from fixation (and regression) to this stage
4	Latency phase	5-6 years to 12 years	Oedipus (and Electra) complex is usually resolved at the beginning of this stage. This is a stage of relative sexual quiescence. *Super-ego* is formed at this stage. Sexual drive is channelised into socially appropriate goals such as development of interpersonal relationships, sports, school, work, etc.	Neurotic disorders
5	Genital phase	12 years onwards)	Adult sexuality develops with capacity for intimacy (during puberty) and respect for others. Gradual release from parental controls with more influence of peer group. True self-identity develops.	Neurotic disorders

The normal development described here is a simplified account of Sigmund Freud's theory of psychosexual development. Till date, it remains a theory; there is no empirical evidence for, say, Oedipus complex or contribution of these stages to development of psychiatric symptoms or syndromes.

Theory of Dreams

Dream interpretation has been a major component of psychoanalysis. Beginning with his own dream experiences, Freud analysed dreams as "the royal road to the unconscious". He believed dreams to be conscious expression of unconscious fantasies or impulses which are not accessible to the individual in wakefulness, thereby providing gratification by wish fulfilment.

Since expression of unconscious forbidden fantasies can evoke considerable anxiety, these fantasies are considerably modified so as to preserve sleep on the one hand and provide gratification of the fantasies on the other. This modification is known as *dream work*.

Here the unconscious forbidden fantasies or wishes which threaten to break sleep constitute the *latent dream content*, whereas the dream content modified by dream work constitutes the *manifest dream content*. According to Freud, the aim of dream interpretation is to get to the latent dream content from manifest dream content, via free association, in order to understand the 'real meaning' of the dream experience.

According to this theory, the dream work consists of the following mechanisms:
1. Symbolism
2. Displacement
3. Condensation
4. Projection
5. Secondary elaboration (since dream content consists of *primary process thinking,* secondary elaboration is used to introduce logical thinking or *secondary process thinking* in the dream content).

In addition to the unconscious impulses, wishes and fantasies, the dream content is also influenced by:
1. Nocturnal sensory stimuli (e.g. thirst, hunger, full bladder).
2. Day residue (residue of day experiences of previous one or several days).

Psychoanalysis and Psychoanalytical Psychotherapy

Psychoanalysis and psychoanalytical psychotherapy as treatment methods are briefly discussed in Chapter 18.

Chapter 18 — Psychological Treatments

PSYCHOTHERAPY

Psychotherapy can be defined (modified from Wolberg) as, the treatment by psychological means, of the problems of an emotional nature, in which a therapist deliberately establishes a professional relationship with the patient to,
1. Remove, modify or retard existing symptoms,
2. Mediate disturbed patterns of behaviour, and/or
3. Promote positive personality growth and development.

Psychotherapy can be conducted by either verbal or non-verbal means. There are several different kinds of psychotherapies. The important types include the following (Table 18.1).

Psychoanalysis and Psychoanalytical Psychotherapy

These psychotherapeutic methods are based primarily on Sigmund Freud's work, although many other techniques developed by other important workers (such as Carl Jung, Alfred Adler, Erich Fromm, Harry Stack Sullivan, Karen Horney, Melanie Klein, Otto Rank, Wilhelm Reich and many others) are also in use.

A detailed discussion of Freudian psychoanalysis is not attempted here (see Chapter 17) and a very brief outline of therapy is presented.

Classical Psychoanalysis

Freudian psychoanalysis typically needs 2-5 visits/ week by the patient for a period of 3-5 years (even

Table 18.1: Psychosocial Therapies

	Therapy/School	Proponent(s)
1.	Psychoanalysis	Sigmund Freud
2.	Analytical psychology	Carl Gustav Jung
3.	Behaviourism	John Broadus Watson
4.	Character analysis	Wilhelm Reich
5.	Classical conditioning	Ivan Petrovich Pavlov
6.	Client-centred psychotherapy	Carl R Rogers
7.	Cognitive behaviour therapy	Donald Meichenbaum
8.	Cognitive therapy	Aaron T Beck
9.	Dual sex therapy	William Masters and Virginia Johnson
10.	Existential logotherapy	Victor E Frankl
11.	Gestalt therapy	Frederich Perls
12.	Group therapy	Joseph Pratt
13.	Hypnosis	James Braid
14.	Operant conditioning	Burrhus Frederic Skinner
15.	Primal therapy	Arthur Janov
16.	Progressive muscular relaxation	E. Jacobson
17.	Psychodrama	Jacob L Moreno
18.	Rational emotive therapy	Albert Ellis
19.	Reciprocal inhibition	Joseph Wolpe
20.	Therapeutic community	Maxwell Jones
21.	Token economy	Ayllon and Azrin
22.	Transactional analysis	Eric Berne
23.	Will therapy	Otto Rank

longer). No detailed history taking, mental status examination, or formalised psychiatric diagnosis is attempted. The patient is allowed to communicate unguided, by using 'free association'.

The therapist remains passive with a non-directive approach; however, the therapist constantly challenges the existing *defenses* and interprets *resistance* (during the therapy) and *transference* (patient's feelings, behaviours and relationship with the therapist).

No direct advice is ever given to the patient. The crux of the therapy is on interpretation. During the therapy, the patient typically lies on the couch, with the therapist sitting just out of vision. No other therapy is usually used as adjunct.

Psychoanalytically-oriented (Psychodynamic) Psychotherapy

Psychoanalytically-oriented, psychodynamic psycho-therapy is a much more direct form of psychoanalysis. The duration of therapy is much briefer and advice is given to the patient occasionally. The patient and the therapist may sit face-to-face or else couch is used. The rest of technique is nearly the same as psychoanalysis. However, additional modes of treatment, including drug therapy can be used.

The indications for both psychoanalysis and psychoanalytically-oriented psychotherapy are not usually based on any psychiatric diagnoses. The most important indication is the presence of long-standing mental conflicts which, although are unconscious, produce significant symptomatology.

The prerequisites of therapy are that the patient should be motivated for therapy, should have strong 'ego-structure' (which can bear frustrations of impulses during the therapy), should be psychologically-minded and should not have recent significant life stressors.

It is usually used for the treatment of neurotic disorders and personality disorders (or characterological difficulties).

Behaviour Therapy

Behaviour therapy is a type of psychotherapy (broadly defined) which is based on theories of learning, and aims at modifying maladaptive behaviour and substituting it with adaptive behaviour.

Although there are many theories of learning, majority of behaviour therapy techniques are based on *operant conditioning model* (Skinner) and *classical conditioning model* (Pavlov). Many of the ideas actually seem like (and are) common sense principles. The learning theories assume that all behaviour is *learned behaviour*. The behaviour that is followed by a reward is more likely to occur again (*operant model*), and that behaviour is learned more easily if taught in small steps.

Behaviour therapy is typically a short duration therapy; therapists are easy to train and it is usually cost-effective. The total duration of therapy is usually 6-8 weeks. Initial sessions are scheduled daily but the later sessions are more spaced out. A behavioural analysis is usually carried out before planning behaviour therapy. One of the simplest methods of behaviour analysis is called as ABC charting, which involves a close look at the:

i. Antecedent (e.g. circumstances under which the behaviour began; who, if any, were present; other details),
ii. Behaviour (description of the behaviour in detail), and
iii. Consequence (what happened afterwards; what factors helped to maintain behaviour).

Some of the important behavioural techniques are described briefly.

Systematic Desensitisation

Systematic desensitisation (SD) is based on the principle of reciprocal inhibition, described by Wolpe. The principle states that if a response incompatible with anxiety is made to occur at the same time as an anxiety-provoking stimulus, anxiety is reduced by reciprocal inhibition.

This consists of three main steps:
i. *Relaxation training* (described later).
ii. *Hierarchy construction*: Here the patient is asked to list all the conditions which provoke anxiety. Then, he is asked to list them in a descending order of anxiety provocation. Thus,

a hierarchy of anxiety-producing stimuli is prepared.

iii. *Systematic desensitisation proper*: This can be done either in imagery (SD-I) or in reality/*in vivo* (SD-R). At first, the lowest item in hierarchy is confronted (in reality or in imagery). The patient is advised to signal whenever anxiety occurs. With each signal, he is asked to relax (Step-I). After a few trials, patient is able to control his anxiety. Thus, gradually the hierarchy is climbed till the maximum anxiety-provoking stimulus can be faced in the absence of anxiety.

SD is a treatment of choice in phobias and obsessive-compulsive disorders.

Aversion Therapy

Aversion therapy is used for the treatment of conditions which are pleasant but felt undesirable by the patient, e.g. alcohol dependence, transvestism, ego dystonic homosexuality, other sexual deviations.

The underlying principle is pairing of the pleasant stimulus (such as alcohol) with an unpleasant response (such as brief electrical stimulus), so that even in absence of unpleasant response (after the therapy is over), the pleasant stimulus becomes unpleasant by association. The unpleasant aversion can be produced by electric stimulus (low voltage), drugs (such as apomorphine and disulfiram) or even by fantasy (when it is called as *covert sensitisation*).

Typically, 20-40 sessions are needed, with each session lasting about 1 hour. After completion of treatment, booster sessions may be given. The current use of aversion therapy has declined sharply in the Western world (and also elsewhere) as it is felt by many that it may violate the human rights of the patient.

Operant Conditioning Procedures for Increasing Behaviour

The common methods for augmenting an adaptive behaviour include:

i. *Positive reinforcement*: Here, the desirable behaviour is reinforced by a reward, either material or symbolic.

ii. *Negative reinforcement*: Here, on performance of the desirable behaviour, punishment can be avoided.

iii. *Modelling*: The person is exposed to 'model' behaviour and is induced to copy it. This can also be used to avoid certain behaviours.

Flooding

This is usually the method used in the treatment of phobias. Here, the person is directly exposed to the phobic stimulus, but escape is made impossible. By prolonged contact with the phobic stimulus, therapist's guidance and encouragement, and therapist's modelling behaviour, anxiety decreases and the phobic behaviour diminishes.

Operant Conditioning Procedures for Decreasing Behaviour

These methods include:

i. *Time-out*: Here, the reinforcement is withdrawn for some time, contingent upon the undesired response. Time-out is often used in therapy with children.

ii. *Punishment*: Aversive stimulus is here presented, contingent upon undesired response (i.e. whenever undesired response occurs, punishment is given).

iii. *Satiation*: The undesired response is positively reinforced, so that tiring occurs. A similar technique is *negative practice procedure*.

Other Behavioural Techniques

Many other techniques such as *token economy* (for hospitalised patients), *social-skills training* (for patients with social difficulties), family therapy, marital therapy, and cognitive behavioural therapy are available. The interested reader is referred to the Reading List.

Cognitive Therapy or Cognitive Behaviour Therapy

Cognitive behaviour therapy (CBT) is a type of psychotherapy which aims at correcting the maladaptive methods of thinking, thus providing relief from con-

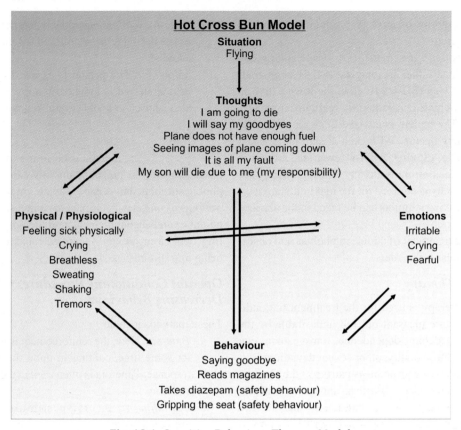

Fig. 18.1: Cognitive Behaviour Therapy Model

sequent symptoms. The therapist plays an active role, unlike in psychoanalysis.

Developed separately by Beck and Meichenbaum, it is used for treatment of depression, anxiety disorder, panic disorder, phobias, eating disorders, anticipatory anxiety, and also for teaching problem-solving methods. Some centres also use CBT for management of psychotic symptoms such as delusions and hallucinations.

Figure 18.1 illustrates the hot cross bun model of cognitive behaviour therapy.

A typical cognitive therapy schedule consists of about 15 visits over a three-month period. Some important techniques in CBT are:

i. *Cognitive techniques* such as recognising and correcting negative automatic thoughts, teaching reattribution techniques, increasing objec-

tivity in perspectives, identifying and testing maladaptive assumptions, and decentering,

ii. *Behavioural techniques* such as activity scheduling, homework assignments, graded task assignment, behavioural rehearsal, role playing, and diversion techniques, and

iii. *Teaching problem-solving skills.*

iv. *Mindfulness*, originally a Buddhist technique, can also be combined with CBT.

Supportive Psychotherapy

This is a very directive method of psychotherapy, with the focus clearly on existing symptoms and/or current life situations. The aims of the therapy are:

i. Correction of the situational problem.

ii. Symptom rectification.

iii. Restoring or strengthening defenses.

iv. Prevention of emotional breakdown.

v. Teaching new coping skills.

The aim is achieved by a conglomeration of techniques which include guidance, suggestion, environmental manipulation, reassurance, persuasion, development of a doctor-patient relationship, diversion, and even hospitalisation and medication. This is a highly skilled method of psychotherapy which can provide excellent results when used judiciously.

Family and Marital Therapy

In family therapy and marital therapy (also called as couples therapy), the focus of intervention is not on the individual but is instead on the family as a unit or the marital unit.

There are several varieties of family and marital therapies, such as those based on psychodynamic, behavioural or systemic principles. Whenever there are relational problems within a family or marital unit (either primarily or secondary to a psychiatric disorder), family and/or marital therapy is indicated. For example, in a behavioural marital therapy, components of therapy may include problem solving, training in communication skills, writing a behavioural marital contract, and home-work assignments.

Group Therapy

Group therapy (or group psychotherapy) is a less time-consuming procedure, in which usually 8-10 people can be treated at one time. This was first used by Joseph Pratt (an internist) in 1905, for patients suffering from tuberculosis.

Now, it is known that group therapy is not only time-saving but also especially beneficial for certain group of patients. Group therapy offers patients (and their relatives) an opportunity to realise that many others have and share problems which are very similar to their own problems, and that they are not alone in their suffering.

Typically, sessions are held once or twice a week, with each session lasting 1-2 hours (often 1½ hours). The patients usually sit in a circle, with equal opportunities for interaction. Group therapy may utilize psychoanalytic, supportive, transactional or behavioural approaches.

Over the years, many types of group therapies have emerged such as self-help groups (Alcoholics Anonymous for alcoholics, Weight Watchers for obese, Phoenix-House for opiate dependent individuals), Transactional Analysis groups (Eric Berne), Training groups (Kurt Lewin), Psychodrama (Jacob Moreno) and the like.

Suggestion

Although an integral part of supportive psychotherapy, it is often used alone. It is used by nearly all medical practitioners, without realising or naming it as such. It is suggestion, which is in part responsible for the placebo response. A placebo prescribed confidently by an 'impressive' physician can lead to some improvement in about 33% of patients with most conditions.

Hypnosis

Hypnosis is a state of artificially induced (by self or others) increased suggestibility. There is a constriction in the peripheral awareness with increased focal concentration on task at hand.

Trance phenomena were routinely utilized by Anton Mesmer in 1775 who called 'this force' as animal magnetism. The word hypnotism was first used by James Braid in the 19th century.

Not everyone can be hypnotised. The capacity for hypnosis is called *hypnotisability*, which can be measured in a person by using tests such as the eye roll sign or hand levitation test. Basically, these tests measure suggestibility.

About 60% of the general population can be hypnotised but only 5-10% reach deep hypnotic trance. A wide variety of techniques are available for the induction of hypnosis.

Following changes occur commonly during the hypnotic trance:

i. The person under hypnosis becomes highly suggestible to commands of hypnotist, without understanding their nature.

ii. Dissociation of a part of body or emotions from the remainder may occur.

iii. There is a partial or complete amnesia for the events occurring during the hypnotic trance.

iv. There is an ability to produce or remove symptoms, perceptions and/or movements.

v. Post-hypnotic suggestion can be given just after the trance and it is followed by the hypnotised person.

Persons who are hypnotisable are in no way abnormal as compared to the rest of the population.

Indications in Psychiatry

i. As an adjunct to psychotherapy.

ii. To abreact past experiences.

The conditions in which hypnosis can help in treatment are many. The most important ones are listed below.

i. Psychosomatic disorders

ii. Conversion disorder (hysteria)

iii. Dissociative disorder (hysteria)

iv. Eating disorders (anorexia nervosa, bulimia nervosa and obesity)

v. Habit disorders (smoking)

vi. Pain

vii. Anxiety disorder.

Abreaction

Abreaction is an important procedure which brings to conscious awareness, for the first time, unconscious conflicts and associated emotions.

The release of emotions is therapeutic. Although abreaction is an integral part of psychoanalysis and hypnosis, it can be used independently also. Abreaction can be done with or without the use of medication.

Abreaction with Medication

Earlier amphetamines, ether, nitrous oxide and lysergic acid diethylamide (LSD) have been used for abreaction. Particularly, intravenous amphetamines were very successful as they lead to a marked increase in productivity of speech, thus facilitating release of unconscious ideas and emotions. These agents are no longer commonly used in clinical practice, due to risk of dependence (in case of amphetamines and LSD) and/or side effects.

Another method is the use of 5% solution of sodium amobarbital (amytal) or thiopentone sodium (pentothal), infused at a rate no faster than 1 cc/min to prevent sleep as well as respiratory depression. *This procedure must always be done very carefully with support from an anaesthetist who should be physically present.*

The abreactive procedure is begun with neutral topics at first, gradually approaching area(s) of conflicts. Usually about 150-350 mg (3-7 cc.) of amytal is sufficient for the purpose. In elderly and patients with organic brain disorder, even 75 mg of amytal may produce excessive drowsiness.

The indications of amytal interview include:

i. Abreaction (mainly) e.g. in hysteria.

ii. Interview with a mute patient.

iii. Diagnostic test in catatonic syndrome.

iv. Differentiating test in stupor (for differential diagnosis of depression, schizophrenia, hysteria and organic brain disorder).

There are certain contraindications for the use of amytal interview:

i. Airway disease including upper respiratory tract infection.

ii. Severe renal or hepatic disease.

iii. History of porphyria.

iv. Hypotension.

v. Dependence on barbiturates.

vi. Psychosis (except for catatonia or stupor).

The other medications which have been used successfully for abreaction include diazepam and ketamine. The use of abreaction has declined considerably in the last three decades and the current practice and guidelines do not encourage its routine use.

Relaxation Therapies

The aim of these therapies is to induce muscular relaxation. Since anxiety produces muscular tension, which in turn reinforces (and thus increases) anxiety, any relaxation technique would decrease both anxiety and muscular tension.

Relaxation techniques are an integral part of a majority of behaviour therapies, such as systematic desensitisation. There are many methods which can be used to induce relaxation and these include:

A. *Jacobson's progressive muscular relaxation*: This is the most frequently used technique. The patient first tenses and then relaxes major muscle groups of the body in a prefixed and systematic order, usually beginning at the top of the body and progressing downwards.

B. Hypnosis

C. Transcendental meditation (TM) or Yoga

D. 'Shavasna' ('The corpse posture'): Similar to progressive relaxation but the sequence of progression is below upwards.

E. Yog Nindra, Pranayama and Vipasna are other Indian methods.

F. Biofeedback.

Biofeedback

Biofeedback (introduced for the first time in 1969) is the use of an instrument (usually electronic), which provides immediate feedback to the patient regarding his physiological activities normally not available to the conscious mind, such as ECG, EEG, pulse rate, blood pressure, EMG, and galvanic skin response (GSR).

The feedback helps the patient, apparently to control these responses. Relaxation is easily achieved by this method. A simpler form (*relaxometer*) uses only one parameter, the GSR.

The other uses of biofeedback include treatment of enuresis, migraine headaches, tension headache, idiopathic hypertension, incontinence, cardiac arrhythmias, uncontrolled generalised tonic clonic seizures, and also for neuromuscular rehabilitation.

Rehabilitation

Psychiatric rehabilitation is defined as restoration of the fullest physical, mental, social, vocational, and economic usefulness of which the person suffering from psychiatric disorder is capable.

A large number of patients with psychiatric disorders (such as schizophrenia) may have a poor quality of life, residual symptoms, and long-term disability. Although early recognition and treatment is the cornerstone of preventing long-term disability, a substantial number of patients may need rehabilitation.

There are several components and methods available for rehabilitation, depending on the type and/or stage of disorder and the type of support available to the patient. Necessarily, a comprehensive assessment is needed before deciding on the individualized rehabilitation for a particular patient.

Some of the methods used for psychiatric rehabilitation include housing placement (such as half way homes, supervised housing), vocational training and rehabilitation (such as activity therapy, sheltered workshop, transitional or supported employment, vocational guidance, occupational therapy), and treatment (such as ensuring compliance with medication, social skills therapy, family therapy, cognitive remediation).

There is an acute shortage of psychiatric rehabilitation facilities in most parts of India. The Persons with Disabilities (Equal Opportunities, Protection of Rights, and Full Participation) Act (PDA), 1995 is a step forward, as it includes psychiatric disorders and mental retardation.

Indian Perspective

Just about the time Freud was practicing psychoanalysis, Girindra Shekhar Bose was using his own version of psychoanalysis in Calcutta. However, currently psychoanalysis is not widely used in India.

It is believed by some that most Indian patients, as compared to patients in western, developed countries, are not psychologically minded and are unable to introspect. They lack verbal fluency and have more physical symptoms.

The Indian patients have difficulty in maintaining one-to-one relationship with the physician-psychiatrist, as they believe him to be a healer who is of higher status than them (something like a Guru). The Guru-Chela relationship in the patient-doctor interaction was first described by JS Neki.

Psychoanalysis (which avoids giving direct advice) is difficult, as patients expect the therapist to guide them and make decisions for them. The patients are also often fatalistic ('this had to happen'; 'it is the result of destiny and past karma') and often have magical expectations of cure.

Most psychotherapists in India agree that Western models of psychotherapy cannot be directly transplanted in the Indian setting. Psychotherapy in a majority of Indian patients should be preferably brief, direct, crisis-oriented, with the therapist playing an active role. However, in psychologically minded and educated Indian patients, western models can be used with or without modification.

The commonest type of psychotherapy used in India is probably supportive psychotherapy though use of CBT has increased substantially over the last few years.

Chapter 19

Emergency Psychiatry

An *emergency* is defined as an unforeseen combination of circumstances which calls for an immediate action.

A *medical emergency* is defined as a medical condition which endangers life and/or causes great suffering to the individual. A *psychiatric emergency* is a disturbance in thought, mood and/or action which causes sudden distress to the individual (or to significant others) and/or sudden disability, thus requiring immediate management. A similar term *crisis* means a situation that presents a challenge to the patient, the family and/or the community.

TYPES OF PSYCHIATRIC EMERGENCIES

A psychiatric emergency can be one or more of the following:
1. A new psychiatric disorder with an acute onset.
2. A chronic psychiatric disorder with a relapse.
3. An organic psychiatric disorder.
4. An abnormal response to a stressful situation.
5. Iatrogenic emergencies.
   i. Side effects or toxicity of psychotropic medication(s).
   ii. Psychiatric symptomatology as a side effect or toxicity of other medication(s).
6. Alcohol or drug dependence.
   i. Withdrawal syndrome.
   ii. Intoxication or overdose.
   iii. Complications.
7. Deliberate harm to self or others.

EXAMINATION

When faced with a psychiatric emergency, it is often important to combine speed with obtaining of 'comprehensive' or 'adequate' information. A scheme for the typical emergency psychiatric evaluation is presented here:

Psychiatric History

It is important to 'always' obtain history from both the patient and the informant(s). Informant(s) may be more coherent and may provide more relevant information in emergency situation(s).
   i. *Chief complaint*: elaborate, with emphasis on dating of onset and progression.
   ii. *Recent life-changes*, such as any losses (real or imagined); any physical illnesses.
   iii. *Level of adjustment,* prior to the psychiatric emergency.
   iv. *Past history* (briefly) of any physical or psychiatric disorder(s).
   v. *Family history* (briefly) of any physical or psychiatric disorder(s).
   vi. *Drug and alcohol history,* prescription drugs, street drug(s) or alcohol dependence/abuse.

Detailed General Physical and Neurological Examination

It is essential to rule out (or diagnose) secondary psychiatric disorders, with particular emphasis on the presence of any head injury.

Mental Status Examination

i. Screen for *organicity* (most important). Test for higher mental (or cognitive) functions, such as consciousness, orientation, attention, concentration, memory, intelligence, abstract thinking, insight and judgement.

ii. Brief mental status examination, to diagnose or rule out any psychiatric disorder(s).

iii. Particular emphasis should be placed on the presence of ideas of self-harm or suicide, or of harming others.

COMMON PSYCHIATRIC EMERGENCIES

Suicide

Suicide is the model of psychiatric emergencies and is also the commonest cause of death among the psychiatric patients. Some common themes in suicide are listed in Table 19.1.

Suicide is a type of *deliberate self-harm* (DSH) and is defined as a human act of self-intentioned and self-inflicted cessation (death). It ends with a fatal outcome. DSH is an act of intentionally injuring oneself, irrespective of the actual outcome.

An *attempted suicide* is an unsuccessful suicidal act with a nonfatal outcome. It is believed that 2-10% of all persons who attempt suicide, eventually complete suicide in the next 10 years.

A *suicidal gesture*, on the other hand, is an *attempted suicide* where the person performing the action never intends to die by the act. However, some of these persons may accidentally die during the act. Attempted suicide is more common in women while completed suicide is 2-4 times commoner in men.

Epidemiology

Suicide is among the top 10 causes of death in India and most other countries. The official suicide rate in India in 2008 was 10.8/100,000 population/year (9.7 in 1995; 6.3 in 1980). In 2000, the rate in men was 12.2/100,000 and in women 9.1/100,000) with an overall male to female ratio of 64:36 in 2008 (NCRB). However, as there is considerable under-reporting of

Table 19.1: Some Common Themes in Suicide

1. A crisis that causes intense suffering with feelings of hopelessness and helplessness
2. Conflict between unbearable stress and survival
3. Narrowing of the person's perceived options
4. Wish to escape (it can often be an escape, rather than a going-towards)
5. Often a wish to punish self and/or punish significant others with guilt

suicidal behaviour, the probable suicide rate per year in India would be around 15/100,000 population.

According to the National Crime Records Bureau (NCRB), there were 125,017 suicides in India in 2008, which is an increase of 1.95 over the previous year. In 2003, there were about 300 suicides per day or one suicide every 5 minutes. The comparable period prevalence rate for suicide throughout world ranges from 5/100,000 population/year to 30/100,000 population/year. The World Health Report, 2001, estimates that every year one million people worldwide commit suicide (100,000 suicides per year in India out of 1 million suicides in the world every year), while 10-20 million people attempt suicide. Thus, the ratio of attempted suicide to completed suicide is 10-20:1.

In India, the highest suicide rate is in the age group of 15-29 years. Some of the highest numbers of suicide in India are reported from West Bengal (11.9% of all cases), Tamil Nadu, Maharashtra, Andhra Pradesh and Karnataka. These five states account for 56.2% of all suicides in the country (NCRB 2008). There are some recent reports of high rates of suicide in teenage girls (15-19 years old) in some parts of Tamil Nadu and farmers in some areas of Andhra Pradesh.

However, suicide rate per 100,000 population (as opposed to number of suicides) was highest in Sikkim (48.2 as compared to national average of 10.7/100,000 population/year) and followed by Pondicherry (46.9) (NCRB 2008).

Some important risk factors are summarised in Table 19.2. Table 19.3 lists an example of biopsychosocial summary of risk and protective factors for suicide in a given case.

Aetiology

Some of the common causes of suicide include:

Psychiatric Disorders

Psychiatric disorders are a major cause of suicide; for example:

Table 19.2: Risk Factors for Suicide

The presence of following factors increases the risk of completed suicide:
1. Age > 40 years
2. Male gender
3. Staying single
4. Previous suicidal attempt(s)
5. Depression (risk about 25 times more than usual)
   i. Presence of guilt, self-accusation, agitation, nihilistic ideation, worthlessness, hypochondriacal delusions and/or severe insomnia
   ii. Risk is usually higher at the beginning or towards the end of a depressive episode
   iii. Risk can often be higher soon after response to treatment rather at the peak of depression; this applies to all forms of treatment but particularly so with antidepressant treatment
   iv. There is a higher risk of suicide in the week after discharge from a psychiatric inpatient unit
6. Suicidal preoccupation (for example, a written 'suicide note' and/or detailed plans are made for committing suicide)
7. Alcohol or drug dependence
8. Severe, disabling, painful or untreatable physical illness
9. Recent serious loss or major stressful life event
10. Social isolation
11. Higher degree of impulsivity

1. Depression
   i. Major depression.
   ii. Depression secondary to a serious physical illness.
   iii. Reactive depression, secondary to life stressors, e.g. family and/or marital disputes, failure in goal achievement, occupational and financial difficulties, and death of significant others.
2. Alcoholism and drug dependence.
3. Schizophrenia.

Genetic factors (a concordance rate of 18% in monozygotic twins) and biochemical factors (low levels of 5-HIAA) are important in some cases of suicide.

Physical Disorders

Patients with incurable or painful physical disorders, such as cancer and AIDS, often commit suicide (21.9% of all suicides in India; NCRB 2008).

Psychosocial Factors

Psychosocial factors are a very important cause of suicide. Some of the examples are failure in an examination, love affairs (3%), dowry difficulties (2.4%), marital difficulties, 'illegitimate' pregnancy, family problems (23.8% of all suicides in India) or family psychopathology, loss of a loved object by death or otherwise, occupational and financial difficulties (bankruptcy 2.4%; poverty 2.4%), and social isolation (data from NCRB 2008). In about 16% cases, no obvious causes were found (NCRB 2008).

Methods Used

In India (NCRB 2008), the commonest modes of committing suicide are ingestion of poison (34.8%)

Table 19.3: An Example of Summary of Risks and Protective Factors for Suicide

Factors	Biological	Psychological	Social
Predisposing	Genetic factors	Early childhood trauma	Poor social support
	Male gender	Personality traits	Unemployment
	Older age		
Precipitating	Discontinuation of antidepressant	Separation from spouse	Financial difficulties
	Psychiatric diagnosis	Hopelessness	Easy availability of lethal means
		Worthlessness	
Perpetuating	Alcohol and drug misuse	Poor self-esteem	Poor social support
Protective	Children; elderly parents; religious and moral values; good engagement with treatment		

followed by hanging (32.2%), burning (about 8.8%), drowning (about 6.7%), jumping in front of a train or another vehicle (3%) and 'alcoholism' (1.2%). There were also about 3038 'dowry deaths' in a year in 2008. Men often tend to use more violent methods for suicide as compared with women.

Medicolegal Aspects

Under the Indian law, suicide and attempted suicide are punishable offenses. Section 309 of IPC (Indian Penal Court) states that "whoever attempts to commit suicide and does any act towards the commission of such offense, shall be punishable with simple imprisonment for a term which may extend to one year and shall also be liable to fine".

It was argued that the law esteems the lives of men as not only valuable to their own possessors but also valuable to the State which protects them and for the protection of which the State exists. The State, therefore, had the right to prevent persons from taking their own lives. However, it compounded the sufferings of a person who survived after a suicide attempt by making him/her a punishable offender.

The Section 309 of IPC was repealed by the Supreme Court of India in 1994. However, in March 1996, a five judge Constitution Bench of the Supreme Court again made the 'attempt to suicide' a punishable offense. So, the Section 309 IPC continues to be valid at present.

Management

Once suicide is committed, it is obviously no longer treatable. The management of suicide, therefore, lies in preventing the act. This can be done at suicide prevention centres, crisis intervention centres (both of these are not available as yet on a large scale in India), psychiatric emergency services, medical emergency services, social welfare centres (such as Samaritans, Sanjivini, Maitri, Sumaitri, Befrienders International) or even at home of the patient.

There are several misconceptions about suicide and these are briefly enumerated in Table 19.4.

Some important steps for preventing suicide include:

1. Take all the suicidal threats, gestures and/or attempts seriously and notify a psychiatrist or a mental health professional.
2. Psychiatrist (or a mental health professional) should quantify the seriousness of the situation (a proper risk assessment) and take remedial precautionary measures.
   i. Inspect physical surroundings and remove all means of committing suicide, such as sharp objects, ropes, drugs, firearms, etc. Also, search the patient thoroughly.
   ii. Surveillance, depending on the severity of risk.
3. Acute psychiatric emergency interview.
4. Counselling and guidance
   i. to deal with the desire to attempt suicide.
   ii. to deal with on-going life stressors, and teaching coping skills and interpersonal skills.
5. Treatment of the psychiatric disorder(s) with medication, psychotherapy and/or ECT.
   ECT is the treatment of choice for patients with major depression with suicidal risk. It should also be used for the treatment of suicidal risk associated

Table 19.4: Common Misconceptions about Suicide (Modified after Shneidman and Farberow, 1961)

	Misconceptions	Facts
1.	People who talk about suicide, do not commit suicide	Nearly 80% of persons who commit suicide, give definite warnings and/or clues about their suicidal intentions
2.	Suicide happens without warning	
3.	Suicidal persons are fully intent on dying	Most suicidal persons are undecided about dying or living
4.	Once a person is suicidal, he/she is suicidal forever	Suicidal person is usually suicidal only for a limited period of time
5.	All suicidal persons are mentally ill or psychotic	Although a suicidal person is often extremely unhappy, he/she is not necessarily mentally ill

with psychotic disorders. Follow-up care is very important to prevent future suicidal attempts or suicide.

Stupor and Catatonic Syndrome

Stupor is a common condition which presents at the emergency services. It is defined as a clinical syndrome of *akinesis* and *mutism* but with relative preservation of conscious awareness.

The term stupor, traditionally, has a psychiatric connotation, but a careful analysis of the stuporous patients shows that a large majority of them have an underlying organic cerebral cause. Stupor is often associated with catatonic signs and symptoms (catatonic withdrawal or *catatonic stupor*). Catatonic syndrome is any disorder which presents with at least two catatonic signs. Catatonia can be either excited or withdrawn (or mixed). Only catatonic withdrawal is associated with stupor.

The various catatonic signs include mutism, negativism, stupor, ambitendency, echolalia, echopraxia, automatic obedience, posturing, mannerisms, stereotypies, excitement (not goal-directed), impulsiveness, combativeness or nudism.

Aetiology

A wide variety of disorders can cause catatonic stupor. Some of the important causes are listed in Table 19.5.

Differential Diagnosis

It is of foremost importance to differentiate between organic stupor and psychogenic (or so called 'functional') stupor. This can be done on the basis of antecedent medical and psychiatric history, mode of onset, and detailed physical and neurological examination.

The important differentiating points between an organic and a psychogenic stupor are tabulated in Table 19.6. If a diagnosis of organic catatonic stupor is made, a search for underlying cause should be made. On the other hand, if the pentothal/amytal/diazepam interview reveals psychopathology, appropriate treatment can be instituted.

Table 19.5: Some Causes of Catatonic Stupor

1. Neurological Disorders
   i. Post-encephalitic parkinsonism
   ii. Limbic encephalitis
   iii. Surgical procedures on basal ganglia
   iv. Neoplasms in diencephalon, frontal lobe and limbic system
   v. Subacute sclerosing panencephalitis (SSPE)
   vi. General paresis of insane (GPI)
   vii. Petit mal status
   viii. Post-ictal phase of epilepsy
   ix. Subdural haematoma
   x. Cerebral malaria
   xi. Cortical venous thrombosis
2. Systemic and Metabolic Disorders
   i. Diabetic ketoacidosis
   ii. Acute intermittent porphyria
   iii. Hyperparathyroidism causing hypercalcaemia
   iv. Pellagra
   v. Hepatic encephalopathy
   vi. Systemic lupus erythematosis
   vii. Homocystinuria
   viii. Membranous glomerulonephritis
3. Drugs and Poisoning
   i. Organic alkaloids
   ii. Antipsychotics
   iii. ACTH (therapeutic doses)
   iv. Aspirin
   v. Illuminating gas
   vi. Ethyl alcohol (large doses)
   vii. Levodopa
   viii. Disulfiram
   ix. CO poisoning
   x. Lithium toxicity
   xi. Methylphenidate
   xii. Phencyclidine (large doses)
   xiii. Mescaline
4. Psychiatric Disorders
   i. Catatonic schizophrenia
   ii. Depressive stupor
   iii. Manic stupor
   iv. Periodic catatonia
   v. Conversion and dissociative disorder
   vi. Reactive psychosis
   vii. During hypnosis.

Table 19.6: Organic and Psychogenic Stupor

Features	Organic Stupor	Psychogenic Stupor
1. Previous psychiatric illness	Usually absent	Usually present
2. Previous medical illness	Usually present	Usually absent
3. Previous history of stupor	About 10% of cases	24-33% of cases
4. Precipitating stressor	Usually absent	Usually present
5. Frequency	Much more common	Not so common (3-5% of all stupor cases)
6. Onset	Sudden or insidious	Often sudden
7. Course	Longer	Shorter. Recovery usually within 7 days
8. Protective reflexes (Blepharospasm, menace reflex, protective response)	Absent	Present
9. Resistance to eye opening	Absent	Usually present
10. Doll's head eye phenomenon (Oculocephalic reflex)	Usually present	Absent (may avoid the gaze of examiner)
11. Meaningful posture and/or facial expressions	Absent	May be present
12. Urinary/faecal incontinence	Usually present	Unlikely
13. Neurological signs and deficits	May be present	Absent
14. Abnormal EEG	More often	Less often
15. Oculovestibular reflex	Absent	Present
16. Pentothal/amytal interview*	Low dose (100-150 mg) increases stupor and neurological signs develop or increase	High dose (300-400 mg) increases alertness and a mental status examination can often be conducted
17. Mortality	About 35%	0-3%

*Pentothal/amytal interview is no longer carried out routinely in clinical practice

Examination

The examination consists of the following steps:

1. History and physical examination, with special emphasis on neurological examination.
2. Level of consciousness should ideally be rated on the Glasgow Coma Scale. This scale consists of three main categories of activity, namely eye opening (1-4), motor response (1-5) and verbal response (1-5). The rating is done on a scale from 3 to 14.
3. Pentothal/amytal/diazepam interview is sometimes very helpful in differentiating organic and psychogenic catatonic stupor. It should however be noted that pentothal/amytal/diazepam interview is not routinely administered in clinical practice, and the emphasis has recently shifted to making this distinction on a clinical basis.
4. Investigations: Blood glucose, blood urea, serum creatinine, serum electrolytes, blood (arterial) gas analysis, ECG, blood and urine examination for drugs and poisons, blood and urine culture, and peripheral smear for malarial parasite.

Also routine bloods including haemoglobin, total leucocyte count (TC), differential leucocyte count (DC), ESR, urine (routine and microscopic) examination, thyroid and adrenal functions, liver function tests, CSF examination, gastric lavage with examination of aspirate, EEG and CT scan/MRI scan brain (if indicated).

Management

Since psychogenic stupor may easily be mistaken for organic stupor and coma, certain steps must be taken even before a detailed examination is undertaken, to prevent irreversible brain damage and death which may otherwise occur. These steps should be taken in the management of any unconscious patient.

1. Ensure the patency of airway; and provide ventilatory support with oxygen (for possible hypoxia).
2. Check cardiac rhythm and stabilise it (if needed).
3. Maintain circulation; insert IV (intravenous) line and give fluids (for possible fluid and electrolyte imbalance).
4. Investigations; withdraw blood, CSF and urine samples, before instituting any treatment.
5. 50 ml of 50% dextrose (2 ml/kg body weight for a child) should be given IV (for possible hypoglycaemia).
6. Administer:
   Naloxone 0.4 mg IV (if morphine poisoning is suspected);
   Physostigmine 1-2 mg IV (if anticholinergic poisoning is suspected);
   Thiamine 100 mg IV (if Wernicke's encephalopathy or delirium tremens is suspected);
   Hydrocortisone 100 mg IV (if adrenal crisis is suspected);
   L-Thyroxin 200-500 µg IV (if myxoedema coma is suspected);
   Flumazenil 0.2 mg IV (if benzodiazepine overdose is suspected).

This should be followed by a detailed work-up. The underlying medical or psychiatric cause of stupor should be searched for and treated. The importance of supportive care during the period of stupor cannot be overemphasised.

Excited Behaviour and Violence

Excitement is a common reason for a referral to an emergency psychiatry setting. Although a large majority of psychiatric patients are not dangerously violent, some patients can indeed be aggressive especially during the acute phase of the illness.

Aetiology

Some common causes of excited behaviour are listed below.

I. Organic psychiatric disorders
   1. Delirium (acute organic brain syndrome), e.g. delirium tremens.
   2. Dementia, e.g. catastrophic reaction, loss of control.
   3. Wernicke-Korsakoff's psychosis.
II. Nonorganic psychiatric disorders
   1. Schizophrenia and other psychoses.
      i. Schizophreniform psychosis.
      ii. Catatonic (excited) schizophrenia.
      iii. Paranoid schizophrenia.
      iv. Acute psychotic disorder.
   2. Mania.
      Although excitement is common, violence occurs usually only when the patient is prevented from engaging in his activities, or when he is irritable. Similarly, patients with dysphoric mania or mixed affective states may occasionally present similarly.
   3. Depression: Agitated depression may present with excitement. Occasionally aggressive, violent behaviour may occur if the patient is irritable and agitated.
   4. Drug and alcohol dependence: Excitement and violence may occur in:
      i. Intoxication.
      ii. Withdrawal syndrome.
      iii. Comorbid psychiatric disorder(s).
   5. Epilepsy.
      i. Complex partial seizures.
      ii. Postictal confusion.
      iii. Epileptic furore.
   6. Acute stress reaction.
   7. Neurotic disorders.
      i. Panic disorder.
      ii. Agoraphobia with panic attacks.

Marked excitement can occur during a panic attack but violent behaviour does not usually occur.

8. Impulsive violent behaviour.
   i. Borderline personality disorder.
   ii. Intermittent explosive disorder.
9. Reactive psychosis.

Management

The patient is examined according to the guidelines suggested earlier in this chapter. The physician, psychiatrist or another mental health professional, examining an excited patient, must demonstrate an attitude of empathy but at the same time must be firm and should exude confidence.

The measures which can be adopted to handle excited or violent behaviour include:

1. *Reassurance*: In case of emergency, it rarely works alone but must be tried first.
2. *Sedation*: Diazepam 5-10 mg parenterally slowly (or lorazepam 1-2 mg parenterally slowly) can be given. In the presence of psychosis, haloperidol 2-10 mg parenterally (with or without 5-10 mg diazepam or 50 mg of promethazine) can be given. It is really important to exercise care in administering parenteral antipsychotics to any patient, but particularly one who is treatment (antipsychotic) naïve. Oral antipsychotics are preferable to parenteral antipsychotic in routine clinical practice.
3. *Restraint*: Restraint should always be used as a last resort, but when needed, it should not be delayed. Restraint should always be done in a humane way, after taking (preferably) written consent from the attendant relatives/carers. A second opinion from another mental health professional is helpful.

Restraint is usually followed by compulsory hospitalisation and parenteral medication. It is rarely ever necessary to continue restraint for more than a few hours and restraint should be removed at the earliest possible time.

Electroconvulsive therapy (ECT) is not a treatment for excitement or violence per se. When used, there should be a clear indication for the use of ECT, which should be clearly recorded in the case notes.

Other Psychiatric Emergencies

The list of possible psychiatric emergencies is long. A few psychiatric emergencies are listed below, some of which have already been discussed in the book.

1. *Severe depression* (Chapter 6): Apart from presenting as a suicide/suicidal attempt and/or agitation, the depressed patient may come to casualty because of a refusal to eat and drink, leading to dehydration or because of refusal to take medication (for example, secondary to hopelessness).
2. *Hyperventilation syndrome* (Chapter 8).
3. *Side effects of psychotropic medication*, e.g. acute dystonia (promptly relieved by promethazine 25-50 mg parenterally), akathisia, neuroleptic malignant syndrome (Chapter 15).
4. *Psychiatric complications of medical and surgical diseases*, procedures and medication (e.g. ICU syndrome, hypomania caused by steroids).
5. Severe *insomnia* (Chapter 11).
6. *Pseudo seizures* (conversion and/or dissociation hysteria) (Chapter 8).
7. *Anorexia nervosa* (usually presenting with dehydration and/or cachexia) (Chapter 12).
8. *Battered child syndrome* or *child abuse*.
9. *Grief and bereavement* (Chapter 12).
10. *Psychosocial crises* (e.g. marital conflict, occupational and financial difficulties).
11. *Drug or alcohol use disorders* (Chapter 4).
12. *Panic disorder* (Chapter 8).
13. *Acute psychosis* (Chapter 7).

Psychiatric patients, especially when excited or emotionally disturbed, often arouse anxiety in the treating physicians as well as other patients in the casualty. So, it is necessary to have an 'emergency psychiatry room' or 'psychiatric holding area' near the casualty, where the patients can be interviewed and treated.

An ideal place for treating psychiatric emergencies is a separate 'psychiatric intensive care unit' (PICU) or 'crisis intervention centre' (CIC) attached to a psychiatric unit in a general hospital or to a psychiatric hospital or nursing home.

Chapter 20

Legal and Ethical Issues in Psychiatry

Forensic psychiatry deals with the legal aspects of psychiatry. Law comes in contact with psychiatry at many points; for example, admission of a mentally ill person in a mental hospital, crime committed by a mentally ill person, validity of marriage, witness, will, consent, right to vote, and drug dependence.

The various legal aspects of psychiatry are briefly discussed below.

CRIMINAL RESPONSIBILITY

In January 1843, a young Scotsman, Daniel McNaughten shot dead Edward Drummond, the secretary to the British Prime Minister Sir Robert Peel. He had intended to kill the Prime Minister but Drummond was assassinated by mistake.

The Jury, after testification by nine physicians, found McNaughten *not guilty by reasons of insanity*. Queen Victoria, Sir Robert Peel and other prominent persons were outraged. Following this, 15 prominent judges were invited by the House of Lords. They were asked to respond to a series of questions on criminal responsibility. The answers, which are immortalised in the history of forensic psychiatry, have now come to be known as *McNaughten Rule(s)*.

The *McNaughten Rule* is used in a slightly modified form in many countries even now. In India, Section 84 of the Indian Penal Code (Act 45 of 1860) states that 'nothing is an offense, which is done by a person, who at the time of doing it, by reason of unsoundness of mind, is incapable of knowing the nature of the act or that he is doing what is either wrong or contrary to law'.

So a mentally ill person is not protected *ipso facto*. He must satisfy the above mentioned rule. A mentally retarded person (called 'idiot' in law) is not considered liable under Indian criminal law.

The Law generally classifies *criminal lunatics* into three classes: an under-trial who cannot stand trial because of mental illness; guilty but insane; and criminals who later become mentally ill. A Class II 'criminal lunatic' is acquitted under the law but is detained in a mental hospital (asylum) for further treatment.

CIVIL RESPONSIBILITY

There is usually a presumption in the favour of sanity and the contrary must be proved. This applies both to the civil and criminal proceedings in the court of law.

Marriage

The Hindu Marriage Act (Act 25 of 1955) provides for conditions for a Hindu marriage under Section 5. One of the conditions, i.e. Section 5 (ii) introduced by Act 68 of 1976, states that 'at the time of the marriage, neither party,

a. is incapable of giving a valid consent... (due to)... unsoundness of mind; or

b. though capable of giving consent, has been suffering from mental disorder of such a kind or to such an extent as to be unfit for marriage and the procreation of children; or

c. has been subject to recurrent attacks of insanity or epilepsy.'

Any marriage solemnised in the contravention to this condition shall be voidable and may be annulled by a decree of nullity under Section 12 of the Act. Another ground of nullity under the same section is the fact that the consent for marriage was obtained by 'fraud'...'as to any material fact or circumstance concerning the respondent', for example, the fact of mental illness or treatment for the same.

Divorce can be granted under Section 13 of the Act on a petition presented by either spouse on the ground that the other party 'has been incurably of unsound mind, or has been suffering continuously or intermittently from mental disorder of such kind and to such an extent that the petitioner cannot reasonably be expected to live with the respondent' (Section 13 (iii) inserted by Act 68 of 1976).

Here, the term mental disorder means 'mental illness, arrested or incomplete development of mind, psychopathic disorder or any other disorder or disability of mind and includes schizophrenia'. The term psychopathic disorder means 'a persistent disorder or disability of mind (whether or not including subnormality of intelligence) which results in abnormally aggressive or seriously irresponsible conduct on the part of the other party, and whether or not it requires or is susceptible to medical treatment'.

Under the dissolution of Muslim Marriages Act 1939, a woman married under Muslim law is entitled to obtain a decree for the dissolution of marriage on the ground of her husband being insane for a period of 2 years. The husband under the Muslim law has the power to pronounce divorce (*talak*) at anytime, anywhere, and without assigning any reason.

Any married person may be granted divorce, under the Parsi Marriage and Divorce Act 1936, on the ground that the other party had been of unsound mind at the time of marriage (and the petitioner was ignorant of the fact) and has been habitually so till the date of petition, which should be within 3 years of the date of marriage.

Adoption

Under the Hindu Adoptions and Maintenance Act (Act 78 of 1956), any Hindu male 'who is of sound mind and is not a minor' can adopt a child, with the consent of his wife unless '...(she) has been declared by a court...to be of unsound mind' (Section 7).

Similarly, any Hindu female 'who is of sound mind', is not a minor, and is not married, can adopt a child. If she is married, 'then her husband is dead, or has ...renounced the world, or ...ceased to be a Hindu, or ...has been declared by a court ...to be of unsound mind' (Section 8).

In addition, the person capable of giving in adoption of a child should be of sound mind.

Witness

Under the Indian Evidence Act 1872, a 'lunatic' is not competent to give evidence if he is prevented by virtue of his 'lunacy' from understanding the questions put to him and giving rational answers to them (Section 118).

However, such a person can give evidence during a lucid interval on discretion of the judge (and the jury).

Testamentary Capacity

Testamentary disposition is regulated by the Indian Succession Act (Act 39 of 1925). Some of the salient points regarding testamentary disposition are as follows:

1. A will must be in writing, though it need not be registered.
2. It must be signed by testator in the presence of at least two witnesses.
3. A legatee cannot attest a will.
4. An executor(s) is appointed under the will by the testator to carry out its terms after his death.
5. A will can be revoked or modified any time before the death of the testator.
6. A will comes into effect after the death of the testator. It is said to speak from grave and to be 'ambulatory'.
7. The testator must be of a 'sound and disposing mind'. Section 59 of the Act states that 'every person of sound mind, not being a minor, may dispose of his property by will'.

Explanation 4 of this section states that 'no person can make a will while he is in such a state of mind, whether arising from intoxication or from illnesses or from any other cause, that he does not know what he is doing'.

If a medical practitioner is called to examine a testator as to his fitness to make a valid will, the following points must be kept in mind:

1. Testamentary capacity consists of:
   i. an understanding of the nature of the will,
   ii. a knowledge of the property to be disposed of, and
   iii. an ability to recognize those who may have justifiable claims on his property.
2. The testator should be tested on the above mentioned points by thorough questioning.
3. If the testator is seriously ill, he must be made to read out aloud the will in the presence of the doctor.
4. A will is invalid if it is executed under undue influence of any other person. If there is reason to suspect that such is the case, the testator should be questioned when he is alone.
5. A will is invalid under the following conditions (for example):
   i. imbecility arising from advanced age or by excessive drinking.
   ii. insane delusions making the testator incapable of rational views and judgement.
6. A will is valid under the following conditions (for example):
   i. deaf, dumb or blind persons who are not thereby incapacitated for making a will and are able to know what they do by it.
   ii. lucid intervals.
   iii. if testator commits suicide immediately after making the will, in the absence of evidence of mental disorder.
   iv. presence of delusions not affecting in any way the disposal of the property or the persons affected by the will.
7. A will may be declared invalid if the testator disposes his property in a way which he would not have done under normal conditions.

Transfer of Property

Under the Transfer of Property Act 1882 (Section 7), only persons competent to contract, are authorised to transfer property.

Contract

Under the Indian Contract Act 1872 (Section 11), every person to be competent to contract must be a major and of sound mind.

A person is said to be of sound mind for the purposes of a contract, if at the time of making a contract he is capable of understanding it and of forming a rational judgement as to its effect upon his interests.

Driving

It is important that advice be given regarding driving if there is likelihood that driving can be impaired by the nature of illness, prescribed medication and/or misuse of alcohol or drugs.

INDIAN LUNACY ACT, 1912

The Indian laws related to mental disorders were based on British Acts. For example, the Indian Lunacy Act (ILA), Act 4 of 1912, was based largely on the earlier English Lunacy Act of 1890 and replaced the existing Indian Lunatic Asylums Act, Act 36 of 1858.

The ILA had 8 Chapters. Chapter 1 defined a lunatic as 'an idiot or person of unsound mind'. Defectiveness of reasoning, whether partial or complete, was considered as unsoundness of mind. In Chapter 3, five categories of admission methods were mentioned, namely voluntary, reception order on petition, reception order without petition, inquisition (judicial), and as a criminal lunatic.

There was a 'board of visitors' appointed by the Government which had a role in admission of voluntary patients, interfering with ongoing care and treatment and discharge (except in criminal cases). IG (prisons) was an ex-officio member of this board.

In 1950, three eminent psychiatrists appointed by the Indian Psychiatric Society prepared a draft 'Indian Mental Health Act' and forwarded it to Government of India. There was no action taken on the draft for next ten years and it was only in 1978 that the Mental Health Bill was introduced in Parliament. The bill had to be reintroduced in Lok Sabha in 1981 and was passed by Rajya Sabha in November 1986.

THE MENTAL HEALTH ACT, 1987

The Mental Health Bill became the Act 14 of 1987 on 22nd May 1987. Later, the Government of India issued orders that the Act came in force with effect from April 1, 1993 in all the states and Union territories of India.

The Act is divided into 10 chapters consisting of 98 sections. Chapter I (Preliminary) deals with the various definitions. The Act uses the term 'mentally ill person' instead of 'lunatic' and defines it as 'a person who is in need of treatment by reason of any mental disorder other than mental retardation'.

The term 'mentally ill prisoner' is used instead of 'criminal lunatic'. Other new terms, which are defined in the Chapter 1, are psychiatric hospital (instead of mental hospital), psychiatric nursing home and psychiatrist.

Chapter II provides for establishment of Mental Health Authorities at Centre and State levels. These authorities will regulate and coordinate mental health services under Central and State Government, respectively.

Chapter III lays down the guidelines for establishment and maintenance of psychiatric hospitals and nursing homes. In addition, there is a provision for a Licensing Authority who will process applications for licenses. No private psychiatric hospital or nursing home will be allowed to function without a valid license, which has to be renewed every 5 years.

There is also a provision for an Inspecting Officer who will inspect the psychiatric hospitals and nursing homes to prevent any irregularities.

There is a provision for separate hospitals for:
1. Those under the age of 16 years,
2. Those addicted to alcohol or other drugs which lead to behavioural changes,
3. Mentally ill prisoners, and
4. Any other prescribed class or category.

Chapter IV deals with the procedures of admission and detention in psychiatric hospitals or nursing homes. In addition to the 5 methods allowed by the Indian Lunacy Act of 1912, one more method has been incorporated.

Hence, the admission in a psychiatric hospital or nursing home can be made in one of the following manners:
1. Voluntary Admission.
    i. By the patient's request, if he is a major.
    ii. By the guardian, if a minor (a new provision).
2. Admission under Special Circumstances.
    This is an involuntary hospitalisation when the mentally ill person does not or cannot express his willingness for admission. Admission is made, if a relative or a friend of the mentally ill person applies in writing for admission and the medical officer in-charge of the hospital is satisfied that the admission will be in the interest of the mentally ill person. The duration of admission cannot exceed 90 days.
3. Reception order on application.
4. Reception order without application, on production of mentally ill person (e.g. wandering, dangerous, ill-treated or neglected mentally ill person) before the Magistrate.
5. Admission as inpatient, after judicial inquisition.
6. Admission as a mentally ill prisoner.

In addition, the Magistrate can order detention of an alleged mentally ill person for short periods pending report by medical officer (for a period not exceeding 10 days in aggregate) or pending his removal to psychiatric hospital or psychiatric nursing home (for a period not exceeding 30 days).

Chapter V deals with the inspection, discharge, leave of absence and removal of mentally ill persons. Chapter VI deals with the judicial inquisition regarding the alleged mentally ill person possessing property, custody of his person and management of his property. If the court feels that the alleged mentally ill person is incapable of looking after both himself and his property, an order can be issued for the appointment of a Guardian. If, however, it is felt that the person is only incapable of looking after his property but can look after himself, a Manager can be appointed.

Chapter VII deals with the liability to meet the cost of maintenance of mentally ill persons detained in psychiatric hospitals or nursing homes. Chapter VIII is aimed at the protection of human rights of mentally ill persons. This is a new chapter in the Act. It provides that:

1. No mentally ill person shall be subjected, during treatment, to any indignity (whether physical or mental) or cruelty.
2. No mentally ill person, under treatment, shall be used for the purposes of research, unless
   i. Such research is of direct benefit to him.
   ii. A consent has been obtained in writing from the person (if a voluntary patient) or from the guardian/relative (if admitted involuntarily).
3. No letters or communications sent by or to a mentally ill person shall be intercepted, detained or destroyed.

Chapter IX deals with the penalties and the procedure, while Chapter X provides for miscellaneous sections.

In addition, the State Mental Health Rules, 1990 (which also contains the nine important forms required by the Mental Health Act, 1987) and the Central Mental Health Authority Rules, 1990, have also been passed by the Government of India on December 29, 1990.

Currently consultations are in progress to consider either modifying or updating the current Act.

THE NARCOTIC DRUGS AND PSYCHOTROPIC SUBSTANCES ACT (NDPSA), 1985

The first Act for drug abuse and dependence in India was The Opium Act of 1857. This was revised first in 1878 (The Opium Act, 1878) and then in 1950 (The Opium and Revenue Laws Act, 1950). Another relevant Act was the Dangerous Drug Act of 1930, which included among other drugs, Opium and its alkaloids and Cocaine. This Act provided for a maximum punishment of 3 years.

With the coming in force of the NDPSA, Act 61 of 1985, on 16th September 1985, the above mentioned acts have been repealed. The Act includes narcotic drugs (cannabis, cocaine, coca leaf, opium, poppy straw and all manufactured 'drugs') and psychotropic substances (76 drugs and their derivatives are listed in the schedule, e.g. diazepam, pentazocine, phenobarbital).

The authorities and officers have been suggested in Chapter 2. If any person produces, possesses, transports, imports, exports, sells, purchases, or uses any narcotic drug or psychotropic substance (except 'ganja'), he shall be punishable with,

1. Rigorous imprisonment (RI) for not less than 10 years (which may extend to 20 years), and
2. A fine of not less than 1 Lakh rupees (which may extend to 2 Lakh rupees).

Punishment for a repeat offense is a RI for not less than 15 years (which may extend to 30 years) and a fine of not less than 1.5 Lakh rupees (which may extend to 3 Lakh rupees). Punishment for ganja handling is a RI for 5 years and/or a fine of 0.5 Lakh rupees. For a repeat offense, the imprisonment may extend to 10 years and the fine to 1 Lakh rupees.

However, if a person is carrying 'small quantities' (e.g. 250 mg of heroin, 5 g of Charas, 5 g of opium, 125 mg of cocaine) which were later specified, then the punishment is a simple imprisonment which may extend to 1 year or a fine (unspecified) or both. For ganja (<500 g), imprisonment is up to 6 months.

There is also a provision for detoxification under court order. A later enactment, the Prevention of Illicit Traffic in NDPS Act, 1988 has also been passed (Act 46 of 1988). There is now a provision for preventive detention and seizure of property. The maximum punishment is death penalty, if a person is found to be trafficking more than or equal to 1 kg of pure heroin (for example), twice (despite conviction and warning on the first attempt). The Act was further amended by the Narcotic Drugs and Psychotropic Substances (Amendment) Act, 2001.

A CODE OF ETHICS FOR PSYCHIATRISTS

The Indian Psychiatric Society (IPS) has recommended a code of ethics for psychiatrists (1989) which is summarised here:

Principles

1. A psychiatrist has a clear social responsibility.
2. A psychiatrist must maintain high standards of professional competence and ensure continuing self-education.
3. Benevolence and patient interest precede self interest.
4. A psychiatrist must maintain high moral standards.
5. Patient welfare is of paramount concern to a psychiatrist. It includes not treating cases which are not in his domain, terminating treatment when cannot help the patient, and treating with the best of the ability.
6. Confidentiality of the patient records must be meticulously maintained.

Recommendations

1. Treatment should be given with patient's consent. Every person who is a major and does not appear to have lost ability of reason is capable of consent. If the patient cannot give consent due to mental illness, consent should be taken from a person close to the patient who appears to be clearly interested in patient's welfare. However, treatment can be given without consent in an emergency situation involving immediate threat to the life or health of patient or others.

   For research purposes, consent should be entirely voluntary. The patient can withdraw consent at any stage, without this affecting patient's interest.
2. Hospitalisation should be for patient's welfare, keeping in view the legal and administrative constraints, and social appropriateness.
3. Psychiatric treatment should be started only on clinical consideration for patient welfare and should be humane and never punitive.

   No psychiatrist should refuse to treat in an emergency.
4. No gifts and gratifications should be accepted from patients under treatment.
5. Any sexual advance towards any patient is unethical.
6. In case of doubt and/or unconventional treatment procedures a second opinion must be obtained.
7. It is unethical to force a contract on a patient during treatment.
8. Even if the patient is referred by legal or administrative authority, patient's welfare is paramount and patient should be informed of the purpose for which he is to be examined.
9. The basic human rights of mentally retarded should not be unethically abridged.
10. In the interest of the patient and the society, drug abusers who refuse to give consent may be treated with the consent of their relatives. Effort has to be made to motivate them for accepting treatment voluntarily.

ICMR GUIDELINES FOR RESEARCH, 2000

In 2000, the Indian Council of Medical Research (ICMR) has released 'Ethical guidelines for biomedical research in human subjects'. These guidelines are very similar to the GCP (Good Clinical Practice) guidelines and the prevalent international guidelines. These guidelines regulate all biomedical research in human subjects in India.

MCI CODE OF MEDICAL ETHICS, 2002

All psychiatrists as doctors are also bound by the code of medical ethics of Medical Council of India (MCI). Called as the Indian Medical Council (Professional conduct, Etiquette and Ethics) Regulations, 2002, the code came in to effect from 6th April, 2002. The full code is available at the website of MCI, at http://mohfw.nic.in/code.htm.

Chapter 21

Community Psychiatry

Born in 1963, the community psychiatry movement has been hailed as *the third psychiatric revolution*. The *first revolution* was the age of enlightenment following the middle ages, when mental illness was viewed as a consequence of sin and witchcraft. The *second revolution* was the development of psychoanalysis which offered hope for a causative explanation of psychiatric disorders.

However, the community psychiatry movement was made possible by another revolution, the one ushered by the advent of psychopharmacology. Therefore, it may be more appropriate to refer to community psychiatry as the *fourth* psychiatric revolution.

The *community psychiatry* concept has its antecedents in Clifford Beers' (1908) mental hygiene movement and Adolf Meyer's recommendation (1913) of establishment of treatment centres in the community. The period between 1955 and 1980 was an era of deinstitutionalisation in USA and other Western countries, consisting of discharging mentally ill patients from mental hospitals, to be cared for in the community supported by community mental health centres. This provided an impetus to the development of community psychiatry.

In 1975, the World Health Organization strongly recommended the delivery of mental health services through primary health care system as a policy for the developing countries. In India, attempts to develop models of psychiatric services in the PHC (primary health centre) setting were made nearly simultaneously at PGI, Chandigarh in 1975 (Raipur Rani block of Ambala district, Haryana) and NIMHANS, Bangalore in 1976 (Sakalwara in Karnataka).

The basic model of community mental health was defined by Gerald Caplan in 1967. The predominant characteristics of community psychiatry are:

1. Responsibility to a population for mental health care delivery.
2. Treatment close to the patient in community based centres.
3. Provision of comprehensive services.
4. Multi-disciplinary team approach.
5. Providing continuity of care.
6. Emphasis on prevention as well as treatment.
7. Avoidance of unnecessary hospitalisation.

NATIONAL MENTAL HEALTH PROGRAMME (INDIA)

Mental health is an integral component of health, which is defined as a positive state of well-being (physical, mental and social) and not merely an absence of illness. With this aim in mind, an expert group was formed in 1980. The final draft was submitted to the Central Council of Health and Family Welfare (the highest policy making body for health in the country) on 18-20 August 1982, which recommended its implementation. The National Mental Health Programme (NMHP) appeared almost simultaneously with the National Health Policy (1993).

The objectives of NMHP are:

1. To ensure availability and accessibility of *minimum mental health care for all* in the foreseeable future, particularly to the most vulnerable and underprivileged sections of population.
2. To encourage *application of mental health knowledge* in general health care and in social development.
3. To promote *community participation* in the mental health service development and to stimulate efforts towards self-help in the community.

Three aims are specified in the NMHP in planning mental health services for the country:

1. Prevention and treatment of mental and neurological disorders and their associated disabilities.
2. Use of mental health technology to improve general health services.
3. Application of mental health principles in total national development to improve quality of life.

Two strategies, complementary to each other, were planned for immediate action:

1. *Centre to periphery strategy:* Establishment and strengthening of psychiatric units in all district hospitals, with outpatient clinics and mobile teams reaching the population for mental health services.
2. *Periphery to centre strategy:* Training of an increasing number of different categories of health personnel in basic mental health skills, with primary emphasis towards the poor and the underprivileged, directly benefiting about 200 million people.

The mental health care service was envisaged to include three components or subprogrammes, namely treatment, rehabilitation and prevention.

1. Treatment Subprogramme: Multiple levels were planned.

A. *Village and subcentre level:* Multi-purpose workers (MPW) and health supervisors (HS), under the supervision of medical officer (MO), to be trained for:
   i. Management of psychiatric emergencies.

   ii. Administration and supervision of maintenance treatment for chronic psychiatric disorders.
   iii. Diagnosis and management of grand mal epilepsy, especially in children.
   iv. Liaison with local school teacher and parents regarding mental retardation and behaviour problems in children.
   v. Counselling in problems related to alcohol and drug abuse.

B. *Primary health centre (PHC)*: MO, aided by HS, to be trained for:
   i. Supervision of MPW's performance
   ii. Elementary diagnosis
   iii. Treatment of functional psychosis
   iv. Treatment of uncomplicated cases of psychiatric disorders associated with physical diseases
   v. Management of uncomplicated psychosocial problems
   vi. Epidemiological surveillance of mental morbidity.

C. *District hospital:* It was recognized that there should be at least 1 psychiatrist attached to every district hospital as an integral part of the district health services. The district hospital should have 30-50 psychiatric beds. The psychiatrist in a district hospital was envisaged to devote only a part of his time in clinical care and greater part in training and supervision of non-specialist health workers.

D. *Mental hospitals and teaching psychiatric units:* The major activities of these higher centres of psychiatric care include:
   i. Help in care of 'difficult' cases.
   ii. Teaching.
   iii. Specialised facilities such as occupational therapy units, psychotherapy, counselling and behaviour therapy.

2. Rehabilitation Subprogramme: The components of this subprogramme include maintenance treatment of epileptics and psychotics at the community levels and development of rehabilitation centres at both the district level and the higher referral centres.

3. Prevention Subprogramme: The prevention component is to be community-based, with the initial focus on prevention and control of alcohol-related problems. Later, problems such as addictions, juvenile delinquency and acute adjustment problems such as suicidal attempts are to be addressed.

The other approaches designed to achieve the objectives of the NMHP include:

- Integration of basic mental health care into general health services.
- Mental health training of general medical doctors and paramedical health workers.

A plan of action was outlined in 1982, with the first opportunity to develop it in the 7th-five-year plan starting from 1985, with a plan allocation of Rs. 100 lakhs (10 million). A National Mental Health Advisory Group (NMHAG) was formed in August 1988 and a Mental Health Cell was opened in the Ministry of Health and Family Welfare under a Central Mental Health Authority (MHA).

Various activities were planned under the action plan for implementation of national mental health programme in the 7th-five-year plan, such as community mental health programmes at primary health care level in states and union territories; training of existing PHC personnel for mental health care delivery; development of a state level Mental Health Advisory Committee and state level programme officer; establishment of Regional Centers of community mental health; formation of National Advisory Group on Mental Health; development of task forces for mental hospitals and mental health education for undergraduate medical students; involvement of voluntary agencies in mental health care; identification of priority areas (child mental health, public mental health education and drug dependence); mental health training of at least 1 doctor at every district hospital during the next 5 years; establishment of a department of psychiatry in all medical colleges and strengthening the existing ones; and provision of at least 3-4 essential psychotropic drugs in adequate quantity, at the PHC level.

The District Mental Health Programme (DMHP) was started in 1995 as a component of NMHP. The prototype of the District Mental Health Programme was the Bellary District Programme (in Karnataka, ~320 km from Bangalore). Started in 1985, it caters to a population of 1.5 million. District hospital psychiatry units have been opened in every district of Kerala and Tamil Nadu.

Following the implementation of National Mental Health Programme in India 1982, other neighbouring countries soon followed the example by drawing national programmes for mental health (Sri Lanka 1982; Bangladesh 1982; Pakistan 1986; Nepal 1987).

The revised National Health Policy (NHP-2002) has been released in 2002. Its focus on mental health "envisages a network of decentralised mental health services for ameliorating the more common categories of disorders". At the same time the NMHP 10th-five-year plan was launched, with a plan to extend the DMHP to 100 districts. It also emphasizes the need to broaden the scope of existing curriculum for undergraduate training in psychiatry and to give more exposure to psychiatry in undergraduate years and internship. An essential list of psychotropic drugs was also being prepared.

The emphasis of NMHP-1982 was primarily on the rural sector. It is being realized that the urban mental health needs also need to be addressed under the ambit of NMHP.

During the 11th-five-year plan, an allocation of Rs 1000 crore (Rs 10 billion) has been made for the NMHP. The current focus (2009) is on establishing centres of excellence in mental health, increasing intake capacity and starting postgraduate courses in psychiatry, modernisation of mental hospitals and upgradation of medical college psychiatry departments, focus on non-government organisations (NGOs) and public sector partnerships, media campaign to address stigma, a focus on research, and several other measures (See http://india.gov.in/sectors/health_family/mental_health.php).

Table 21.1: Extent of the Problem and Facilities Available in India

The Problem	Psychiatric beds in India
Population = 1027 million (2001)	Per 10,000 population = 0.25 (World = 1.69;
Prevalence of psychiatric disorders = 58/1000	Median)*
Severe mental illness	
Point prevalence = 10-20/1000 population	**Manpower Available in India**
Incidence = 35/100,000 population	Psychiatrists (qualified) in India
Neuroses and psychosomatic disorders	Numbers = ~3500
Point prevalence = 2-3%	Per 100,000 population = 0.2 (World = 4.15 Mean;
Mental retardation	1.2 Median)
Point prevalence = 0.5-1.0% of all children	Total qualified doctors in India = 503900 (1999)
Psychiatric disorders in children	Clinical psychologists in India
Point prevalence = 1-2% of all children	Numbers = ~1000
Psychiatric OPD attendance in (1990 data)	Per 100,000 population = 0.03 (World = 0.6
Govt. hospitals = 3.63 million/year	Median)*
Private practice = 2.63 million/year	Psychiatric social workers
Total OPD attendance = 6.29 million/year	Numbers = ~1000
(~1% of population)	Per 100,000 population = 0.03 (World = 0.4
Additionally, 15-20% of all help-seekers in the general	Median)*
health services do so for emotional and psychosocial	Psychiatric nurses in India
problems.	Numbers = 800-900
	Per 100,000 population = 0.05 (World = 2.0
Existing Mental Health Services	Median)*
No. of government mental hospitals = 37	Total nurses in India = 737000 (1999)
No. of mental hospital beds = ~19000	Postgraduate centers = ~40 (very few of 140 medical
Private psychiatric hospital beds = 2000-3000	colleges have a psychiatry department)
General hospital psychiatry unit beds (GHPU beds) =	MD/DPM seats (Psychiatrists/year) = ~200 (For com-
4000-5000	parison: Doctors/year = 13,000) (1990)
Total health beds in India = 870161 (1994-95)	

* *Source: Atlas: Mental Health Resources in the World, 2005, WHO*

The extent of mental health problems and facilities available in India are briefly summarised in Table 21.1.

WORLD (MENTAL) HEALTH REPORT 2001

This landmark publication of the WHO was published in 2001 (Editor-in-Chief: RS Murthy). The 2001 World Health Report focused on mental health *(Mental Health: New Understanding, New Hope)*, with a slogan, *Stop Exclusion: Dare to Care.*

The report identified that 'one person in every four will be affected by a mental disorder at some stage of life'. It points out that the psychiatric disorders are estimated to account for 12% of the global burden of disease, yet the mental health budgets of the majority of countries constitute <1% of their total health expenditures.

The WHR-2001 appears along with the *Atlas*, a unique publication of WHO giving a comparative account of the mental health resources in the world. The report identifies that 'mental disorders affect all people in all countries', but the 'people do not get the care they need...because of lack of resources,... because of fear of seeking help, ...and because of lack of (mental health) policies'.

The WHR-2001 makes ten recommendations for action:

1. Provide treatment in primary care.
2. Make psychotropic drugs available.
3. Give care in the community.
4. Educate the public.
5. Involve communities, families and consumers.
6. Establish national policies, programmes and legislation.
7. Develop human resources.
8. Link with other sectors.
9. Monitor community mental health.
10. Support more research.

Appendices

	Nobel Laureates	Major Contributions	Year of Award
1.	**Ivan Petrovich Pavlov** (1849-1936; Russia)	Classical conditioning Physiology of digestion	1904
2.	**Camillo Golgi** (1843-1926; Italy) **Santiago Ramon y Cajal** (1852-1934; Spain)	Structure of CNS	1906
3.	**Julius Wagner von Jauregg** (1857-1940; Austria) (First psychiatrist to receive a Nobel Prize in Physiology or Medicine)	Malarial treatment for GPI (First successful treatment of a major psychosis)	1927
4.	**Antonio Caetano de Abreu Freire Egas Moniz (Egas Moniz)** (1874-1955; Portugal) **Walter Rudolf Hess** (1881-1973; Switzerland)	Psychosurgery (prefrontal leucotomy) Cerebral angiography	1949
5.	**Konrad Lorenz** (1903-1989; Austria) **Karl Von Frisch** (1886-1982; Germany) **Nikolaas Tinbergen** (1907-1988; UK)	Ethology	1973
6.	**Sir Godfrey Newbold Hounsfield** (1919-2004; UK) **Allan Macleod Cormack** (1924-1998; US)	Computerised Tomography Scan	1979
7.	**Stanley B. Prusiner** (1942b; US)	Discovery of *Prions*	1997
8.	**Eric R. Kandel** (1929b; US) **Arvid Carlsson** (1923b; Sweden) **Paul Greengard** (1925b; US)	Signal Transduction in CNS	2000
9.	**Paul C. Lauterbaur** (1929-2007; US) **Sir Peter Mansfield** (1933b; UK)	Magnetic Resonance Imaging	2003

Appendix II: Some Important Contributors in Psychiatry

Contributor	Coined the Term	Special Mention
Adler, Alfred (1870-1937)	Life style Inferiority complex Will to power Creative self	Founder of the school of individual psychology
Alexander, Franz (1891-1964)	—	Sometimes known as the father of psychosomatic medicine
Ayurveda (<4000 BC)	—	Five types of constitution and 3 main types of personality were described. Modernistic descriptions of mental disorders were stated
Beard, George Miller (1839-1883)	Neurasthenia	—
Berne, Eric (1910-1970)	Games Transaction	Founder of transactional analysis (TA). Wrote the book 'Games People Play'
Binet, Alfred (1857-1911)	—	Designed the 1st formal scale of intelligence
Bleuler, Eugen (1857-1939)	Schizophrenia	Described 'cardinal' symptoms of schizophrenia
Braid, James (1795-1860)	Hypnosis	—
Cicero (106-43 BC)	Libido	—
Cullen, William (1710-1790)	Neurosis	—
Delay, Jean PL (b 1907)	Neuroleptic Neuroleptic malignant syndrome (NMS)	1st antipsychotic treatment (chlorpromazine) of psychoses
Dendy, Walter Cooper (1794-1871)	Psychotherapy ('Psychotherapeia')	—
Deniker, Pierre (b 1917)	'Hibernotherapie'	—
Erikson, Erik H (1902-1994)	Psychohistory Identity crisis	Described the stages of life
Esquirol, Jean ED (1772-1840)	Hallucination Monomania	—
Falret, Jean-Pierre (1794-1870)	Mental alienation	Thus, psychiatrists came to be known as alienists
Fechner, Gustav Theodore (1801-1887)	Psychophysics	Founder of experimental and physiological psychology
Feuchtersleben, Ernst von (1806-1849)	Psychosis	—

Contd...

Contd...

Contributor	Coined the Term	Special Mention
Freud, Sigmund (1856-1939)	Free association Psychoanalysis Psychodynamics Oedipus complex Electra complex Penis envy Primal scene Ego defense mechanisms Repression Psychological determinism Pleasure principle Reality principle	Founder of psychoanalysis; some of the significant contributions include: interpretation of dreams, theory of infantile sexuality, structural and topographical model of mind, theory of instincts, psychopathology of everyday life and stages of psychosexual development
Gall, Franz Joseph (1758-1828)	—	Founder of phrenology
Gita Bhagavad (~ 4th Century BC)	—	Probably the 1st recorded evidence of crisis-intervention psychotherapy
Gockel (1547-1628)	Psychology	—
Griesinger, Wilhelm (1817-1868)	Unitary psychosis	Founder of the speciality of neuropsychiatry; 1st full time academic psychiatrist with a medical orientation
Hecker, Ewald (1843-1909)	Hebephrenia	—
Heinroth, Johann C (1773-1843)	Psychosomatic	—
Horney, Karen (1885-1952)	—	American psychoanalyst; Neo-Freudian; Described a theory of neurosis
Janet, Pierre (1859-1947)	Psychasthenia	—
Jones, Maxwell (b 1907)	Therapeutic community	—
Jung, Carl Gustav (1875-1961)	Collective and personal unconscious Complex Introvert and extrovert Archetypes Persona Anima and animus	Founder of the school of analytical psychology

Contd...

Contd...

Contributor	Coined the Term	Special Mention
Kahlbaum, Karl (1828-1899)	Catatonia Symptom complex Cyclothymia	—
Kanner, Leo (1894-1981)	—	Described infantile autism
Klein, Melanie (1882-1960)	Basic trust	Child psychoanalyst
Kraepelin, Emil (1856-1926)	Dementia praecox	Important work on psychiatric nosology and classification
Krafft-Ebing, B Richard von (1840-1902)	Sadism Masochism	Classic description of sexual perversions
Maslow, Abraham (1908-1970)	Self-actualization Self-realization	Humanistic psychology; Described hierarchy of needs
Mesmer, Franz Anton (1734-1815)	Animal magnetism	—
Meyer, Adolf (1866-1950)	—	Founder of psychobiology; Famous for 'common sense psychiatry'
Morel, Benedict-Augustin (1809-1873)	Demence' precoce'	—
Pavlov, Ivan Petrovich (1849-1936)	Classical conditioning	Animal studies on conditioned reflexes
Piaget, Jean (1897-1980)	—	Extensive studies on the nature of children's intellectual development
Pinel, Philippe (1745-1826)	—	Famous for humane and 'moral' treatment of mentally ill
Prichard, James (1786-1848)	Moral insanity	—
Rado, Sandor (1890-1972)	Adaptational psychodynamics	Hungarian psychoanalyst
Rank, Otto (1884-1939)	Birth trauma Will therapy	—
Ray, Issac (1807-1881)	—	Father of American forensic psychiatry
Reil, Johann Christian (1759-1820)	Psychiatry	Founded the 1st psychiatric journal
Rogers, Carl (1902-1987)	Client-centred psychotherapy	American psychologist; Non-directive psychotherapist
Rush, Benjamin (1745-1828)	—	Father of American psychiatry
Skinner, Burrhus Frederic (1904-1990)	—	Founder of operant conditioning model of learning
Sullivan, Harry Stack (1892-1949)	—	Founder of interpersonal school of psychiatry
Tissot, Simon Andre (1728-1797)	Onanism	1st medical description of masturbation

Contd...

Contributor	Coined the Term	Special Mention
Vives, Juan Louis (1492-1540)	—	Wrote the 1st modern textbook of psychology
Watson, John Broadus (1878-1958)	—	Founder of behaviourism
Weyer, Johann (1515-1588)	—	Sometimes known as the father of modern psychiatry
Zacchia, Paolo (1584-1659)	—	Probably the 1st forensic psychiatrist

Appendix III: Glossary of Some Important Terms in Psychiatry

Abstract thinking: Abstract thinking is the ability to assume a mental set voluntarily, shift voluntarily from one aspect of a situation to another, keep in mind simultaneously the various aspects of a situation, grasp the essentials of a 'whole' (e.g. situation or concept), and to break a 'whole' into its parts.

Affect: The outward expression of the immediate *(cross-sectional)* experience of emotion at a given time.

Agitation: Presence of anxiety with severe motor restlessness.

Akinesia: Absence of motor activity.

Alexithymia: Inability to verbally describe one's emotionally feelings.

Ambitendency: Due to ambivalence, tentative actions are made, but no goal directed action occurs.

Ambivalence: Inability to decide for or against, due to co-existence of two opposing impulses for the same thing at the same time in the same person.

Anergia: Lack of energy for day-to-day activities.

Anhedonia: Inability to experience pleasure in previously pleasurable activities.

Anxiety: An unpleasurable emotional state, associated with psycho-physiological changes in response to an intrapsychic conflict.

Blunted affect: Severe reduction in the intensity of affect.

Catalepsy: The person maintains body posture in to which it is placed. Also see *waxy flexibility.*

Cataplexy: Abrupt loss of muscle tone without impairment of consciousness. Often seen in Narcolepsy.

Circumstantiality: Digression in to unnecessary details that distract from the central theme; however, the patient returns back to the original theme after digression (unlike in tangentiality).

Confabulation: A false memory that the patient believes to be true.

Coprolalia: Vocal tics characterised by shouting of obscene words.

Deja entendu: A false sense of familiarity when hearing something new.

Deja vu: A false sense of familiarity with unfamiliar circumstances or scenes.

Delusion: A false, unshakable belief which is not amenable to reasoning, and is not in keeping with the patient's socio-cultural and educational background.

Delusional perception: Normal perception has a private and illogical meaning.

Depersonalization: An alteration in the perception of self, so that the feeling of one's reality is *(as if)* temporarily changed or lost.

Derealization: An alteration in the perception of external world, so that the feeling of the reality of external world is *(as if)* temporarily changed or lost.

Disorientation: A disturbance in orientation in time, place and/or person.

Distractibility: Inability to concentrate or focus attention.

Echolalia: Repetition, echo or mimicking of phrases or words heard.

Echopraxia: Repetition, echo or mimicking of actions observed.

Ecstasy: Very severe elevation of mood (seen in delirious or stuporous mania); Intense sense of rapture or blissfulness.

Elation: Moderate elevation of mood (seen in mania; Stage II); Feeling of confidence and enjoyment along with increased psychomotor activity.

Emotional incontinence: Complete loss of control over affect (represents an extreme form of emotional lability).

Euphoria: Mild elevation of mood (seen in hypomania); Increased sense of psychological well-being and happiness, not in keeping with on-going events.

Euthymia: Normal range of mood, with absence of depressed or elevated mood.

Exaltation: Severe elevation of mood (seen in severe mania; Stage III); Intense elation with delusions of grandeur.

Flight of ideas: Rapid speech with sudden shifts in ideas, without loosing logical connection.

Folie à deux: Delusions shared between two closely connected persons. Also known are folie à trios, folie à quatre, and folie à famille.

Formication: A false sense of insects crawling on one's skin.

Fugue: Physical and psychological flight (wandering) from one's usual place.

Grandiosity: Excessive and exaggerated feeling of one's importance.

Hallucination: A perception that occurs in the absence of a stimulus.

Illusion: A misinterpretation of stimuli arising from external object(s).

Incoherence: Thought process that is disconnected, disorganised, or incomprehensible.

Insight: The ability to understand one's own behaviour and emotions. In the context of psychiatric disorders, it implies the degree of awareness and understanding that the patient has regarding his/her illness.

Intelligence: The ability to think logically, act rationally, and deal effectively with the environment.

Jamais entendu: A sense of unfamiliarity when hearing something familiar.

Jamais vu: A sense of unfamiliarity with familiar circumstances or scenes.

Judgement: An ability to assess a situation correctly and act appropriately within that situation.

Labile affect: Rapid and abrupt changes in affect, unrelated to external stimuli.

Loosening of associations: Thought process characterised by a series of ideas without apparent logical connections.

Mannerisms: Odd, repetitive and goal-directed movements.

Mood: The pervasive feeling tone which is *sustained* (lasts for some length of time) and colours the total experience of the person.

Mutism: Complete absence of speech.

Negativism: An apparently motiveless resistance to all commands and attempts to be moved, or doing just the opposite.

Neologisms: These are idiosyncratically formed new words whose derivation cannot be understood easily.

Panic: An acute, intense, overwhelming episode of anxiety, often associated with feelings of impending doom.

Perplexity: Puzzled bewilderment.

Perseveration: Persistent repetition of words or themes beyond the point of relevance.

Phobia: An irrational fear of an object, situation or activity.

Posturing: Voluntary assumption of an inappropriate and often bizarre posture for long periods of time.

Poverty of speech: Decreased speech production.

Poverty of content of speech: The speech production is adequate, but the content conveys little information.

Pressure of speech: Rapid production of speech output, with a subjective feeling of racing thoughts.

Rigidity (Catatonic): Maintenance of a rigid posture against efforts to be moved.

Somatic passivity: Bodily sensations, especially sensory symptoms, are experienced as imposed on body by some external force.

Somnolence: Inability to maintain a state of alertness without constant stimulation.

Stereotypy: Odd, repetitive and non-goal directed movement (can also be verbal).

Stupor: A clinical syndrome of akinesis and mutism, with relative preservation of conscious awareness.

Suicide: A human act of self-intentioned and self-inflicted cessation (death).

Tangentiality: Sudden and oblique digression in to unnecessary details that completely distract from the central theme; however, the patient never returns back to the original theme after digression (unlike in circumstantiality).

Thinking: Normal thinking is a goal directed flow of ideas, symbols and associations initiated by a problem or a task, characterised by rational connections between successive ideas or thoughts, and leading towards a reality oriented conclusion.

Thought diffusion or Broadcasting: Subject experiences that his thoughts are escaping the confines of his self and are being experienced by others around.

Thought echo: Voices speaking out thoughts aloud; also called as *echo de la pense*.

Thought insertion: Subject experiences thoughts imposed by some external force on his passive mind.

Thought withdrawal: Thoughts cease and subject experiences them as removed by external force.

Tic: Involuntary, sudden, rapid, recurrent, non-rhythmic and stereotyped movement (can also be verbal).

Trance: A sleep like state of reduced consciousness and suggestibility.

Verbigeration: Senseless repetition of same words or phrases over and over again.

Waxy flexibility: Parts of body can be placed in positions that will be maintained for long periods of time, even if very uncomfortable; flexible like wax. The process is called as *waxy flexibility*, while the end result is called as *catalepsy*.

Suggested Further Reading

1. Abse DW. Hysteria and Related Mental Disorders: An Approach to Psychological Medicine. 2nd edn, John Wright, Bristol, 1987.
2. Diagnostic and Statistical Manual of Mental Disorders. 4th edn, Text Revision. American Psychiatric Association, Washington DC, 2000.
3. Task Force Report on Electroconvulsive Therapy. American Psychiatric Association, Washington DC, 1990.
4. The Practice of Electroconvulsive Therapy: Recommendations for Treatment, Training and Privileging. Task Force Report on ECT, American Psychiatric Association, Washington DC, 2001.
5. Arieti S. Interpretation of Schizophrenia. 2nd edn, Basic Books, New York, 1974.
6. Ashton H. Benzodiazepines: How they work and how to withdraw? The Ashton Manual. http://benzo.org.uk/manual/index.htm
7. Bancroft J. Human Sexuality and its Problems. 3rd edn, Churchill Livingstone Elsevier, Edinburgh, 2009.
8. Barlett J, Bridges P, Kelly D. Contemporary indications for psychosurgery. British Journal of Psychiatry 1981;138:507.
9. Beck AT, Rush AJ, Shaw BI, et al. Cognitive Therapy of Depression. Guilford, New York, 1979.
10. Beck AT. Cognitive Therapy and the Emotional Disorders. International Universities Press, New York, 1976.
11. Bellack AS, Hersen M, Kazdin AE. International Handbook of Behavior Modification and Therapy. Plenum Press, New York, 1982.
12. Benson DF, Blumer D. (Eds). Psychiatric Aspects of Neurologic Disease. Grune and Stratton, New York Vol I, 1975 and Vol II, 1982.
13. Benson FD. Aphasia, Alexia and Agraphia. Churchill Livingstone, New York, 1979.
14. Bleuler E. Dementia Precox: The Group of Schizophrenias. International Universities Press, New York, 1950.
15. Bowlby J. Processes of mourning. International Journal of Psycho-Analysis 1961; 42: 317-40.
16. Brown GW, Birley JLT, Wing JK. Influence of family life on the course of schizophrenic disorders: A replication. British Journal of Psychiatry 1972;121:241.
17. Brown JAC. Freud and the Post-Freudians. Penguin, New York, 1978.
18. Cavenar JO, Brodie HKH. (Eds). Signs and Symptoms in Psychiatry. JB Lippincott, Philadelphia, 1983.
19. Chapman JP. The early symptoms of schizophrenia. British Journal of Psychiatry 1966; 112: 225.
20. Ciompi L. Catamnestic long-term studies on the course of life of schizophrenics. Schizophrenia Bulletin 1980;6:606-18.
21. Cleckley H. The Mask of Sanity. 4th edn, Mosby, St. Louis, 1964.
22. Crow TJ. Molecular pathology of schizophrenia: More than one disease process. British Medical Journal 1980; 280: 66-68.
23. David A, Fleminger S, Kopelman M, Lovestone S, Mellors J. Lishman's Organic Psychiatry: A Textbook of Neuropsychiatry. 4th edn, Wiley-Blackwell, Oxford, 2009.
24. Dement WC. Some Must Watch While Some Must Sleep. WH Freeman Co, San Francisco, 1974.
25. Directorate General of Health Services. National Mental Health Programme for India. Directorate General of Health Services, New Delhi, 1982.

26. Editorial. What next with Psychiatric illness? Nature 1988;336:95-96.
27. Fenichel O. The Psychoanalytic Theory of Neurosis. Norton, New York, 1945.
28. Fink M. Convulsive Therapy: Theory and Practice. Raven Press, New York, 1979.
29. Folstein MF, Folstein SE, McHugh PR. Mini-Mental State: A practical method for grading the cognitive state of patients for the clinician. Journal of Psychiatric Research 1975;12:189.
30. Freud A. The Ego and the Mechanisms of Defense. Hogarth Press, London, 1937.
31. Freud S. The Psychopathology of Everyday Life. In: Strachey J (Ed). The Standard Edition of the Complete Psychological Works of Sigmund Freud. Hogarth Press, London, 1960; 6.
32. Gelder M, Mayou R, Cowen P. Shorter Oxford Textbook of Psychiatry. 4th edn, Oxford University Press, New York, 2001.
33. Gelenberg AJ. The catatonic syndrome. Lancet 1976;1:1339.
34. Gottesman II, Shields J. Schizophrenia: The Epigenetic Puzzle. Cambridge University Press, New York, 1982.
35. Government of India. The Mental Health Act 14, 1987.
36. Government of India. The Narcotic Drugs and Psychotropic Substances Act 61, 1985. (Amended in 1989, Act 2 of 1989).
37. Hall CS. A Primer of Freudian Psychology. World Publishing, Cleveland, 1954.
38. Hamilton M. Fish's Clinical Psychopathology. 3rd edn, John Wright, Bristol, 1983.
39. Hamilton M. Fish's Schizophrenia. 3rd edn, John Wright, Bristol, 1986.
40. Heilman KM, Valenstein E (Eds). Clinical Neuropsychology. 2nd edn, Oxford University Press, New York, 1985.
41. Hinsie LE, Campbell RJ. Psychiatric Dictionary. 5th edn, Oxford University Press, New York, 1981.
42. Indian Council of Medical Research. Manual of Mental Health for Medical Officers. NIMHANS, Bengaluru, 1983.
43. Indian Council of Medical Research. Collaborative Study on Phenomenology and Natural History of Acute Psychosis. Report of an ICMR Task Force Study. Indian Council of Medical Research, New Delhi, 1989.
44. Indian Council of Medical Research. Factors Associated with Course and Outcome of Schizophrenia. Report of an ICMR Task Force Study. Indian Council of Medical Research, New Delhi, 1989.
45. Jefferson JW, Griest JH, Ackerman DL. Lithium Encyclopedia for Clinical Practice. American Psychiatric Press, Washington DC, 1983.
46. Jellinek EM. The Disease Concept of Alcoholism. College and University Press, New Haven, 1960.
47. Jones E. The Life and Work of Sigmund Freud. Basic Books, New York, 1957.
48. Kraepelin E. Dementia Praecox and Paraphrenia. GM Robertson (Ed). Huntington. NY: Krieger, 1971.
49. Kraepelin E. Manic-Depressive Insanity and Paranoia. Livingstone, Edinburgh, 1921.
50. Leff JP, Issacs AD. Psychiatric Examination in Clinical Practice. 2nd edn, Blackwell, Oxford, 1981.
51. Lerer B, Weiner RD, Belmaker RH. ECT: Basic Mechanisms. John Libbey, London, 1984.
52. Marks IM. Fears, Phobias and Rituals. Academic Press, New York, 1988.
53. Masters WH, Johnson VE. Human Sexual Inadequacy, Little Brown, Boston, 1966.
54. Masters WH, Johnson VE. Human Sexual Response. Little Brown, Boston, 1966.
55. Mellor CS. First rank symptoms of schizophrenia. British Journal of Psychiatry 1970;117:15.
56. Merksey H. The Analysis of Hysteria. Bailliére Tindall, London, 1979.
57. Ministry of Health and Family Welfare. National Mental Health Programme Booklet. DGHS, New Delhi, 1982.
58. Morgan C, Bhugra D (Eds). Principles of Social Psychiatry. 2nd edn, Chichester: Wiley-Blackwell, 2010.

59. Murthy RS, Wig NN. The WHO Collaborative Study on Strategies for Extending Mental Health care. American Journal of Psychiatry 1983;140:1486.

60. Murthy RS. National Mental Health Programme in India (1982-1989): Mid-point appraisal. Indian Journal of Psychiatry 1989;31:267.

61. National Collaborating Centre for Mental Health. Borderline Personality Disorder: The NICE Guideline on Treatment and Management. National Clinical Practice Guideline No. 78. British Psychological Society and Royal College of Psychiatrists, 2009.

62. National Institute for Health and Clinical Excellence. Core Interventions in the Treatment and Management of Schizophrenia in Adults in Primary and Secondary care. NICE Clinical Guideline 82. National Collaborating Centre for Mental Health, 2009.

63. National Crime Records Bureau. 2008. Suicides in 2008. http://ncrb.nic.in/ADSI2008/suicides-08.pdf

64. Neki JS. Guru-Chela relationship: The possibility of a therapeutic paradigm. American Journal of Orthopsychiatry 1973;3:755-66.

65. Noshpitz JD (Ed). Basic Handbook of Child Psychiatry. Vol I-IV. Basic Books, New York, 1979.

66. Oyebode F. Sims's Symptoms in the Mind: An Introduction to Descriptive Psychopathology. 4th edn, Elsevier Saunders, 2008.

67. Padesky CA, Greenberger D. Mind over Mood: Change How You Feel by Changing the Way You Think. Guilford Press, 1995.

68. Perry JC, Jacobs D. Overview: Clinical applications of the amytal interview in psychiatric emergency settings. American Journal of Psychiatry 1982;139:552.

69. Pincus J, Tucker GJ. Behavioral Neurology. 3rd edn, Oxford University Press, New York, 1985.

70. Plum F, Posner C. The Diagnosis of Stupor and Coma. 3rd edn, FA Davis, Philadelphia, 1980.

71. Sachdev PS, Keshavan MS (Eds). Secondary Schizophrenia. Cambridge University Press, Cambridge: 2010.

72. Sadock BJ, Sadock VA, Ruiz P (Eds). Comprehensive Textbook of Psychiatry. 9th edn, Lippincott Williams and Wilkins, 2009.

73. Sadock BJ, Sadock VA. Kaplan and Sadock's Synopsis of Psychiatry. 10th edn, Lippincott Williams and Wilkins, 2007.

74. Schreiber FR. Sybil. New York: Warner Books, 1973.

75. Scott AIF (Ed). The ECT Handbook, 2nd edn, Council Report CR128. Royal College of Psychiatrists, 2004.

76. Sharma SD. Mental Hospitals in India. DGHS, New Delhi, 1990.

77. Shneidman ES, Farberow NL. Some Facts about Suicide. PHS Publication No 852, US Government. Printing Officem, Washington DC, 1961.

78. Singh G, Tewari SK. Morbid grief: Its clinical manifestations and proposed classification. Indian Journal of Psychiatry 1980; 22: 74-80.

79. Slater E, Roth M. Clinical Psychiatry (Mayer-Gross). 3rd edn, JPB Publishers, New Delhi, 1986.

80. Strub RL, Black FW. The Mental Status Examination in Neurology. 2nd edn, FA Davis, Philadelphia, 1985, reprinted by JPB Publishers, New Delhi, 1991.

81. Taylor D, Paton C, Kapur S. The Maudsley Prescribing Guidelines. 10th edn, Informa Health care, London, 2009.

82. Thigpen CH, Cleckley HM. The Three Faces of Eve. New York: McGraw Hill, 1957.

83. Varma VK. Psychotherapy in a Traditional Society: Context, Concept and Practice. JPB Publishers, New Delhi, 2008.

84. Vaughn C, Leff J. The measurement of expressed emotion in the families of psychiatric patients. British Journal of Social and Clinical Psychology 1976;15:157-65.

85. Watson JB, Rayner R. Conditioned emotional responses. Journal of Experimental Psychology 1920;3:1-14.

86. Wolberg LR. The Technique of Psychotherapy. Vol I and II. Secker and Warburg with Heinemann, London, 1989.

87. World Health Organization. The ICD-10 Classification of Mental and Behavioural Disorders: Clinical descriptions and diagnostic guidelines. World Health Organization, Geneva, 1992.

88. World Health Organization. Definition of Health. Accessed May 2010. See http://www.who.int/about/definition/en/print.html/

89. World Health Organization. Report of the International Pilot Study of Schizophrenia (IPSS). Geneva: WHO, 1973.

90. World Health Organization. Schizophrenia: An International Follow-up Study, Wiley, New York, 1979.

91. The World Health Report: 2001. Mental Health: New Understanding, New Hope, World Health Organization, Geneva, 2001.

92. Atlas: Mental Health Resources in the World. World Health Organization, Geneva, 2005. http://www.who.int/mental_health/evidence/atlas/en/

93. Zilboorg GA, Henry GW. A History of Medical Psychology. Norton, 1941.

94. Zubin J, Spring B. Vulnerability: A new view of schizophrenia. Journal of Abnormal Psychology 1977;86,103-26.

Index